The European Experience of Declining Fertility

Studies in Social Discontinuity

General Editor: Charles Tilly, The New School for Social Research

Studies in Social Discontinuity began in 1972 under the imprint of Academic Press. In its first 15 years, 53 titles were published in the series, including important volumes in the areas of historical sociology, political economy, and social history.

Revived in 1989 by Blackwell Publishers, the series will continue to include volumes emphasizing social changes and non-Western historical experience as well as translations of major works.

Published:

The Perilous Frontier
Nomadic Empires and China
Thomas J. Barfield

Regents and Rebels
The Revolutionary World of an Eighteenth-Century Dutch City
Wayne Ph. te Brake

The Word and the Sword
How Techniques of Information and Violence Have Shaped Our World
Leonard M. Dudley

Coffee, Contention, and Change
in the Making of Modern Brazil
Mauricio Font

Nascent Proletarians
Class Formation in Post-Revolutionary France
Michael P. Hanagan

Social Evolutionism
A Critical History
Stephen K. Sanderson

Coercion, Capital, and European States
AD 990−1990
Charles Tilly

Anti-Semitism in France
A Political History from Léon Blum to the Present
Pierre Birnbaum

In preparation:

Forget the Family
David Levine

The European Experience of Declining Fertility, 1850–1970

The Quiet Revolution

Edited by

JOHN R. GILLIS, LOUISE A. TILLY,
AND DAVID LEVINE

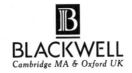

BLACKWELL
Cambridge MA & Oxford UK

Copyright © John R. Gillis, Louise A. Tilly, and David Levine 1992

First published 1992

Blackwell Publishers
Three Cambridge Center
Cambridge, Massachusetts 02142
USA

108 Cowley Road
Oxford OX4 1JF
UK

Library of Congress Cataloging-in-Publication Data

The European experience of declining fertility, 1850–1970 / edited by
John R. Gillis, Louise A. Tilly, David Levine.
p.   cm. – (Studies in social discontinuity)
Includes bibliographical references and index.
ISBN 1–55786–122–6
1. Fertility, Human – Europe – History.   I. Gillis, John R.
II. Tilly, Louise A.   III. Levine, David, 1946–   .   IV. Series:
Studies in social discontinuity (Blackwell Publishers)
HB991.E97   1992
304.6′32′094–dc20   91–37246
                                                      CIP

British Library Cataloguing in Publication Data

A CIP catalogue record for this book is available from the British Library.

Typeset in 10½ on 12pt Ehrhardt
by Graphicraft Typesetters Ltd, Hong Kong
Printed in the United States of America

This book is printed on acid-free paper.

Contents

Postscript
Moments in Time: A Historian's Context of Declining
Fertility   326
David Levine

Contributors

George Alter   *Department of History, Indiana University*
John R. Gillis   *Department of History, Rutgers University*
Michael R. Haines   *Department of Economics, Colgate University*
Michael Hanagan   *Committee on Historical Studies, New School for Social Research*

Lynn Hollen Lees   *Department of History, University of Pennsylvania*
David Levine   *Department of History, Ontario Institute for Studies in Education, Toronto*

Mary Jo Maynes   *Department of History, University of Minnesota*
Angus McLaren   *Department of History, University of Victoria, British Columbia*

Leslie Page Moch   *Department of History, University of Michigan–Flint*

Ellen Ross   *School of Social Science, Ramapo College*
Chiara Saraceno   *Dipartimento de Scienze Sociali, Universita degli Studi di Torino*

Jane Schneider   *Anthropology Department, Graduate Center of the City University of New York*

Peter Schneider   *Division of Social Sciences, Fordham University*
Wally Seccombe   *Department of Sociology, Ontario Institute for Studies in Education, Toronto*

Martine Segalen   *Centre d'Ethnologie Française, Paris*
Louise A. Tilly   *Committee on Historical Studies, New School for Social Research*

Susan Cotts Watkins   *Department of Sociology, University of Pennsylvania*
Jay M. Winter   *Pembroke College, University of Cambridge*

Series Editor's Preface

THIS SERIES

Studies in Social Discontinuity presents historically grounded analyses of important social transformations, ruptures, conflicts, and contradictions. Although we of Blackwell Publishers interpret that mission broadly, leave room for many points of view, and absolve authors of any responsibility for proselytization on behalf of our intellectual program, the series as a whole demonstrates the relevance of well-crafted historical work for the understanding of contemporary social structures and processes. Books in the series pursue one or more of four varieties of historical analysis: (1) using evidence from past times and places systematically to identify regularities in processes and structures that transcend those particular times and places; (2) reconstructing critical episodes in the past for the light they shed on important eras, peoples, or social phenomena; (3) tracing the origins or previous phases of significant social processes that continue into our own time; and (4) examining the ways that social action at a given point in time leaves residues that limit the possibilities of subsequent social action.

The fourth theme is at once the least familiar and the most general. Social analysts have trouble seeing that history matters precisely because social interaction takes place in well-defined times and places, and occurs within constraints offered by those times and places, producing social relations and artifacts that are themselves spatiotemporal and whose existence and distribution constrain subsequent social interaction. The construction of a city in a given place and time affects urban growth in adjacent areas and subsequent times. Where and when industrialization occurs affects how it occurs. Initial visions of victory announce a war's likely outcomes. A person's successive migrations have cumulative effects on his or her subsequent mobility through such simple matters as the presence or absence of information about new opportunities in different places and the presence or absence of social ties to possible destinations. A population's past experience with wars, baby booms, and migrations haunts it in the form of bulging or empty cohorts and unequal gender ratios. All of these matters are profoundly historical, even when they occur in the present; time and place are of their essence. They form the core of Studies in Social Discontinuity.

Edward Shorter, Stanley Holwitz, and I plotted Studies in Social Discontinuity in 1970–1; the first book, William Christian's *Person and God in a Spanish Valley*, appeared in 1972. Over the years Academic Press published more than 50 titles in the series. But during the early 1980s publication slowed, then ceased. In 1988 Blackwell Publishers agreed to revive the series under my editorship. *The European Experience of Declining Fertility* arrives as the ninth book of the renewed series.

THIS BOOK

This book falls chiefly into our third category of analysis: tracing the origins or previous phases of significant social processes that continue into our own time. Editors John R. Gillis, Louise A. Tilly, and David Levine and their contributing authors take up one of the deepest social processes – the vexing but little-resolved question of how to explain sustained fertility declines in large populations. The rate at which populations produce children obviously interacts with rates of mortality and migration to govern how fast those populations grow or shrink. Less obvious, however, is that this fertility rate also interacts with how much of their lives women spend in pregnancy and childbearing, what sorts of domestic and commercial work women do, the length of childhood and adolescence, male and female sexual practices, beliefs about family life, definitions of gender differences, and opportunities for romantic love. Gillis, Tilly, Levine, and their collaborators deal with all these questions, and more.

Chapters of *The European Experience of Declining Fertility* resemble the roots of a great oak: they all meet at a common trunk, but from there each goes its own way to search for sustenance. These 15 chapters discuss not only abortion, contraception, sexual practices, marriage, husband-wife relations, and parenthood, but also war, state policy, social class, occupations, and long-distance migration. A reader can find in this study, for example, evidence that advocates of voluntary contraception frequently sought to discourage previously widespread abortion, that whole populations practiced coitus interruptus quite effectively, that total war moved governments toward vigorous promotion of rewards for childbearing. Collectively these essays survey much of the most challenging work researchers are now doing on the historical context of demographic change. As a small encyclopedia of inquiries now in progress, this book has much to recommend it.

The chapters of this volume constitute at once an aftermath and a prologue to the study of fertility decline. The quarter century following 1965 began in the midst of a great resurgence in fertility – the famous baby boom of Western Europe and North America – but ended with fertility levels that were low in comparison with previous centuries throughout the West. It also began with many students of population defending, against the apparent counter-evidence of the baby boom, a theory of demographic transition that saw a shift toward low fertility as a relatively direct, inevitable, and irreversible consequence of industrialization, urbanization, and rising income levels. Since the 1960s many researchers in Europe and North America have sought to put twentieth-century changes in perspective and to challenge or refine theories of demographic transition by conducting detailed historical studies of populations in which long-term fertility declines had already occurred. This research included large-scale studies of French fertility change from the eighteenth to the twentieth century initiated by Louis Henry; even more massive analyses of English fertility from the sixteenth to the nineteenth century led by E. A. Wrigley and Roger Schofield; a vast comparison of demographic changes in European regions during the nineteenth and twentieth centuries coordinated by Ansley Coale; and a plethora of smaller-scale analyses by demographers, historians, and economists.

The quarter century's results badly shook the old theory of demographic transition but did not construct a widely accepted alternative. Instead, these results left students of fertility decline with a much clearer account of what had to be explained, a catalog of failed hypotheses, a variety of competing new hypotheses, considerable skepticism about the directness of connections between industrialization and fertility decline, and a widespread conviction that something called "culture" played a large part in the transition from high to low fertility. This book comes as an aftermath to that set of conclusions: in the first chapter George Alter lays out the history and impact of that research with exemplary clarity.

The authors recruited by Gillis, Tilly, and Levine concern themselves especially with the findings of the Princeton University study conducted by Ansley Coale and associates. These findings provide not only a timetable but also a geography of fertility change during the nineteenth and twentieth centuries for small political subdivisions through much of Europe. They establish unequivocally the rapidity and definitiveness of European child-bearing rates after 1870 or so and deny any neat correspondence of that decline to industrialization and urbanization. They also provide substantial indications that the populations of entire countries and of regions of two or more adjacent countries with similar religions and/or languages tended to experience fertility decline together. Following up on these indications, this book's authors examine the historical record for clues to the actual relationships of cultural differences to fertility patterns.

In this regard *The European Experience of Declining Fertility* is also a prologue. Overall, its contributors study the middle ground between broad transformations such as industrialization and fine changes in fertility-affecting behavior. Although the authors vary somewhat in their proportions of materialism and idealism, they are on the whole dissatisfied with leaving "culture" the unexplained cause of all social behavior. In general they conceive of culture as socially shared understandings and the objectifications thereof. As a group they search for concrete connections between culturally informed practices and the range of action that immediately affects fertility – notably marriage, sexual relations, and contraception. (Nutrition and disease, to take two other powerful factors in fertility, come in for very little attention here.) Without making great claims or proposing grand theories, the authors aim toward new models of fertility change in which alterations and variations in socially shared understandings and their objectifications strongly affect the rates at which whole populations produce children. They are writing an invitation to a bold new inquiry.

CHARLES TILLY

Acknowledgments

This volume owes much to a variety of people and places. It is the product of three working sessions, the first at the Continuing Education Center of Rutgers University, the second at the Ontario Institute for Studies in Education in Toronto, and the third at Pembroke College, Cambridge. Bringing an international group of scholars together would not have been possible without the financial support of the Council of European Studies, the Western European Committee of the Social Science Research Council, the Social Sciences and Humanities Research Council of Canada, and the Alfred A. Sloan Foundation. Editing for this volume of essays was completed while Louise Tilly was a Fellow at the Center for Advanced Study in the Behavioral Sciences, Stanford, California. She is grateful for financial support provided by National Endowment for the Humanities # RA-20037-88 and the Andrew W. Mellon Foundation.

The number of persons who have encouraged, guided, and critiqued our work at various stages is legion, but we would like to make special mention of Dr. Michael Teitelbaum of the Alfred A. Sloan Foundation, Professors Tony Wrigley and Richard Wall of the Cambridge Group for the Study of Population and Social Structure, and Professor Charles Tilly of the New School for Social Research. Not least, we would like to thank Barbara Sutton for her meticulous editing of our collective work.

John R. Gillis
Louise A. Tilly
David Levine

In memory of

Zachary Glendon-Ross
(1982–1989)

Benjamin Robert Gillis
(1965–1991)

INTRODUCTION

The Quiet Revolution

John R. Gillis, Louise A. Tilly, and David Levine

Some revolutions begin with the roar of cannons and are commemorated with parades and fireworks. Others take place without fanfare and run so silently that they are ignored even by historians charged with recording great social changes. The rapid and comprehensive fertility decline that began in Europe in the 1870s had an effect every bit as dramatic as two other great transformations, urbanization and industrialization, with which it is usually associated and, simplistically, conflated. Yet educated people and historians alike have taken the fertility decline for granted as an unexamined feature of modern society, requiring no further explanation.

The prevalent reproduction pattern across Europe (and in North America) today is one of the unique and distinctive developments of modern times. Although urbanization and industrialization were well under way by the latter part of the nineteenth century, the kind of family limitation all Europeans now practice was confined to a few isolated groups before the 1870s. Some elements of the aristocracy and certain urban bourgeoisies had started to stop having large families earlier, but only in France had family limitation in the modern sense already been initiated on a broader social scale (Livi-Bacci, 1986, pp. 182–200). There fertility had already fallen by 10 percent by 1827, but in the rest of Europe old patterns persisted until the last third of the century. Then, with remarkable simultaneity and speed, European fertility began its unprecedented plunge. Between 1890 and 1920, half of Europe's 600 provinces experienced a 10 percent decline in fertility. This began in the Northwest, but the South and East were not slow to follow. Belgium had reached the point of 10 percent decline by 1881, Germany by 1888, Britain (excluding Ireland) by 1910, the Netherlands by 1911. Scandinavia followed by 1912, Italy by 1913. Spain reached the same point in 1920, and European Russia in 1922, the same year as Ireland (Coale and Treadway, 1986, p. 38).

It can be shown that the downward trend was remarkably uniform within nations, disregarding boundaries between town and country, agricultural and industrial areas, regions of high literacy and regions of low literacy. While the pattern of uniformity within national boundaries is striking, the long-term results were much the same regardless of nationality. The fertility decline was not only universal, it was also unrelenting. Once the 10 percent fall was achieved, the trend toward the two-child family has continued with no sign of reversal.

Europe's fertility patterns have fluctuated before, but declines – usually quite limited – were due to changes in the age of marriage or the spacing of births, and they always ended in resumed high fertility. In earlier times, when women had wed later or breast-fed their children longer (thus increasing the intervals between births), they continued to have children until menopause. Beginning in the 1870s, however, women were starting to stop before the end of their fertile years, signalling not only a fundamental strategic change in patterns of family limitation but new attitudes toward fertility itself. In the space of just a few decades, longstanding childbearing patterns changed fundamentally, moving toward the current norm of European fertility: two children born early in the marriage or, as is now the case in some Scandinavian countries, within stable cohabitation.

Today the large families of earlier generations are only a memory, sometimes the object of nostaglia but almost never of emulation. To Europeans, as to most Americans, the two-child family now seems perfectly natural, unquestionably the right way of doing things. If they were told that what they are doing is extraordinary, even revolutionary, they would be quite surprised.

HISTORIANS AND FERTILITY DECLINE

People's reluctance to think of their own reproductive behavior as subject to change can be explained by modern culture's regrettable tendency to mistake the historical for the natural, the variable and particular for the eternal and universal. It is therefore imperative, Roland Barthes reminds us, "to reverse the terms of this very old imposture, constantly to scour nature, its 'laws' and its 'limits' in order to discover History there, and at last to establish Nature itself as historical" (Barthes, 1987, p. 101).

It is particularly regrettable (and inexcusable) that historians have paid so little attention to this quiet revolution. They have been content to let demographers describe and analyze temporal and geographic variation in fertility. We are indeed fortunate that the quantitative dimensions of fertility decline have been superbly laid out and discussed by Ansley Coale and his historical demographer colleagues in the the Princeton European Fertility Project. Without their early posing of the problem, their systematic investigation for hundreds of European provinces, and their long labor of analysis, the spatial and temporal dimensions of the quiet revolution would be only imperfectly known.*

Historians have been slow to recognize the contributions of historical demographers. And even when they acknowledge the historicity of fertility decline, they only rarely integrate this into their master narrative of political, economic, and cultural changes. Fertility decline has instead been permitted to stand in splendid isolation, in that "facts-of-life" category which requires no further explanation. Reproduction is thus placed outside history, in the realm of biology and nature, governed by a logic different from other large-scale changes with which historians feel more comfortable.

To date, the fertility revolution is not one of those subjects like World War I or the Great Depression that is regarded as integral to the explanation of how Europe came to be what it is today. This volume is an effort to change that, to suggest the ways in which fertility decline was connected with the political and economic as well as the social and cultural changes that make up the broad sweep of modern European history.

Demography is too important to be left to the demographers. As George Alter's introductory essay points out, their methods and objectives are not necessarily those of historians, even when they are dealing with historical materials. The results of the Princeton project are critically important, but, because they have collected data at the province level rather than from smaller units such as the parish or the household, they cannot possibly answer all the questions about personal and social behavior that historians would pose.

Furthermore, demographers are also more likely to be satisfied with inference from statistical correlations, while many historians look for causes at the level of intentional behavior, which is best explored with qualitative sources. Historians think in terms of contingencies – events such as wars, depressions, intellectual movements – allowing for the play of structures and forces of change, whereas demographers think in terms of transcultural, transnational processes – industrialization, urbanization, modernization – which tend not only to neglect the particular but also to obscure human agency.

Demographers themselves have begun to question whether such crude variables should be used to explain the fertility decline and are now talking about culture as the key to new explanation (Watkins, 1986). Most historians, however, would regard their concept of culture as insufficiently specified, still so reified as to deny the kind of contingency and agency that is typically central to historical narrative.

It would be wrong to fault demographers, however, for what are really historians' failings to engage themselves with a subject so central to the development of European society. Historians have paid surprisingly little attention

---

* Results summarized in Coale and Watkins, 1986.

to the ways in which fertility decline has affected the labor force and consumer economy, and how it has shaped the welfare, education, and military
policies of modern nation-states. The quiet revolution's connection with class,
gender, and generational change has also been largely neglected. The absence
of a synthetic treatment that would establish the significance of fertility for
the shape of modern European society is something for which historians
have only themselves to blame.

We do not claim to have remedied this lacuna in a systematic way. What
the essays in this collection provide is, *first*, insight into the experience of
fertility decline in the public as well as private lives of Europeans, and,
second, analysis of the fertility decline as both cause and consequence of
other processes of large-scale structural change. We are concerned here with
reintegrating the story of fertility decline with modern European history
generally. We do not claim to have constructed a final synthesis; nor do we
pretend to provide a complete account of either cause or effect. Several of
our studies look at aggregate fertility as it is related to large-scale structural
change. For example, Susan Cotts Watkins effectively demonstrates some of
the ways in which aggregate fertility decline has been related to state formation and national development, and Michael R. Haines looks at occupation
and fertility cross-nationally. Most of our authors are concerned, however,
with microprocesses and small-scale settings in which the focus is how
fertility decline was actually experienced by the millions of woman and men
who participated in the quiet revolution. Here the essays by John R. Gillis,
Angus McLaren, Mary Jo Maynes, Ellen Ross, Chiara Saraceno, Wally
Seccombe, and Martine Segalen are exemplary. Still other contributors, such
as Jane and Peter Schneider, combine an acute sense of large-scale political
and economic change with community ethnography and class analysis.
Several chapters concern ways in which fertility decline has affected the
shape of modern Europe: Lynn Hollen Lees, for example, examines the
effect of declining fertility on education and welfare policies, and Michael
Hanagan discusses its interaction with labor relations and workers' collective
action. Other contributors, such as Leslie Page Moch, show the ways in
which migration tended to reduce urban/rural differences during the nineteenth century, and J. M. Winter, who surveys the consequences of two
world wars for fertility, looks at the relation of world historical events to
reproductive practice. None of our contributors confronts global questions
of cause; they are more concerned with the conditions under which the
quiet revolution came about than with making a final statement of why it
happened.

Thus we offer no grand theory about why Europe started to limit births so
uniformly. Our research reveals the many patterns subsumed in the overall
decline, how that decline is related to other large-scale changes, and how, in
turn, its consequences have shaped European history since 1870 and have
been shaped by it. Together, these essays make a convincing case for placing

fertility decline as both cause and effect at the center of any analysis of the conditions under which Europe assumed its present political, economic, and social characteristics.

TOWARD AN EXPLANATION

The relative simultaneity of fertility decline both among various social groups within particular nation-states and across Europe would seem to suggest a singular process, if not a single cause. But in this case the uniformity of outcomes obscures the variety and complexity of the many local processes that contributed to the remarkable result. When demographers study fertility at aggregated levels (the nation, or even the province) they seek causes in large structural changes. When the same events are studied at the village or household level, however, it is not uniformity but diversity, not one cause but many, which emerge. As this volume shows, the quiet revolution is not one story but many. The results in various nation-states may be similar, but they were arrived at in quite dissimilar ways.

We have found it useful to think of a mechanism for fertility change in terms of "cultures of contraception," specific to place and to time, constantly changing even as they contributed to the quiet revolution. The cultures of contraception were specific to class, gender, and community. Angus McLaren's research demonstrates that the method of birth control chosen in Britain was strongly influenced by class culture. The middle-class preference for mechanical devices owed not only to the fact that the affluent could afford such devices, but to a class culture than promoted conjugal intimacy and encouraged men and women to cooperate in sexual matters. A sharper division between husbands and wives prevalent in working-class marriages meant that, in Britain, the women of that class were more likely to choose abortion as the first line of fertility control so that they did not have to rely on male cooperation. What the middle class condemned as irrational and immoral, working-class women found satisfactory and well justified. In peasant agricultural societies and in nominally Catholic urban Italy, coitus interruptus, which required male participation, was more acceptable. The medical profession and advocates of birth control played a part in shaping cultures of conception and the norms of sexuality as well, but there was no one pattern by which reproductive norms were transmitted between classes, genders, or generations.

We emphasize, then, the degree to which the European fertility decline was the product of conscious choice, but we do not want to suggest by this that the range of options open to women and men was unlimited. On the contrary, factors of class weighed heavily, and power relations between the sexes determined the timing and methods by which reductions in births were achieved. The cultures of contraception some of our authors describe were rarely consensual and were often hotly contested. At times the quiet revolution produced quite violent public debates over abortion and other issues. In the private sphere as well, it was often accompanied by conflict and violence.

Social and cultural factors are important in understanding fertility decline. The Princeton project showed that the broad outlines of fertility decline tended to conform to cultural boundaries rather than run along urban/rural or agricultural/industrial divisions. Susan Watkins has demonstrated that, in country after country, "after controlling for modernization, those provinces that were contiguous, and especially those that could be said to share a language, religion, or ethnic identification, or more generally a cultural as well as spatial location, were similar to each other" (1986, p. 441). In her essay for this volume, Watkins suggests that mass education, the nationalization of media (including advertising), and the emergence of national consumer markets had the powerful effect of eroding provincial differences within national boundaries.

Leslie Moch's study of migration provides additional insight into why urban and rural cultures of contraception were less different than might be expected. In a similar manner, Michael Hanagan demonstrates the permeability of agrarian and industrial boundaries in France, thus providing concrete evidence of why abstract concepts like industrialization no longer have the credibility sometimes attributed to them.

There is no question but that, in the nineteenth century and the first half of the twentieth, national boundaries became increasingly important culturally and economically. As J. M. Winter suggests, one aspect of this process was mass mobilization for war, which in turn affected fertility patterns. While pronatalist governments such as Fascist Italy have been generally unsuccessful in controlling reproductive behavior directly, without question state power has, as David Levine points out, altered the experience of fertility decline in subtle and often indirect ways.

At the same time, our studies also suggest that cultures of contraception remain essentially local and highly particular with respect to class and gender. Martine Segalen's work shows that cultures of contraception could vary from region to region within Brittany. As the Schneiders' study of Sicily shows, people living in the same village practiced family limitation in different ways, with the timing of their adoption of control varying according to their class. The gentry were the first to stop, followed by better-off artisans, and only much later the poorest rural wage laborers. This convergence was not simply a matter of diffusion. People began to limit births because they had decided for themselves when and with what means to stop having more children.

Contraceptive practice varied not only by class, however; cultures of contraception were – and are – gendered. Wally Seccombe shows how gender relationships changed before coitus interruptus could become an effective means of limiting fertility. The couple is not always an appropriate unit of analysis when it comes to explaining reproductive behavior. Among the English working class in particular, there existed quite separate male and female cultures of contraception, and responsibility for fertility control was unevenly distributed, with the greater burden falling on the woman. Among peasant groups studied by Segalen and the Schneiders, cooperation in contraceptive practice paralleled the shared enterprise of the peasant household; some urban groups, like the Milanese examined by Chiara Saraceno, also shared responsibility.

Abstract notions of motherhood and fatherhood are inadequate, John Gillis argues, to the task of interpreting gender-specific experiences of parenthood. These have been shaped by changing definitions of masculinity and femininity, and have varied historically during the modern period. Gillis shows how changing gender conceptions among the British middle class transformed the meaning of motherhood, which in turn had important consequences for fertility. Ellen Ross also demonstrates how changing notions of maternity affected, albeit in a quite different way, the experience of fertility among the London working classes, while Saraceno's research confirms the importance of changing gender conceptions in altering attitudes toward family life in Italy.

Fertility decline was not just a matter of changing notions of femininity, as these affected motherhood. Understanding men's experience and changing motivation is necessary to any complete analysis of reproductive behavior. The timing and method of family limitation were dependent also on changing views of masculinity. Saraceno's study shows that for coitus interruptus to work, the concept of the good husband also had to change significantly.

Our studies do not address directly the notion of rational parents planning family size based on the costs and benefits of children. They do show, however, that views on ideal family size are invariably mediated by a variety of social, cultural, and economic considerations. When couples started to stop having more children they did not necessarily make numeric calculations, and in some cases the value of sons or daughters varied according to prevailing gender conceptions.

Different groups held very different views of what constituted a proper family. Much depended on the way they perceived fatherhood and motherhood and appropriate parent-child relationships, but variable concepts of childhood played a part in fertility decline. The ways childhood was experienced – or, better yet, how that experience was later constructed – had important consequences for adult attitudes toward childbearing. The enormous stress that large families placed on working-class families in the late nineteenth and early twentieth centuries had consequences that have been felt well into our own times. Mary Jo Maynes's study of German and French autobiographies suggests that a generation's decisions about family size were not just a matter of objective calculations of future costs and benefits;

subjectively constructed memories of childhood abundance or deprivation also shape notions of ideal family size.

* * *

If *demographic transition* is defined as a universal pattern that first occurred in the Western world and, under similar circumstances, will also transpire in other world regions, then our understanding of European fertility decline does not fit well with the conventional notion. Our findings will not provide much support to those who think that a particular mix of industrialization and urbanization or a special educational program will result in fertility decline elsewhere in the world.

The period before fertility decline began in the 1870s is often presented as dominated by fatalism, governed by biology or yoked to the past through custom and tradition. A sharp contrast is usually drawn between an unreflective, hidebound fertility behavior in the past and self-conscious, future-oriented modes of thinking in the present. The variety of cultures of contraception we have explored cannot be neatly arranged along a continuum from traditionalism to instrumental rationality. As Angus McLaren (1984) has shown, women and men of the past were by no means passive about their fertility, even though they did not always have the means to regulate it except at great sacrifice.

Nor do men and women today necessarily act rationally when it comes to reproduction. In the case of Breton villagers studied by Martine Segalen, the decision to have fewer children sometimes conflicted with the needs of the family farm, suggesting that modern birth controllers are not necessarily better calculators than their forebears. In fact, the very unrevolutionary idea of tradition figures prominently in Europe's quiet revolution. Desire to uphold beloved traditions was often one of the motivations for fertility reduction.

When people decide how many children they wish to have they are simultaneously deciding how they understand themselves and how they wish to represent themselves to the world. We have found that it is impossible to separate biological from cultural reproduction. Childbearing and child raising remains one of modern Europeans' most important symbolic activities, contributing to the way they think about themselves, communicate with one another, and construct their gender, class, and communal identities.

Within the present organization of scholarship the study of population change is an independent discipline, leaving the impression that fertility is separable from other human concerns and activities, that it has its own special logic, more closely linked to economic interests than to cultural values. But decisions about fertility are always embedded in class, gender, and community concerns. No purely rational or functional approach can possibly capture all that was involved in Europe's quiet revolution.

The experience – the causes and the consequences of fertility decline – is best approached through interdisciplinary efforts. Our working group consists of anthropologists, sociologists, historians, economists, and demographers. Among our historian colleagues are several interested in political and military as well as social change, in the cultural as well as the economic dimensions of the past. In the course of the three meetings that led to this volume, we have stretched the categories of analysis, opened up new perspectives, and, while complicating the subject, enriched its analysis and enhanced its relevance to many areas of modern European history.

We do not claim to provide a complete picture of the European experience of fertility decline. Our geographical coverage is incomplete, considering only some of the national, regional, and social groupings of Western Europe. Many dimensions of the fertility decline we have barely touched on. For instance, we have not explored in depth the relationship of fertility to developments in medicine, to changing conceptions of the body, or to the history of housing. If these essays convince the reader of the centrality of fertility decline to modern European history, if they provide new ways of understanding phenomena previously seen in isolation, if they provide models for future research in other countries, then the book will have served the purposes for which it was intended.

I

The Debate about European Fertility Decline

I

Theories of Fertility Decline:
A Nonspecialist's Guide to the Current Debate

George Alter

Historical research on human fertility has been closely linked to the current controversies over international and national population policies. The European fertility transition during the nineteenth century was the inspiration for the most widely held theory of demographic change, and it continues to be used as a model for developing and testing hypotheses. There is a noteworthy interchange between historical studies and research on contemporary populations. Major demographers have written on historical themes, and historians have been quick to recognize new theories in the demographic literature. Despite the abundance of demographic studies of non-European societies, there is still an important role for historical demography in this debate.

In the last 20 years the field's dominant consensus, the theory of the demographic transition, has been dramatically shattered. This consensus was largely a generalization about European experience, and historical research on Europe was responsible for discrediting it. The result has been a period of retrenchment and the gradual emergence of new styles of reasoning. The policy implications of these new positions significantly differ from the earlier consensus and from each other. Readers who approach this literature with a different perspective may have difficulty seeing why some distinctions are considered important by specialists in the field. Indeed, historians may ultimately question whether it is necessary to choose among these competing theories at all.

In this essay I examine three leading theories of fertility decline that are widely cited by demographers concerned with both historical and contemporary demographic problems. My goal is not to evaluate the evidence in support of each theory but rather to identify the central assumptions and propositions underlying each school of thought. I shall try to show that these schools can be characterized by their answers to two fundamental questions: Do fertility transitions result from changes in parents' motivation to limit family size or from changes in attitudes and access to birth control? If changes in motivation are the determining factor, to what extent are these changes linked to socioeconomic change, or are key attitudes about the family and children spread independently of prevailing structural conditions?

DEFINING THE PROBLEM

Although much has been written about fertility transitions, it is easy to become lost in technical details and lose sight of the central issue. It is helpful, therefore, to pose the question in its simplest terms – that is, What behavior characterizes a population that has undergone a fertility transition? The answer is that post-transitional populations are ones in which many couples decide not to have any additional children before the end of their childbearing years. In any historical moment the decision every couple faces is whether to have another child. Theories of fertility more often pose the question in terms of a desired family size rather than a decision to continue childbearing, and it may be that couples enter marriage with a target size in mind. Nevertheless, each couple can always choose to have another child at any moment as long as both wife and husband remain fecund. The fertility decision, therefore, is always ultimately the decision to have or not to have one more child.

Despite the apparent simplicity of this definition of the problem, it precludes alternative forms of population control that have drawn the attention of historical demographers in recent years. The first alternative involves strategies of controlling fertility by limiting the proportion of the population who are married. Malthus drew attention to delayed marriage as a way of reducing family size, and English historical demographers have continued to attach considerable importance to the role of marriage (both age at marriage and proportion never marrying) in the regulation of preindustrial population growth (Hajnal, 1965, 1983; Wrigley and Schofield, 1981, chap. 11). In Europe the fertility transition represents a shift in the mechanism of population control from restriction of marriage to limitation of childbearing within marriage.

The role of "spacing" versus "stopping" in early stages of the fertility transition is also controversial. Because a woman's childbearing years are limited, completed family size can be reduced by increasing the intervals between children. Couples could have created lower fertility by substantially increasing the intervals between children without deciding to stop childbearing completely at any given point. Thus contraception may be used in one of two ways to achieve a family of a certain size: couples may not use it until a target number of children has been reached and then try to prevent any additional births, or they may use it more or less continuously from the beginning of marriage to reduce overall family size by extending the intervals between all births. Although some researchers have adduced evidence that appears to show some role for spacing, most of the evidence points to "stopping" as the main strategy of family limitation (Henry, 1961, 1977; Coale and Trussell, 1974; cf. Anderton and Bean, 1985). If we look at the problem from a broader perspective, "spacing" could have been no more than a temporary stage. In the twentieth century the intervals between births were reduced, as couples compressed childbearing into a smaller amount of time.

Demography has a tradition of taking as the problem the decision to avert the next birth rather than the decision to have another child. This manner of posing the question is based upon long-held assumptions. Demographers begin with the position that a minimal rate of sexual intercourse between married couples is unavoidable. This assumption can be traced backward at least to Malthus (1959, pp. 4-5), who is commonly regarded as one of the founding fathers of demography. While Malthus emphasized delayed entry to marriage as the most effective control on fertility, demographers since the late nineteenth century have typically looked to neo-Malthusian controls such as contraception and abortion.

Complete sexual abstinence within marriage has never been widely advocated, although Paul A. David and Warren C. Sanderson (1976) have argued that reducing the frequency of intercourse may have played an important role in some social groups. Nor is there extensive evidence of population control after birth (i.e., infanticide). Although some historians have asserted that infanticide was common, historical cases of infanticide can almost always be traced to unwed mothers. Even these women were rarely convicted of murder (Higginbotham, 1985, pp. 218-47; Leboutte, 1983). Some authors, however, argue that practices such as wet-nursing and child abandonment were thinly veiled forms of infanticide, and others believe that more or less deliberate neglect contributed to high infant mortality before the fertility transition (Shorter, 1977, chap. 5).

Given this definition of the problem, we must explain family limitation, not fertility itself. Since childbearing will continue at some "natural" rate under the impulse of sexual attraction, the problem to be explained is why couples go to the trouble to prevent another birth. The essence of the problem, therefore, is that some couples decide to stop after they have reached a family size that their parents had generally surpassed.

ECONOMIC AND NONECONOMIC ASPECTS OF FAMILY SIZE DECISIONS

In simple terms, couples must weigh the costs and benefits of life with one more child against the costs and benefits of life without another child *plus* the costs of preventing the birth of the next child. Simple terms, however, are often misleading, and in this debate seemingly economic terms often hide arguments about subjective states and values. Many of the costs and benefits of children are subjective, nonmonetary considerations. Parents must assess how highly they value the satisfaction and pride that they derive from a child, as well as the many opportunities that they must forego because of childrearing. Economic terminology like "costs" and "wealth" are used to describe changes in preferences and life-styles that are fundamentally non-economic in origin.

The most important example of this problem is the question of the "costs of children." It is frequently argued that children have become more expens-ive. Subjects in surveys and interviews overwhelmingly report that children cost more now than they did in the past (Knodel, Chamratrithirong, and Debavalya, 1987, chap. 7). On close examination, however, they are not describing a change in the costs of children as much as a change in their own definition of appropriate childrearing. The money cost of a child is the sum of the prices of the commodities that children consume and the quantities of these commodities consumed. In economic analysis it is important to distinguish between prices and quantities in the cost of a child, because they imply different definitions of parental behavior. Changes in prices are beyond the family's control. The quantities consumed at a given price level are within the parents' control, however, and a change in their behavior represents a change in their subjective preferences, not in the economic environment.

Historically, children have become expensive not because the prices of commodities consumed by children have risen, but rather because parents have decided to invest more in goods and services for their children. Parents in each generation have chosen to educate their children more than their forebears had, often in advance of prodding from the state. Although longer education has dramatically increased the cost of rearing a child, this change has little to do with the price of a year of education. Even if the price of a given level of education did rise relative to other prices, it certainly did not rise faster than real incomes in Europe. In effect, parents have chosen to raise one or two highly educated children rather than four or five less ex-pensive children. Economists refer to this as a preference for child "quality" rather than child "quantity" (Becker and Lewis, 1973; Sanderson, 1976).

There is more here than a dispute over terminology and language. When rising young professionals decide to buy Volvos rather than Fiats, we do not say that automobiles have become more expensive. Yet both historical and contemporary accounts suggest that parents believe that the rising costs of raising children are outside their control. Childrearing is an area in which the enforcement of behavioral standards is often overt, and parents may well believe that they have little choice but to adhere to the norms of their social groups. Children do become more expensive under these conditions, but this is the result of a cultural change, not an economic change. James S.

Duesenberry remarked in an early debate on this issue: "Economics is all about how people make choices. Sociology is all about why they don't have any choices to make" (1960, p. 223).[1]

EASTERLIN'S "SUPPLY-DEMAND" FRAMEWORK

The differences among competing theories can be more easily understood by relating them to a common framework. Richard Easterlin (1978; Easterlin and Crimmins, 1985) has proposed a useful framework for analyzing fertility decisions in which all three of the theories examined here can be expressed. In Easterlin's model, the fertility decision involves two kinds of choices. Couples implicitly have in mind a desired family size. They compare the costs and benefits of children to the costs and benefits of alternative lifestyles available to them within the limitations imposed by their expected future income. Desired family size is an expression of both the relative costs of childrearing compared with other activities and parents' subjective preferences within the constraints imposed by income. Desired family size, called parents' "demand" for children, must also be compared with the "supply" of children that will be produced in the absence of fertility control measures. The "supply" of children depends on the biological and social determinants of fertility (fecundity, frequency of intercourse, duration of lactation) and on the mortality of children. When mortality is high, parents must plan on a large number of births to achieve a desired number of surviving children.

Parents subjectively evaluate the costs and benefits of the family that they will have if they do not employ birth control. Easterlin characterizes the difference between the subjective evaluations of this "natural fertility" family size and the desired family as the "motivation for fertility control." When desired family size is larger than the natural family size, motivation for family limitation will be lacking.

An "excess supply" of children does not immediately result in a fertility transition, however. Family limitation is not costless, and parents must compare the costs of exceeding their target family size with the costs of regulating their fertility. Several different types of costs are associated with birth control. First, knowledge about methods must be acquired. This information may be very difficult to find when family limitation is not widespread. Second, some contraceptive methods involve money expenditures. (i.e., for condoms, pills). Finally, couples must evaluate the subjective costs of fertility control, in terms of inconvenience, interference with sexual gratification, and their religious and moral beliefs. Couples may decide that the disadvantages of reducing fertility are more distasteful than the costs of additional children.[2]

The Easterlin framework identifies the three major aspects of fertility decision-making that are reflected in competing theories of fertility decline: desired family size, the supply of children, and the costs of birth control. Desired family size may change because of (a) changes in the prices of goods and services associated with childrearing relative to prices of other kinds of expenditures, (b) family incomes, or (c) preferences regarding childrearing and competing activities. The supply of children depends on the determinants of fertility in the absence of fertility limitation and child mortality. The costs of birth control involve the diffusion of information, monetary costs, and cultural values. The major theories of European fertility transition differ in which of these aspects is emphasized.

THE THEORY OF THE DEMOGRAPHIC TRANSITION

For many years discussion of fertility decline was dominated by a set of interrelated propositions known as the theory of the demographic transition. This theory grew out of a description of demographic change in nineteenth-century Europe, and it has always been difficult to distinguish demographic transition as a theory from the historical generalizations based on European experience.[3] Classic statements of the theory are found in Adolphe Landry (1933) and Frank W. Notestein (1953). Like other forms of "modernization theory" popular in the 1950s and 1960s, demographic transition theory assumed that modernization was a complex and multifaceted process. Although societies might differ in timing, each would come under the sway of a common set of forces associated with the rise of industry and the diffusion of education.

The theory held that from the demographic history of Europe we could discern a common sequence of events that were the key to predicting future developments elsewhere in the world. Advances in technology and science beginning in the eighteenth century led to a rising standard of living and improved medical care. These forces reduced the level of mortality and consequently increased the rate of population growth in the nineteenth century. At first fertility remained at preindustrial levels, but forces that reduced fertility as well were soon at work. On one hand, lower mortality increased the survival, and thus the supply, of children. On the other hand, industrialization and urbanization introduced new life-styles reducing the demand for children. The price of food was higher in cities than in the countryside, and children had fewer opportunities to contribute income to the family in an industrial society than they had in peasant agriculture. Furthermore, the new society created alternatives to the family-oriented life-style of previous generations – alternatives that competed for parents' time and money. By the late nineteenth century fertility was falling, and in the twentieth century an equilibrium between fertility and mortality was reestablished. William Petersen summarized the process in this way:

Industrialization loosens the social structure of an agrarian society: the sharp increase in both geographical and social mobility means that more and more persons are removed from the influence and control of the extended kin group to the relatively anonymous life of the large city. The normative system of the agrarian society (religious values, family sentiments, etc.) may also be weakened by this loss of its institutional base, which is challenged as well by the higher valuation of rationality in an industrial urban setting. Fertility, in brief, tends to be associated with social structure, technological standards, and specific prescriptions or taboos; all three of these determinants have been markedly changed by industrialization. (1969, p. 194)

The all-encompassing nature of the societal changes described by demographic transition theory have been a source of both weakness and strength. Critics have charged that it is not a theory at all, but only a description of a vague set of empirical correlations. It is not clear whether the changes described are economic or social in origin. Do modern people make modern societies, or do modern societies make modern* people? This lack of specificity is in its own way a strength, because it does seem to fit one of the obvious aspects of fertility decline. All currently developed societies have undergone a fertility transition, despite differences in timing and culture. Thus, a variety of specific incentives for lower fertility can be related to the general process of economic development. In the late 1960s and early 1970s it was popular to say that "economic development is the best birth control pill."

In terms of the major factors in fertility decision-making, the theory of the demographic transition emphasizes the two factors affecting motivation for fertility control: the supply and demand of children. Transition theory was based on the observation that mortality declined before fertility, and a contemporary advocate of transition theory, Jean Claude Chesnais, attacks evidence that fertility sometimes declined before mortality (1986, p. 11). Transition theory also argues that desired family size was falling, as parents assumed life-styles developed for the new, urban, industrial society. Pre-transition populations did not practice family limitation, because their desired family size was at least as large as the small number of their children who would survive.

The costs of birth control were not viewed as a limiting factor in this scenario. In the 1930s Norman Himes (1936) showed that some knowledge of birth control had been present in every historical period. Furthermore, the early fertility decline in France showed that some method of control, presumably coitus interruptus, was available from at least the eighteenth century.

It has become common to emphasize versions of the theory of the demographic transition in which structural changes in the economy and society are

characterized as the causes of fertility. A quick review of three demography textbooks found that all associated fertility decline with industrialization, urbanization, and education, although each had some reservations
(Bogue, 1969, pp. 676–7; W. Peterson, 1969; Matras, 1973, p. 26). There
can be no question that authors in this tradition believed that economic
change would provoke changes in the demand for children. But they were
not simply economic determinists, as they are sometimes depicted. Economic
change was believed to bring about a profound cultural change with important implications for fertility. A decline in desired family size was as much the
product of cultural factors as economic factors. Indeed, Landry comments
on the speed with which attitudes (*moeurs*) producing family limitation can
be transmitted from one country to another (1933, p. 361).

THE EUROPEAN FERTILITY PROJECT

In 1963 Ansley Coale began to assemble a group of researchers at the Office
of Population Research at Princeton University to reconstruct the course of
fertility decline in nineteenth-century Europe. More than 20 years later the
Princeton European Fertility Project has given us a clear picture of the onset
and diffusion of fertility control at the aggregate level in all the countries of
Europe. With an output of at least eight books, numerous articles, and
a very valuable data base, this has been one of the largest undertakings in
historical demography. The legacy of the European Fertility Project is in
many respects a "negative result." The project was designed under the influence of the theory of the demographic transition, and most people interpret
its findings as a contradiction of that theory. It would be incorrect, however,
to view the work of those on the project as purely descriptive. The later
writings of the Princeton group, especially a well-known summary article by
John Knodel and Etienne van de Walle (1979), adopt a very strong theoretical position on fertility decline that emphasizes the costs of birth control.

The strong role given to economic modernization in transition theory led
to the inference that fertility decline would occur earlier in urban/industrial
areas than it would in rural/agricultural areas. Cross-sectional data from the
twentieth century clearly point in this direction, because fertility has been
notably lower in cities than in the countryside. The European Fertility Project set out to verify propositions of this sort by collecting all data on fertility
and indicators of economic development for all European countries. Most
European countries have had reasonably accurate census and vital statistics
data since the middle of the nineteenth century, and these were tabulated
and published at the province level. Coale and his associates developed a set
of indices (I_f, I_g, I_m, I_h) to control for differences in age structure and to
identify trends in marriage, marital fertility, and nonmarital fertility.

As each volume describing the course of fertility in a European country was published, a mosaic of levels and trends in fertility decline began to emerge. While urbanization and industrialization were not without importance, they explained relatively little of the pattern of fertility decline. Soon after the project began, Paul Demeny (1968) drew attention to the similarity in the timing of fertility decline in England and Hungary in the 1870s. Fertility transitions occurred only a few years apart in the world's most advanced industrial economy and one of the most undeveloped countries in Europe. Urbanization and industrialization were found to play some role in explaining local differences in fertility, but they contribute little to explaining the timing of declines in countries and major regions.

Another major finding of the European Fertility Project was beginning to emerge before the project even began. In dissertation research supervised by Coale, J. William Leasure (1962) discovered that regional patterns of fertility decline in Spain conformed very closely to linguistic regions with little relation to indicators of economic development. This finding has since been verified throughout Europe. Fertility patterns in nineteenth-century Europe closely followed the language and dialect boundaries established centuries earlier. In a dramatic demonstration of this principle, Ron Lesthaeghe matched pairs of Belgian villages on either side of the linguistic frontier (1977, pp. 111–14). Even though the villages were nearly identical in economic characteristics and less than ten kilometers apart, the Walloon villages underwent the fertility transition much earlier than the Flemish villages. Each set of villages followed the timing of the linguistic region to which it belonged.

The importance of linguistic regions clearly points to a cultural interpretation of fertility decline in contrast to the economic factors emphasized by the theory of the demographic transition. Unfortunately, the European Fertility Project was not designed well enough to examine a cultural hypothesis. The data base does not include indicators of culture, and participants in the project have yet to explain what it is about linguistic regions that determines the timing of fertility decline. All of Europe's linguistic regions ultimately underwent a demographic transition, so we must ask why language affected its timing. How did the cultures of European linguistic groups differ, and what aspects of those cultures delayed or accelerated fertility decline? Indeed, did the content of these cultures matter at all, or did linguistic regions simply reflect lines of communication? So far no attempt has been made to characterize the cultural differences between linguistic regions. Lesthaeghe's analysis of socialist voting and fertility comes the closest to proposing a set of beliefs that may have affected the timing of fertility decline (Lesthaeghe, 1983; Lesthaeghe and Wilson, 1986).

It would be incorrect, however, to infer that the only contribution of the European Fertility Project has been the empirical contradiction of the theory of the demographic transition. Participants in the project have adopted a clear and distinctive theoretical position, although they have refrained from stating it as such. In a 1973 article, Ansley Coale described three preconditions for fertility decline: (a) fertility must be "within the calculus of conscious choice," (b) parents must want smaller families, and (c) the means to limit fertility must be available (p. 65). Researchers associated with the project have generally interpreted their evidence as demonstrating the absence of the first of these preconditions. They have argued that neither motivation nor means were lacking, but that the idea of intervening in the process of childbearing was not part of the worldview of nineteenth-century Europeans.

The argument that parents before the fertility transition would not even consider the possibility of birth control was proposed in a 1960 article by Philippe Ariès. Describing the origins of French fertility decline in the eighteenth century, Ariès argued that family limitation could not occur until parents saw fertility as a process subject to human control. In the worldview of early modern Europe, childbearing was considered a part of the natural world: one would no more seek to restrict fertility than try to stop the sun from shining. Fertility control was simply "unthinkable." Other authors have pointed to the results of surveys in developing countries as confirmation of this view. When African women are asked how many children they would prefer to have, they sometimes laugh at the question and respond, "It is up to God." Some demographers view this as evidence that they do not have a desired family size and are unable to even consider controlling their fertility. For Ariès the Enlightenment and the growing belief in science undermined this unified worldview. Just as physicians began to view the human body as a machine subject to physical laws and human manipulation, common people began to assert control over their own reproduction (Ariès, 1960).

It is interesting to note that writers who ascribe to this point of view do not argue that methods of birth control were lacking. Techniques were either known or could be invented (i.e., coitus interruptus). Condoms, in particular, were not unknown, but they were associated with prostitution and protection against venereal disease during illicit sexual activity (van de Walle, 1980, p. 152). A husband would not think of treating his wife like a prostitute by introducing these practices within marriage.

In terms of the three main factors in fertility decision-making I have described, the "unthinkability" hypothesis is an argument pointing to changes in the costs of birth control. A noneconomic argument such as this can be squeezed into an economic model of choice in several ways. We could say that birth control had an infinitely high "psychic" cost, or that parental preferences assured that any alternative other than fertility regulation would be chosen. In addition, this argument implies that the first couples who do consider family limitation an acceptable choice will find information about birth control difficult and expensive to acquire. The more important point is that the unthinkability hypothesis does not attribute a role to changes in the supply of or demand for children in the initiation of fertility decline. By implication, parents had a desire for smaller families, but they did not know that such an alternative could be achieved.

Knodel and van de Walle (1979) have recognized this aspect of the argument and have pointed to evidence of unwanted fertility in pretransitional populations. They emphasize findings that mortality sometimes declined after or at the same time as fertility. In such cases, fertility decline cannot be attributed to an increasing supply of children. Indeed, Knodel and van de Walle suggest that high infant and child mortality may have been prolonged by parental behavior growing out of frustration with excess fertility. In their view, more or less conscious neglect contributed to the persistence of high mortality. Practices such as wet-nursing and child abandonment, which were frequently fatal to children, were thinly veiled forms of infanticide by parents who could see no other alternative.

Lesthaeghe and Wilson (1986) take a somewhat different view. They argue that changes in modes of production affected both the role of children in the family economy and undermined traditional worldviews. Early industrialization did not always result in a desire for smaller families, because some forms of industry put a premium on family labor supply. But capitalist production did provoke a change in the relationship between man and nature and a new secular worldview. These new attitudes are apparent in the growing conflict in Catholic countries where the Church offered more resistance to these ideas than the Protestant clergy. In this explanation, motivation for fertility control was rising in the nineteenth century, but again attitudes about birth control were the determining factor in the timing and speed of fertility decline.

An interesting contrast to the "unthinkability" hypothesis has been offered by Angus McLaren (1984) in his history of "reproductive rituals." McLaren argues that attempts to control fertility, both enhancing and limiting, were in fact widespread in early modern England. Folklore and traditional medicine had numerous references to contraceptives and abortifacients, some of which may have even been effective. The idea of birth control was therefore not incompatible with a traditional worldview. On the contrary, magic and superstition prescribed ways in which fertility could be regulated. The desired result was not always achieved, but that was hardly surprising to people who believe themselves surrounded by mysterious and powerful forces. If McLaren is correct, the idea of fertility control was present, but motivation was generally lacking.

WEALTH-FLOWS THEORY

In 1976 John Caldwell offered a restatement of demographic transition theory that emphasized the role of cultural changes. Caldwell associates the fertility transition with a change in the direction of "intergenerational flows of wealth." In pretransition populations, he argues, "wealth" tends to flow from children to parents, making large families and unrestricted fertility advantageous to parents. Low-fertility societies are characterized by the heavy investments that parents make in the education and support of their children. The fertility transition occurs when the net flow of wealth shifts direction.

Caldwell's terminology has sometimes caused confusion about the character of wealth flows, and economists are likely to object to his definitions of terms. "Wealth" in this model is not a purely economic category. In addition to property, income, goods, and services, Caldwell includes intangible, non-economic benefits among the benefits that parents derive from children. For example, he argues that men in traditional societies derive satisfaction from the deference of their children and social prestige from being the heads of large families. Both deference and prestige are part of the flow of wealth from children to parents. Caldwell does argue that children are economic assets in preindustrial economies, but these economic benefits are only a part of the overall flow of services that parents derive from their children.

Intergenerational wealth flows are linked to modes of production. In peasant society, the familial organization of production reinforced male control over resources as well as reproduction. This control was weakened by the transition from familial to capitalist production, which undermined the economic power of the kin networks on which peasant society is based. The "decisive" change, however, was the rise in the cost of children as education expanded in the nineteenth century: "School children needed and demanded more expenditure, had less time for household chores, and were more resistant to working....Growing parental wealth and the waning influence of religious creeds proclaiming virtue in child austerity and child labour reinforced the tendency to spend more on children and demand less from them. Consequently the net intergenerational flow of wealth changed direction from upward to downward" (Caldwell, 1982, p. 176). In his description of the timing of fertility change in Australia, Caldwell places special emphasis on rising aspirations for education as well as other new consumer goods.

Although economic change is a large part of the historical explanation of fertility decline among European populations, Caldwell's theory is fundamentally a cultural model, not an economic one. His description of the potential for demographic change in Africa and Asia points to the central role of "Westernization," the spread of European concepts of family relationships and life-styles. These ideas are spread widely in developing countries by radio, film, and the advertisement of consumer products without any correspondence to local economic circumstances. Caldwell has been strongly critical of the standard demographic focus on economic and social structure, and he advocates the adoption of anthropological techniques for studying local cultures. His work emphasizes the importance of patriarchy and the subordinate role of women as cultural factors supporting high fertility (Caldwell, Reddy, and Caldwell, 1988).

Thus Caldwell's revised version of demographic transition theory is compatible with the evidence of cultural diffusion produced by the European Fertility Project, but his historical analysis stresses the importance of changing attitudes toward education. Economic modernization can be the immediate cause of new attitudes, as earlier transition theorists have argued, but these attitudes can also be spread by literature and popular culture independently of economic conditions.

Caldwell clearly does not share the Princeton group's focus on attitudes toward fertility regulation. The wealth-flows model points to a change in the motivation for family limitation. Fertility is high in pretransitional populations because parents, in particular fathers, see advantages in large families. A fertility transition begins when this cultural support for fertility is removed.

POLICY IMPLICATIONS

Historical research has continued to attract the attention of demographers interested in contemporary problems because the three major theories here have important policy implications for population planning in developing countries. The main area of concern is the efficacy of family-planning efforts in reducing the birth rate. Each of these theories offers a different answer to this question. The theory of the demographic transition implies that family-planning programs could do little to create a fertility transition, although such services might increase the speed of fertility decline after the transition had begun. Since fertility decline was dependent on economic and social change, economic development programs would eventually have a favorable impact on the birth rate. The European Fertility Project weakened the link between economic development and fertility decline and strengthened the case for family planning. Economic development per se would not necessarily reduce fertility. Family-planning programs, however, could provide birth control information and supplies to couples who were already motivated to reduce their fertility. Perhaps more important, publicity campaigns associated with family-planning efforts could provide cultural legitimacy for fertility regulation and make family limitation thinkable.

The implications of Caldwell's argument fall between these two extremes. Economic development would likely bring with it changes in the economic functions of the family and erode the basis for intergenerational flows of wealth from children to parents. Governments may attempt to alter attitudes toward the family, but it is not clear that they will be able to change strongly held cultural values. However, cultural change and Westernization are likely to proceed with or without government intervention as international communication and contact increase.

It is fair to say that the arguments about socioeconomic structures emphasized by transition theory are no longer persuasive, but it is difficult to choose between cultural explanations focusing on the acceptability of birth control and those emphasizing changes in the demand for children. Both cultural models are consistent with evidence pointing to the diffusion of ideas within culturally defined regions and to other research findings, such as earlier fertility declines in the middle and upper classes. It is also difficult to rule out situationally specific versions of transition theory that focus on the roles of children in certain types of industries or the interaction between family customs and new legal institutions. It would be comforting to conclude that a change as pervasive and widespread as the fertility transition obeyed a common set of social rules, but many different fertility transitions may have occurred, each with its own explanation. Indeed, modernization theory was based on an assumption that a complex constellation of ideas and attitudes tended to be acquired together, and the unthinkability of birth control may have been challenged at the same time that parents began to see their children in a new light.

NOTES

1   This dilemma is reflected in the economics literature itself. Gary Becker proposes an interaction between income and child quality. In his model parents with higher incomes automatically choose higher-quality children. Becker views this as an effect of income, even though he is positing a change in preferences – that is, parents could use their extra income to purchase more lower-quality children. Richard Easterlin argues that this should be viewed as a change in preferences. See Becker and Lewis (1973), G. Becker (1981), and Sanderson (1976).

2   Knodel, Chamratrithirong, and Debavalya (1987, p. 111) use the concept "latent demand for birth control" to refer to unfulfilled demand for fertility control in a period immediately preceding the fertility decline. This term is somewhat unfortunately chosen. The demand for any commodity is always to some extent "latent." In economic theory, demand at the individual level is determined by prices and income, as well as individual preferences, and demand in a market is the aggregate result of these individual "demand curves." At any prevailing price, there are almost always some people who would consume more if the price were lower. (My demand for a Rolls-Royce will remain "latent" until my income rises or the price of Rolls-Royces falls considerably.) Thus the existence of "latent demand" only means that the price of the good, in this case contraception, is greater than zero. Even where modern methods of fertility control are unknown, people are often aware of other methods, which they regard as either ineffective or unacceptable for other reasons. Abortion, for example, is usually known but often rejected because it is dangerous or culturally forbidden. This means that the cost of contraception is high, in either monetary or "psychic" terms. As Knodel, Chamratrithirong, and Debavalya point out, their concept implies that birth control will be adopted when its costs are reduced. In terms of the Easterlin framework used here, "latent demand for contraception" simply means that achieved family sizes are larger than desired family sizes.

The important issue is not whether "latent demand" existed, but the strength of the motivation to reduce family size. On one hand, it is likely that cost-free contraception would reduce family sizes in most societies, but it is not clear how much reduction would be achieved. On the other hand, an increase in the motivation to limit family sizes might lead couples to adopt contraceptive methods that were previously viewed as too costly. For example, Schneider and Schneider (in this volume) find that the postwar fertility decline among Sicilian agricultural laborers was achieved by the practice of withdrawal, a method that had been rejected a generation earlier. One of the costs of fertility control in a pre-transition society is the cost of acquiring information about methods. As motivation to reduce family sizes increases, some individuals will be willing to bear the costs of seeking this information, and the efforts of these pioneers reduce the costs for everyone else.

3   American writers cite Warren S. Thompson's 1929 article as the original statement of the demographic transition model.

II

Family and Gender

2

Gender and Fertility Decline among the British Middle Classes

John R. Gillis

Neither demographers nor social historians have paid much attention to the cultural history of fertility. We know a great deal about reproductive behavior but little about its meaning. The demographers' counterpart to the economists' mythic economic man is *the parent*, that class-, age-, and gender-neutral creature, who, regardless of time, place, or culture, reacts to the opportunities and costs of children with wondrous invariability (Busfield, 1987, p. 67). Especially troubling is the neutering process that obliterates the place of gender in the history of family and reproduction.[1] And it is time that the strongly gendered and historically specific meanings of both motherhood and fatherhood be reintegrated into all accounts of reproduction.

Fathers and mothers not only behave, they signify. They give not only life but meaning to life. Demographers and family historians have tended to treat the symbolic dimension of motherhood and fatherhood as merely epiphenomenal, the reflection of some deeper reality, when, in fact, the rituals and symbols of family life have a history and an agency in their own right. As Virginia Tufte and Barbara Myerhoff remind us, we not only think *about* but we think *with* the family, "using it as an object in our cultural work of self-definition" (1979, p. 15). And the way we think *with* motherhood, fatherhood, and childhood has had a direct effect on the way we reproduce ourselves biologically as well as culturally.

The meanings of fatherhood and motherhood are never stable or transparent but forever contested and changing. Whatever the underlying biological continuity of conception, pregnancy, and birth, virility has no fixed relationship to fatherhood, and fecundity no predetermined relationship to motherhood. The practice of giving up one's own children, common from late antiquity right through the eighteenth century and sanctioned by the Judeo-Christian tradition, should be sufficient reminder that bonds between parents and children have no predetermined meanings.[2] Patrescence and matrescence, the processes of becoming fathers and mothers, vary enormously by place and time (Raphael, 1975, pp. 65–71). The history of father-hood, motherhood, childhood, and family itself is always directly related to cultural definitions of manhood and womanhood – that is, to gender.

Gender is not the same thing as sexual difference but rather the differ-ences attributed to sex. In Joan Wallach Scott's useful definition, gender is "knowledge about sexual difference....Knowledge refers not only to ideas but institutions and structures, everyday practices as well as specialized rituals, all of which constitute social relationships. Knowledge is a way of ordering the world; as such it is not prior to social organization, it is insepar-able from social organization" (1988, p. 2). It is important to add that men and women are perceived as being different not only in relationship to one another but also in the way they relate to children. Femininity and mascu-linity constitute knowledge not just of sex, but of generation.

Changing understandings of patrescence and matrescence affected the fertility of important segments of the British middle classes during the nine-teenth century. On one hand, the definition of a father's responsibility narrowed from that of provision for all the members of the household to support only of the nuclear family. Simultaneously, an earlier understanding of mothering as something all women could do by virtue of their place within the household was being gradually replaced by an individualized, highly linear notion of motherhood in which only the event of birth itself could make a mother, and only perpetual symbolic interaction with her children could sustain that identity. A definition of motherhood that had previously been defined by space (the household) was seen by the mid-nineteenth century as an individualized relationship between the woman and her children.

The new understandings of motherhood and fatherhood involved not only a sharper division of labor between the sexes but a new division among women, reinforcing the boundaries between family and nonfamily, between mothers and nonmothers. *Mothering* – something that had been extended and shared out – was now transformed into *motherhood*, a personal identity so integral to a woman's femininity that to share it constituted a loss of self and forfeit of the claim to true womanhood. Inherent and linear, motherhood had become by 1850 middle-class women's equivalent to the masculine career, but without the option of retirement.

It was at this very moment of epistemological shift that fertility among the upper and middle classes began its historic decline. It would seem paradoxi-cal that when motherhood came to define adult femininity the numbers of children per marriage would begin to fall, but we must keep in mind that maternity is a culturally rather than biologically constructed phenomenon. The crucial cultural shift was from an understanding of motherhood as child-bearing to an understanding of motherhood as childrearing. This change was reflected in the prescriptive literature of motherhood, but also in new symbols and rituals of maternity.

Changes in middle-class fertility were closely bound with new notions of femininity and masculinity, which shaped the meanings of parenthood and childhood and were in turn shaped by them. As the understanding of what it meant to be a father, mother, or child changed, so too did reproductive behavior. In the case of the British middle classes, cultural change seems to have preceded and prepared the way for a reduction in the desired numbers of children. And it is this connection between gender and fertility that this essay aims to illuminate.

TRADITIONS OF MATERNITY AND PATERNITY

Judged by today's gender terms, eighteenth-century women achieved an impossible reconciliation of high productivity with high reproductivity. The prevailing productivist definition of good womanhood – the helpmeet and house mistress – would seem to have been incompatible with the large numbers of live and stillbirths experienced by married women in the seventeenth and eighteenth centuries. However, the prevailing understanding of the female, which defined good motherhood as childbearing rather than as childrearing, served to resolve these contradictions, at least at the symbolic level.

The rituals of childbirth operated to reconcile what seems to us to be the irreconcilable. And here it is important to keep in mind that rituals are not mere reflections of social organization but an integral part of that organization. They not only reflect gender but construct it. As Sherry Ortner has pointed out, rituals are sites of a society's cultural work where apparently intractable contradictions are dealt with: "Rituals do not begin with eternal verities, but arrive at them. They begin with some cultural premises (or several at once), stated or unstated, and then work various operations upon it, arriving at 'solutions' – reorganizations and reinterpretations of the elements that produce a newly meaningful whole" (1978, p. 3).

The birthing rites of the eighteenth century were a way of "solving" the apparently impossible contradiction of a woman's obligation to high productivity and high reproductivity. They did so by representing pregnancy and maternity as something that happened to a woman, as an episode in her life rather than the essence of her sex. Birth itself was represented as more an end than a beginning, the returning of a woman to her normal activities rather than propelling her into a separate state of being. Thinking of maternity as childbearing rather than childrearing, women were able to reconcile high fertility with contemporary notions of high female productivity.

The traditional ritual treatment of fertility allowed women to think about multiple births (including stillbirths) as exceptional events – dangerous episodes that were essentially discontinuous with the rest of a woman's life. What today we celebrate as the fulfillment of womanhood, the moment of new beginnings when a family is created, a time of unambiguous joy and exaltation, was then symbolized and ritualized as so threatening to family and community that it required that the new mother be virtually quarantined until the dangers had passed.

As Arnold van Gennep has pointed out, traditional birthing rites "separate the pregnant woman from society, from her family group, and sometimes even from her sex" (1960, p. 41). Until the late eighteenth century, pregnancy was universally understood as polluting and dangerous.[3] Many menstrual taboos also applied, although these interfered only minimally with female productivity.[4] There was no such thing as antenatal care in the modern sense, although diet and behavior were powerfully prescribed. Pregnant women were encouraged to remain active in everyday tasks, not because they were considered normal but because they were considered imbalanced, or plethoric, requiring leaner diets, more exercise, and extensive bloodletting (Eccles, 1982, pp. 45–7, 60–65; Oakley, 1984, pp. 22–4).[5]

Birthing rites varied in detail by class, but whether the birthing took place under the guidance of the village midwife or a high-society accoucheur, the pattern of separation and isolation followed by reincorporation was the same (Wilson, 1985, pp. 132–5; Shorter, 1982, pp. 48–56; Houlbrooke, 1984, 129–30). Men regarded expectant women as dangerous, and doctors intervened only when life was threatened (Shorter, 1982, pp. 293–4).[6] But pregnancy separated a woman as much from her own sex as from men. Pregnancy was referred to as "breeding," associating mothers with baser forms of life.[7] As birth neared, the episodic nature of maternity was symbolized by the removal of the woman from her own house. Despite the cost and fatigue of travel, many women felt compelled to leave home to give birth. Some, like Ralph Josselin's daughters, returned to their mothers, and there appears to have been a good deal of ritualized mobility at the time of birth at all class levels (Macfarlane, 1970, p. 85). Aristocratic women "went to Town," London being the favorite place to await delivery (J. S. Lewis, 1986, pp. 52–4, 156–8).

Those who could not afford to travel separated themselves symbolically from the household and all familiar routines. The "lying-in chamber" was closed off, the doors shut and the windows draped so that none of the normal sounds, smells, or activities of the household could penetrate (Eccles, 1982, pp. 94–5; Wilson, 1985, p. 135). If a bedroom was chosen, it was completely rearranged so as to deconstruct its familiar features. Few women gave birth in their own beds, for, among the rich as well as the poor, it was normal to substitute a special cot or birthing chair to complete the symbolic separation of the mother from the wife (J. S. Lewis, 1986, p. 161; Wilson, 1985, p. 135; Shorter, 1982, p. 145; Eccles, 1982, p. 92).

Subject to a special food and drink (a caudle of either hot wine or spiced porridge), deliberately cut off from family and friends, the expectant woman was as isolated as if she had been removed to a birthing hut in the African rain forest. Every effort was made to prevent husbands from seeing or hearing what was often a painful and lethal process. They awaited news in the company of male friends, drinking the "groaning malt," drowning the fears that birth invariably evoked in men (Wilson, 1985, pp. 133–6).[8]

The absence of husbands from the birthing room might suggest the absence of a concept of paternity, but in reality the opposite was the case. According to the contemporary understanding of conception, male seed was endowed with as much, if not more, creativity than the female ovum, which had only recently been discovered. The position of intercourse was said to determine the sex of the child, and men believed they could tell at ejaculation whether or not conception had occurred (Eccles, 1982, pp. 24–6, 60; McLaren, 1984, chaps. 1 and 2).[9] Men were also said to feel a pregnancy, sharing their wives' morning sickness and toothaches, even experiencing their labor pains.[10] The fact that until 1839 British fathers had absolute legal possession of their children (including infants) only reinforced a strong notion of paternal connection with the child (Lowe, 1982, pp. 26–8; Riley, 1968, 105–13).[11]

The common language of the time – "with child," "brought to bed," "lying-in" – reflected the notion that both pregnancy and delivery were something that happened to a woman, as if she were an object rather than a subject in her own right (Riley, 1968, pp. 3–4; J. S. Lewis, 1986, p. 72).[12] The fact that the attendants were women did not mean that they were more caring or sensitive to the mother's wishes. There was no notion of natural childbirth, and midwives could be as brutally interventionist as any male physician (Wilson, 1985, pp. 129–30, 144; Shorter, 1982, pp. 38–9).

Birth practices reflected the Christian understanding of birth as the "curse of Eve" and of the suffering involved as inevitable and redemptive (J. S. Lewis, 1986, p. 59). Birth reenacted Eve's fall from grace, explained her polluted and dangerous condition, and justified her isolation. Maternal death was not so frequent as many historians have believed, yet all birth mothers underwent a kind of symbolic death as prelude to their rebirth into a woman's normal productive activities (Schofield, 1986).

And the child was born so polluted that it too had to be symbolically reborn. Ralph Josselin wrote at the birth of his first child in 1642, "God wash it from it[s] corruption and sanctify it and make it his owne." This was the function of church baptism, but even before the child was brought to the font it had ordinarily undergone several folk rites of purification, symbolically separating it from the mother and the dangers associated with her. Great ritual attention was paid to the cutting of the umbilical cord, and the child's head was then physically shaped, as if it had to be remade in a human image.[13] Swaddling served similar symbolic purposes, for it "was these clothes which made the child human, just as the wider ceremony of childbirth of which swaddling was a part made the delivery act of culture, not merely of nature" (Wilson, 1985, p. 137).

The haste to baptize newborns was a reflection of the same idea. Baptism was thought of as prophylactic, protecting as well as purifying the child. When a child was sickly, midwives did not wait upon the recovery of the mother to carry it to the church (Houlbrooke, 1984, pp. 130–31; Berry and Schofield, 1971, pp. 453–63; Thomas, 1971, pp. 36–7, 56). Symbolically, it was the church and the community that gave the child life and health. Christenings were increasingly delayed during the eighteenth century, but these were not yet the big family celebrations they were to become in the mid-nineteenth century. Mothers, still confined to the lying-in chamber by the strict conventions of the day, were rarely present at eighteenth-century baptisms (Wilson, 1985, p. 138).

The rites of passage of mother and child were quite separate, a symbolic dissociation that reinforced a social as opposed to individual notion of motherhood. Birth itself was insufficient to endow either mother or child with the full attributes of humanity. The physical and psychological processes that today we regard as "naturally" productive of womanliness and the bonding between mother and child were seen as dangerous, requiring cultural intervention. The child underwent a series of ritual acts culminating in baptism; the mother followed another set of rites, also ending in "churching," the final stage of her restoration to pure womanhood. Restoring a new mother to the fullness of womanhood required several weeks, often called "her month." For the first week the mother remained immobilized in bed, drinking the special caudle and still subject to dietary restrictions. She would receive a carefully orchestrated series of visitors, women relations first, later female friends, sharing caudle with them. This was not so much a reflection of female bonding as a highly ritualized restoration of a polluted person to a state of social acceptability in which women served as the bridges back to humanity (Eccles, 1982, pp. 95–7; Wilson, 1985, pp. 137–8; J. S. Lewis, 1986, pp. 194–9; van Gennep, 1960, p. 48). Husbands were the first males to enter the lying-in chamber, but it was thought dangerous to have sex during "her month," a taboo that may have been carried over to the entire period a woman was breastfeeding. What later generations were to think of as natural and even erotic attributes of motherhood were still associated with danger (Pollock, 1983, p. 215; Eccles, 1982, p. 98).[14]

Gradually the lying-in chamber would be opened up and restored to its original order (Wilson, 1985, p. 138; J. S. Lewis, 1986, pp. 195–7). The mother would venture into the other rooms of the house but would not leave it until the day of her churching. So dangerous was the unchurched mother that she was thought to kill the grass she stepped on, induce unwanted pregnancies, and bewitch both people and animals (Thomas, 1971, pp. 38–9).[15] Traditionally, churching involved public procession to church, the veiled mother surrounded by a crowd of women who protected others from her contact and gaze. In Henry Barrow's hostile account, it is not until a woman had received the priest's blessing that "she may now put off her veiling kerchief, and look her husband and neighbors in the face again."[16] According to John Brand's eighteenth-century description, "It was most unhappy for a Woman, after bringing forth a Child, to offer a visit, or for her Neighbors to receive it, till she had been duly churched....On the day when such a Woman was Churched, every Family, favoured with a call, were bound to set Meat and Drink before her" (1877, p. 338).

Churching remained popular among women of all classes throughout the eighteenth century. The upper classes differed from the lower only in their preference that it be a private ceremony, performed at home (J. S. Lewis, 1986, pp. 201–2). For all women, however, it signaled return to true woman-hood, to the central identity of house mistress, to which motherhood was secondary. Today we think of birth (and especially first birth) as new begin-ning, initiating motherhood and "starting" a family, initiating a woman into the fullness of her femininity. In this understanding of the female life cycle, menopause is experienced as an ending, as loss. But in the seventeenth and eighteenth centuries the end of a woman's childbearing capacity was by no means the end of her womanhood if she remained mistress of a household.[17]

Traditional treatment of fertility had a powerful impact on social behavior. It rendered the the relationship between mother and child less individual-ized. Mothers were able to see their children as separate from themselves and mothering as episodic and situational, less integral to their personal identities than their productive activities. This is not to say that parents did not care deeply about their children. There is evidence that early nine-teenth-century middle-class fathers were deeply involved with their children, even retiring from business early so as to promote their guidance and instruction (Davidoff and Hall, 1987, pp. 225–8). Furthermore, it was pre-cisely because parents were concerned about the health and well being of their offspring that they were willing to entrust them to the kindness of strangers (Pollock, 1983, pp. 111–13; Boswell, 1987, pp. 428–34). It was this caring that sanctioned practices like swaddling and wet-nursing (Fildes, 1986, pp. 398–401). Parents were willing to entrust their teenage children to surrogate fathers and mothers because they trusted in social rather than biological definition of fatherhood and motherhood (Gillis, 1985, p. 81). An adult woman's identity was not yet centered on childrearing. Taking care of children (her own and others) was central to a mistress's duties but was not necessarily perceived as all-consuming. It was not until the epistemology of motherhood began to shift that childrearing came into conflict with childbearing.

NEW MOTHERHOOD AND FATHERHOOD

We can see the beginnings of this change in the language of maternity adopted by the educated elites at the end of the eighteenth century. In 1791 the *Gentleman's Magazine* reported, "All our mothers and grandmothers, used in due course to become *with child* or as Shakespeare has it, *round-wombed*...but it is very well known that no female, above the degree of chambermaid or laundress, had been with child these ten years past...nor is she ever *brought to bed*, or *delivered*, but merely at the end of nine months, has an accouchement; antecedent to which she informs her friends that a certain time she will be *confined*" (quoted in J. S. Lewis, 1986, p. 72). Lady Sarah Napier could write in 1818, "No one can say 'breeding' or 'with child' or 'lying-in' without being thought indelicate....'In the family way' and 'confinement' have taken their place" (quoted in J. S. Lewis, 1986, p. 72).

New language reflected an epistemological transition, which involved the transformation of the meaning not just of manhood and womanhood but of family as well. In educated circles "family" ceased to mean all members of the household. As the traditional image of the house gave way to the new symbolism of the home, the definition of family narrowed to the nuclear core, excluding resident kin as well as servants and other live-in workers. The shift was more perceptual than compositional, for the membership of most households remained far more diverse than the new imagery suggests. Nevertheless, in educated circles the definition of family underwent an epochal shift.[18]

Simultaneously, the representation of men and women was transformed. Whether or not they worked outside the house, men became strangers in their own homes, forever returning home to be never quite at home (Gillis, 1989). While men became symbolically associated with work, women's productivity suddenly became invisible.[19] Elite women were the first to abandon the title *Mistress* and, in the terminology increasingly popular among middle-class circles of the early nineteenth century, became *Mrs.*, previously a courtesy title for spinsters as well as married women, but now confined to the latter (Davidoff and Hall, 1987, p. 273).

In the eighteenth century marriage had been associated with the assumption of household responsibilities and had endowed the wife with a full measure of what was then defined as adult femininity. In the nineteenth century, however, many middle-class women experienced marriage as loss (sometimes referred to as "marriage trauma") rather than as gain. The brief period of "coming out" just before marriage allowed one brief and very limited period of personal autonomy, which ended abruptly with engagement and marriage (Davidoff, 1973, pp. 49–51). The bride had lost her virginity and innocence and would not regain a full measure of femininity until the arrival of her first child. In this new understanding of womanhood, pregnancy was therefore wholly redefined as the one thing that guaranteed full femininity; maternity was no longer a decentering experience but the fulfillment of womanhood.

In the course of the late eighteenth and early nineteenth centuries, the treatment of prospective mothers had changed dramatically. If pregnant women were now advised to refrain from travel and exercise, this was not because they were seen as unhealthy, but because they were were no longer thought of as plethoric. Bloodletting and heroic interventions diminished significantly as childbearing was gradually removed from the realm of culture to that of "nature." As P. H. Chavasse argued, "Nature is perfectly competent to bring without the assistance of man, a child into the world....Assist Nature! Can anything be more absurd?" (quoted in Oakley, 1984, p. 13).[20]

While working-class women had no choice but to continue their everyday activities, their upper-class counterparts now stayed home more and rarely showed themselves pregnant in public. This was not because they considered themselves polluting, for had this been the case, the home, which now stood for purity and order, would have been the last place for either pregnancy or childbirth. On the contrary, among the educated classes the fertile woman now became the symbol of the natural, seductive rather than repulsive, comforting rather than dangerous. As Ludmilla Jordanova has observed, "Women were the carriers and givers of life, and as a result, a pregnant woman was both the quintessence of life and an erotic object" (1986, p. 106).

The old separation rites gave way to home birth, with mothers now coming to daughters (J. S. Lewis, 1986, pp. 53–4). Understood as natural, fertility was no longer seen as polluting or disruptive. The lying-in chamber was a thing of the past. Special preparations were now more hygienic than symbolic. The birthing room was kept as nearly as possible in a normal state, with doors and windows open. There was no rearrangement of furniture, but rather an effort was made to maintain the usual conditions of domestic life, to normalize childbirth as far as this was socially and medically possible (pp. 53–4).[21] The conjugal bed now served as the maternal bed, not only emphasizing the compatibility between the roles of wife and mother but also minimizing the mysterious and the threatening features of the female body (Shorter, 1982, p. 145).

Among the educated classes, birth ceased to be a public event and became a family occasion with close relations in attendance. By mid-century the midwife had been displaced by the doctor, and, with the exception of the trained nurse, female attendants were much more likely to be chosen on the basis of consanguinity, with mothers and sisters preferred. For the first time, husbands were welcomed into the birthing chamber along with doctors (Suitor, 1981, pp. 278–93; Shorter, 1982, p. 294; J. S. Lewis, 1986, pp. 171–3; Walsh, 1857, p. 558).[22]

Later, hygienic concerns would once again remove husbands from the birthing scene, but these men were moved not only by a deep concern for their wives' physical and emotional condition but also by a felt need to establish their own paternity, which was now no longer assured by law or reinforced by notions of sexual reproduction that by then assigned much more capacity to the female ovum than the male seed. Educated men stopped thinking they could tell when conception had occurred, and men feeling pregnant became something that only working-class people believed in (Oakley, 1984, pp. 12–15). Abandoning the tradition of the "groaning malt," middle-class men felt themselves drawn to birth, as guilt replaced fear as their primary emotional reaction (Miller, 1978, pp. 34–6; Riley, 1968, pp. 113–23). For William Gladstone, the birth of his first child in 1840 was "a new scene & lesson in human life....I have seen her endure today...yet six times as much bodily pain as I have undergone in my whole life....How many thoughts does this agony excite....Certainly the woman has this bless-ing that she may as a member of Christ behold in these pains certain especially means of her purification with a willing mind, & so the more cheerfully hallow them by willing endurance into a thank offering" (quoted in Poovey, 1987, p. 157).

Birth itself become a redeeming experience, a ritual performance in which the new mother was now the central actor. "Labour is a drama, painful to the individual, and exerting a painful interest in those around her," wrote W. Tyler Smith in the 1848 *London Lancet* (quoted in Poovey, 1987, p. 157). By that time, however, birth among the upper and middle classes was beginning to be rendered less physically painful by the introduction of chloroform. Even as anesthetics made mother as childbearer the inert object of new medical practice and male imagination, it created the possibility that the new mother could respond to the newborn with a new kind of sensibility that by now had come to be seen as the essence of motherhood.

In this transformed cultural representation of birth, the women's body became an object, but her feelings were given heightened dramatic possibi-lities.[23] Previously, maternity was something that happened to a woman, her maximum moment of vulnerability and suffering. Henceforth, the test of true womanhood was not how well a woman bore physical suffering but how she responded emotionally to the newborn. This shift coincided precisely with the redefinition of women as the more delicate, more feeling sex, and the consequent spiritualization of motherhood (J. S. Lewis, 1986, pp. 58–9, 71–2; Miller, 1978, pp. 35–9).[24]

Although traditionalists warned that anesthesia was the work of the devil, most women were ready to accept painless delivery, not only because they wished to avoid the physical suffering but because they wanted to experience fully what was now regarded as the beginning of true womanhood. In the flush of the new concern with the emotional condition of mothers, the con-tinuing high rates of maternal mortality tended to be forgotten (Branca, 1975, pp. 89–90). In the advice books written by Mrs. Sarah Ellis and others the physical side of birth ceased to be mentioned. As Judith Lewis has put it, "The experience of motherhood presumably began only after the child's birth – precisely when it was thought to have ended a century earlier" (1986, pp. 73–4).

What mattered now was the symbolic interaction of mother and child, the first magic moments. Melesina Trench described the birth of her first child in 1787 in terms that were to become standard in the next century: "When I looked in my boy's face, when I heard him breathe, when I felt the full pressure of his little fingers, I understood the full force of Voltaire's declaration: – Le chef d'oeuvre d'amour est le coeur d'une mere.... My husband's delight of his son nearly equalled mine" (quoted in Pollock, 1983, p. 206).

In Mrs. Gaskell's novel *Ruth* (1853) first contact is represented in precisely the same terms: "that baby touch called forth her love; the doors of her heart were thrown wide open for the little infant to go in and take possession" (quoted in Miller, 1978, p. 35).[25]

Until this moment a woman's femininity had been only potential; henceforth she was a true woman. Gone was the ritual separation of the child – the umbilical cutting, head shaping, and swaddling. The new mother was no longer a polluting presence to be immobilized and quarantined. The breast, simultaneously naturalized and eroticized, became identified with both nurturance and pleasure (Jordanova, 1980, p. 50ff).[26] Husbands, who had previously viewed breastfeeding as a nuisance and a diminution of their wives' attractiveness, now endorsed the practice. In Victorian novels it is the breast rather than the womb that becomes the central organ of motherhood. David Copperfield dreams that "a baby smile upon her breast might change my child-wife [Dora] into a woman" (quoted in Riley, 1968, p. 5).[27]

In its earlier cultural construction, maternity was something than happened to the woman. In the eighteenth-century story of birth, the wife had "presented" the husband with the child, who in turn re-presented it to the world (Macfarlane, 1971, pp. 88–9; Houlbrooke, 1984, p. 131; Brand, 1877, pp. 340–41). In traditional patriarchal celebrations of the first born, the mother is absent symbolically as well as physically, but in the Victorian period men came to represent their paternity through the indissoluble unity of mother and child. The husband becomes a father when he beholds mother and child together, joined by the powerful symbol of the breast (Riley, 1968, pp. 115–24).

CHANGING MEANINGS OF CHILDREN

Having ceased to be a moment of supernatural if not physical danger, birth was re-presented as a sacramental event with extraordinary powers. Despite high infant and maternal mortality, birth lost its ancient symbolic association with death. An event that in the eighteenth century was invariably approached with foreboding was reinterpreted as a universal moment of joy (Pollock, 1983, pp. 204–8). One reason middle-class women came to prefer doctors to midwives was that the latter were still associated with death, with "laying out" as well as "lying-in."[28]

For the woman it was a new beginning, a clarification of her previously liminal condition and her incorporation into complete femininity. For older women, attendance at births was a perpetual source of renewal of their own sense of womanhood. To Queen Victoria, the prenatal confinements of her own daughters brought back vivid memories and a renewal of what, even for the reigning monarch, was the core of her femininity – being a mother. So strong was her identification that she saw to it that they wore her birthing gown and were confined to the same bed in which they had experienced the first moments of life (Miller, 1978, pp. 37–8).

The old practices of baptism and churching no longer seemed necessary or proper. Infant mortality rates remained relatively high, but among the middle classes the sickly child was no longer hastened away to be given the magical protection of baptism. In the late eighteenth and early nineteenth centuries the spiritual rite was likely to be administered in the home; it was a family and not a community occasion. When christening once again became a church affair in the 1850s and 1860s, it had lost its magical, life-giving power. It was now the baby who brought life to the ceremony, not vice versa (Obelkevich, 1976, pp. 127–30).

Churching went the way of the traditional baptism. Educated women recited prayers of thanksgiving in the privacy of their homes, leaving the public ceremony to the working classes.[29] The presence of mother and child was now seen as sanctifying rather than polluting. Now it was the male, tainted by men's greater association with the world, who required the rites of purification. By the mid-nineteenth century a series of new domestic rituals, including Christmas, provided men with the sanctification they could not find outside the family circle (Gillis, 1989). Birth, previously symbolically associated with death and requiring the external intervention of churching and baptism, had now become its own sacrament (Suitor, 1981, pp. 284–7; Miller, 1978, p. 36).

Changing cultural conceptions of birth were also reflected in fertility behavior of the upper and middle classes. Understood as childrearing, good motherhood ceased to be defined in terms of numbers. A woman's claim to femininity was established by the first birth. Additional children did not add to a woman's status, one of the reasons that, like second marriages, second and third births tended to be less elaborately ritualized than the first (Raphael, 1975, p. 69; Gillis, 1985, pp. 297–9). The bride in white could never be a girl again. Likewise, once a mother, always a mother, with the consequence that motherhood became a full-time calling, with no respites or real retirement.

During the nineteenth century the ancient tradition of sending children out to nurse was terminated by the middle classes. At first wet nurses were brought into the house, but after the 1870s, when bottle-feeding became widely practiced, middle-class mothers dispensed with them also (Branca, 1975, pp. 100–4). While upper-class women employed dry nurses and nannies, most middle-class women now felt fully responsible for the nurturance and training of young children. Children (especially daughters) were staying at home much longer. Boys might be sent away to school, but until they married they were perpetually returning home for the holidays, events around which were now built elaborate homecoming rituals centered on mother (Gillis, 1989).

It was her voice, her smile, her warmth that became the symbolic center of the middle-class construction of family and personal identity. Mothers became the objects of intense nostalgia, particularly among sons whose engagement with an uncertain, fragmented world made the wholeness she stood for so attractive. The multisensory experience of ritualized meals and bedtimes that became a mark of bourgeois respectability in the Victorian era helped create an the image of mother as the fixed point in a changing world, always there, always available: "We find no second mother / We find no second home" (quoted in Gillis, 1985, p. 253).[30] It was her home they returned to on Sunday and at Christmas, and her grave they visited. By 1914 Britain, like America, was ready to consider institutionalizing Mother's Day (Gillis, 1985, pp. 252–3).[31]

The overwhelming symbolic importance of children in the nineteenth century has often been commented on (Coveney, 1957), but the degree to which femininity had come to depend on symbolic interaction with children – not with children in general, but with one's own children – has been ignored. During the nineteenth century stepmothering became more negatively charged. At a time when divorce was becoming acceptable (though not yet widely practiced) a woman could be a wife to more than one husband but a true mother only to her own children (Lowe, 1982, p. 36).[32]

The individualizing of the mother/child relationship meant an intensification of childrearing, transforming it from a part-time occupation, shared extensively, to a lifelong career that did not end even with the empty nest but continued into grandmotherhood. Earlier, childrearing had been understood as a set of tasks – feeding, clothing, teaching – that could be accomplished by a wide range of persons, including men. In the early nineteenth century fatherhood still meant involvement with the spiritual and secular education of children, but by the 1850s this too had become a feminine domain. Good fatherhood was now sustained symbolically as well as materially by what a middle-class man did outside the home. As part of this epochal regendering process, the good father was re-presented as breadwinner, a worldly stranger to domestic life, whose incorporation into the domestic circle now required elaborate rituals of homecoming, yet another task for the good wife and mother (Gillis, 1989).

While it could be argued that physical burdens of childrearing were much diminished from the mid-nineteenth century onwards, the "cultural work" involved increased enormously. Mothers were not only expected to meet the bodily needs of each child but to set the emotional tone of family life, create just the right ambience. Mother became the priestess in charge of the sacred hearth, the chief liturgist of all family occasions.

The demands of motherhood were further increased by the cultural requirement that all children be treated equally. No proper mother could be seen to
be favoring one over another, even sons over daughters. An intrafamily peck-
ing order had existed early in the nineteenth century, with older siblings
caring for younger. Children had then been farmed out to kin, "adopted" by
aunts and uncles when parents became too overburdened (Davidoff and Hall,
1987, pp. 222–5). By the 1850s, however, lineal had replaced lateral forms of
parenting, placing the sole responsibility of bringing up sons and daughters
directly on the natural parents (Banks, 1954, pp. 162–3).

GENDER SYMMETRY AND FERTILITY DECLINE

It is in this context that we can begin to understand the fertility decline that
began in the 1860s and 1870s.[33] It has long been argued that the decline
began when children began to cost more. Variations on this economistic
understanding continued to be used to explain falling birth rates in the last
half of the century (Banks, 1954). However, this argument fails to take into
account the changing meaning of parenthood. Earlier, increased time and
material costs of children had been shifted to other families, related or
unrelated. The significant change was not therefore the changing cost of children but the regendering process that made the old strategy of sharing costs
unthinkable among the respectable classes.

Now that the definition of middle–class manhood was constructed around
the notion of the self-made man, it was no longer possible to admit the aid of
kin, even when such aid was forthcoming in hidden ways.[34] Now the bourgeois male had to appear to support his own children or forfeit his claim to
manliness. Even newlywed males had to appear self-sufficient: "A young
men must plunge into married life at a full gallop; begin where his father
ended" (quoted in Banks, 1954, p. 45).

The regendering of motherhood also contributed to the abandonment
of older strategies of time and cost sharing, but in a different way. Large
numbers of children, previously a sign of good motherhood, now became an
embarrassment. J. A. Banks notes that in the 1850s having few children was
seen as "unnatural," but by the end of the century a mother with many offspring was the object of compassion (1954, p. 167). Here the individual-
ized and intensified notion of motherhood was clearly evident. More children
did not enhance a mother's identity but damaged it.

Equally significant was the fact that the middle classes were talking about
children in gendered terms. It has always been desirable to have a son as
heir, but now it was not the future of the family property that was at stake:
the ambience of family life was at issue. By the 1880s the ideal of the
two–child family was becoming standard, but it is clear that the middle

classes did not think in strictly numeric terms. What is striking is the growing conviction that one girl and one boy constituted the perfect family, symmetrical with respect to gender. The prevailing notion of the dissimilarity but complementarity of the adult sexes carried over to children as well. What Lord Tennyson had observed about marriage was now applied to the family generally:

> seeing in either sex alone
> Is half itself, and true marriage lies
> Nor equal, nor unequal. Each fulfills
> Defect in each[35]

Boys and girls were thought of as bringing very different but equally necessary qualities to family life, so that a family was only complete when it had one of each: "Every woman wanted a son, and a home was incomplete without a daughter, but what need was there for more?"[36] If two sons or two daughters were born, parents might try for a third or fourth child to achieve the right balance, but there was no need to have more once the gender symmetry was achieved. Thinking of children not as equal numeric units but as gendered beings with very different qualities did not preclude larger families, but it did tend to reduce fertility levels to the two-child norm. This gendered understanding of children had clearly spread beyond the middle classes when British parents were surveyed at the time of World War II. Mass Observation found that by that time most people wanted two children but were very explicit that one should be a boy and the other a girl: "As things stand today, first children are mostly born for the sake of the parents; second children often for the sake of the first – to keep it company – and third children in the hope they will be of a different sex from the first two, or by mistake" (1945, pp. 72–3).

More recent surveys have shown a persistent tendency for people to say they favor large families but in practice to stop having children when the gender symmetry is achieved. When asked why they do not have more, the answer is not material cost but the time and energy that children demand (Busfield, 1974, pp. 25–8). What this means is that women remain either entirely consumed by childrearing or, when they also work, are subjected to great strain by the demand that they be simultaneously good mothers and good workers. Contemporary society has not yet found a ritual solution to this particular contradiction. High productivity and high reproductivity remain irreconcilable in both a cultural and practical sense.

Of course these burdens could be reduced in many ways by the sharing of childrearing responsibilities both within and between families. But prevailing gender definitions, reinforced by the symbols and rituals of everyday life, make these alternatives seem unnatural. Given the current meaning of motherhood, which insists that childrearing is the individual woman's responsibility, the only solution is to keep families small. Thus the solution that the middle classes began to employ as early as the 1850s and 1860s has now become the norm across the entire spectrum of social classes.

NOTES

1   On the importance of considering meaning, see Simons (1986), pp. 256–78.
2   On earlier traditions of placement of children, see Boswell (1988); on the varieties of representation of birth, see Callaway (1978), pp. 166–81.
3   A pregnant woman's imagination as well as her actions were thought to affect not only those around her but also the unborn child. See Bouce (1988), pp. 86–100; Shorter (1982), pp. 49–52, 286–7.
4   As late as the 1930s, pregnant women in some rural areas of Britain were not supposed to go near freshly killed pigs. See *Folk-Lore*, 49 (1938); *Notes and Queries for Somerset and Dorset*, 24 (1943–6), p. 277. For middle-class Victorians, pregnancy was seen as one cause of female insanity, although they rejected the idea that women were threats to anyone besides themselves (Showalter, 1987, pp. 55–6).
5   Bleeding was common among the upper classes until the 1840s. See J. S. Lewis (1986), pp. 124–33.
6   On husbands see Houlbroke (1984), p. 130; Macfarlane (1970), p. 85; and van Gennep (1960), p. 48.
7   Ralph Josselin used this language in the seventeenth century (Macfarlane, 1970, pp. 84–5), and it continued among the upper classes until the late eighteenth century. See J. S. Lewis (1986), p. 72; also Riley (1968), p. 4.
8   In the seventeenth century wrapping the new mother in a sheepskin underlined her connection with animal nature (Eccles, 1982, p. 94). The upper classes had abandoned folk practices but still kept the mother isolated (J. S. Lewis, 1986, pp. 198–9). On male confinement parties, see Riley (1968), pp. 105–8; also Tucker (1974), p. 238.
9   On the belief that circumstances of conception affected the child, see Bouce (1988), p. 98.
10 The history of the British couvade is yet to be written, but as late as the 1950s working-class husbands were still said to experience paternity physically. See Newman (1942), p. 142; Dennis, Henrique, and Slaughter (1956), p. 220.
11 On contemporary fatherhood, see Richman (1982), pp. 89–103.
12 On the American experience, see Lewis and Lockridge (1988), pp. 6–14.
13 See Eccles (1982), p. 93; Illick (1974), p. 307. *Notes and Queries*, 5th ser. Sept. 14, 1878, p. 205; Sept. 28, 1878, pp. 255–6.
14 On the notion that a mother's milk could be spoiled by sex, see Fildes (1986) pp. 398–401.
15 In nineteenth-century Oxfordshire it was believed that an unchurched woman could settle a grudge by visiting another woman and getting her pregnant (Percy Manning MS, Bodleian Library, Oxford, Top Oxon d. 191a, f. 26).
16 Barrow was writing in the late sixteenth century (Thomas, 1971, p. 60). For full description, see Wilson (1985), pp. 138–9.
17 On the modern perception of menopause, see Skultans (1970), pp. 639–51. John Demos notes that menopausal women were often associated in seventeenth-century America with mysterious powers, suggesting that menopause may have been experienced as a kind of gain by the women themselves (1982, pp. 155–6).
18 On the continued diversity of middle-class households, see Ruggles (1987).
19 This process in America has been studied by Boydston (1990); see also Cancian (1987), p. 24.

20 For more on the naturalization of childbearing, see Lewis (1986), pp. 123–54; also Conquest (1848), p. 37; Bull (1837), pp. 6–24.

21 This process was evident in the births of Mrs. Francis Place in the 1790s. See Pollock (1987), p. 36; Conquest (1848), pp. 39–46.

22 Walsh thought "men are always in the way at the hour of trial, and the more a husband can be ignored the better" (p. 558), but his remarks suggest that husbands were there nevertheless.

23 Poovey is right that painless birth "silenced" the female body, but she ignores the new subjectivity that accompanied it.

24 Mothers were told to control their emotions, for these, like their health, would affect their children (Conquest, 1837, p. 33). I am indebted to my colleague Jan Lewis for insights on the importance of the emotions in new forms of motherhood during this period.

25 For further literary examples, see Riley (1968), pp. 28–9.

26 Conquest insisted that it made women "more soft and beautiful" (1837, p. 93).

27 On growth of positive ideas toward breastfeeding from 1750 on, see Fildes, (1986), p. 401.

28 The association of birth and death continued in working-class communities well into the twentieth century (Chamberlain and Richardson, 1983, pp. 31–43).

29 On the persistence of churching among the working classes, see Rushton (1983), pp. 118–23; Clark (1982), pp. 115–25.

30 On the importance of the symbol of mother as nurturer and the changing meaning of food, see Brumberg (1988), chap. 5.

31 See also Douglas (1977), pp. 6, 75–6, 110–11.

32 On divorce, see R. Philips (1988), chap. 7.

33 For a suggestive study of some of the cultural factors involved in American middle-class family limitation, see Parkerson and Parkerson (1988), pp. 49–70.

34 Women would admit assistance of kin, but the self-made man could not. On the gender of kinship in contemporary America, see Di Leonardo (1987), pp. 440–53.

35 Tennyson, "The Princess," quoted in Houghton (1957), p. 349.

36 A. S. Swan (1893), quoted in Banks (1954), p. 163.

3

Mothers and the State in Britain, 1904–1914

Ellen Ross

In the decade after 1904, the working-class mothers of London were bombarded with advice, inspections, and regulation by a cluster of governmental bodies and private associations. Health visitors representing borough medical officers or voluntary organizations mailed the women instructions on infant care and were inside their homes within days of a birth. School nurses and doctors examined their children, looking for signs of mothers' failings on their offsprings' clothing and bodies. Public and quasi-public agencies held the mothers responsible for getting children to distant, overcrowded out-patient clinics or for tiresome series of home treatments. "We are constantly calling in the help of every agency, whether official or voluntary, that has the right and the ability to interfere to the children's benefit," wrote one zealous welfare worker in 1912.[1] Mothering had lost its status as an inborn female capacity giving women unchallenged authority over their children and became, at least rhetorically, a profession requiring proper qualifications. Experts called for "mothercraft" training in the public schools and founded special "schools for mothers."

These efforts, and many more akin to them, which contemporaries collectively labeled the Infant Welfare movement, constituted a massive attempt by a loose coalition of agencies and influential individuals to redefine motherhood among the working classes. Raising children was to become a far more demanding project, requiring more actual work and money spent on each child's behalf, and occupying a more central part of an adult woman's life (see also Gillis, in this volume). The reformers wanted working-class mothers, who defined themselves primarily as household *providers and managers*, to make their motherhood – their relationships with their children – the cornerstone of their identity.[2]

My contribution to this collective study of the European fertility decline concentrates on the transmutation of the mother-child bond in Britain, particularly in London, into a relationship calling for more work and new legal responsibilities for mothers. State intervention in motherhood, though it was not specifically intended to lower fertility rates, was nonetheless predicated on women having fewer children – children whom they would care for more intensively. Infant Welfare workers, particularly nurses and doctors, as Wally Seccombe argues in this volume, communicated both directly and by inference their certainty that a woman could never adequately care for more than three or four children, and that each child was a major commitment.

During or around the Infant Welfare years in the early twentieth century much was changing in working-class standards of living: fathers had new obligations, some working-class children could expect better futures, and some working-class incomes were protected by a new national safety net. Clearly these changes impinged too on definitions of motherhood and had something to do with declining working-class fertility rates. The present London case study traces just one motif in a larger mosaic not because Infant Welfare policies have exceptional explanatory power but because they suggest new sets of issues – both public policies and the mother-child bond – that belong in discussions of the fertility decline.

Despite its status as the nation's capital, London was not the object of special government initiatives to improve working-class child health. Certainly the city had been treated to a series of general public health measures in the mid-Victorian years: its sewage system had been constructed by the Metropolitan Board of Works in the 1860s; its water supply, in the hands of private contractors, was not unusually unhealthy; and its mortality figures, not particularly bad in comparison with other British towns, were much superior to those of other European capitals (Thompson, 1967, p. 5; Sheppard, 1971, chap. 7).

The decade under consideration here, from 1904 to World War I, saw fertility rates (the childbearing of married women aged 15 to 45) drop in inner London boroughs more rapidly than in the three previous decades of slower decline. London's rate fell by nearly a third in the 40 years between 1870 and 1910, but the rate was uneven between boroughs and between decades. Looking just at the 20 years between 1880–81 and 1900–1, the decline, for example, in the riverside East London borough of Poplar was only 6 percent. In better-off districts rates had fallen more rapidly: in Kensington the decline was about 21 percent, while in well-off Hampstead the drop was still larger. In a later 20-year interval, though, the declines had become more dramatic and more evenly spread across the metropolitan area. There was a 23 percent decline in Poplar between 1890–91 and 1909–11 and still larger declines in better-off boroughs: 45 percent in Hampstead and 34 percent in Kensington.[3] For inner-London women, clearly it was in the early twentieth century rather than the late-Victorian decades that really dramatic shifts in fertility rates were occurring.

The ideas of the Infant Welfare movement must be viewed as part of the decade of imperialist agitation that preceded World War I. A longstanding debate about national "deterioration" was intensified by General J. F. Maurice's 1902–3 series of apocalyptic journal articles claiming that the British race was so feeble and unhealthy that it was no longer producing enough men qualified to be soldiers. An "Inter-Departmental Committee on Physical Deterioration" made up of civil servants was appointed to investigate the matter and issued its celebrated report in 1904. The report covered all bases but singled out infant mortality as a major national problem, and the issue was also discussed by the registrar-general at some length in his annual report for that year. While infant mortality had long been a concern among British health officials of all kinds, it now became a major national issue (Eyler, 1976; Cullen, 1975; Newsholme, 1935, pp. 138–9, 322–3, 336–7, 349; Soloway, 1982b, pp. 138–48). Infants, children, and mothers were studied with intensity during the next decade, and it was in the interest of lowering infant death rates in poor districts that health-visiting schemes, milk depots, and mothers' and babies' clinics were established, all within a few years, even months, of the 1904 report.

Local and national legislation also followed, some of which, taking advantage of the facilities provided by the schools, involved the care of older children rather than infants. The 1906 Education (Provision of Meals) Act increased the supply of dinners (still means-tested, however) for London schoolchildren. In the early months of World War I, the act was extended considerably, better funded, and, in theory at least, no longer means-tested.[4] The 1907 Education (Administrative Provisions) Act required school authorities to carry out medical examinations twice during children's school careers. In 1907, under the Notification of Births Act, local authorities were empowered to require the announcement of all live births to the district medical officer of health within 36 hours.[5] The London County Council enacted such a measure immediately, and its borough registrars were thus sources of information for the voluntary health-visiting organizations that proliferated in this period. The 1908 Children Act, while it is best known for its creation of a separate system of juvenile justice in England, was a grab bag of middle-class theories about the failings of working-class parents, mothers especially. Among its dizzying number of seemingly unrelated provisions, it outlawed children (under 14) going into pubs, a measure designed in large part to keep their mothers out; it imposed fines or prison terms on parents whose children were killed owing to lack of fireguards in their homes or as a result of overlaying (accidental smothering in the parents' bed) if "at the time of going to bed the person was under the influence of drink," and penalized parental neglect, including failure to provide adequate health care. The National Insurance Act of 1911 with its maternity benefit was also passed in the climate created by the "deterioration" discussions (Gilbert, 1966 and 1965).

The Deterioration Committee and the hundreds of writers who commented on its findings outlined a great many social factors that appeared to contribute to infant deaths: low wages, overcrowding, contaminated milk, hot weather, and inefficient sewage systems among them. Mothers had, of course, only very limited control over many of these factors, but Infant Welfare movement activists endowed women with magical powers to sustain or destroy life. Thus the intellectual machinery was set into motion through which mothers were attributed with superhuman power and, as a corollary, could become targets of extraordinary resentment and blame. The "ignorant" or "feckless" mother was an anchor in "deterioration" discourse. Good mothers could save English babies.

"UNPAID NURSEMAID OF THE STATE"

Political as well as scientific advances in medicine and public health in the late nineteenth century increased the prestige of doctors and health workers who were formulating new definitions of childhood and motherhood. Mothering was to be a paramedical function, and medical personnel were to serve as mothers' helpers and authorities. The confidence with which the new ideas were enunciated was built on a rapidly proliferating body of scientific literature in several fields of human biology. The 1880s, following Robert Koch's discovery of the typhoid bacillus in 1880, was a decade of intense activity in bacteriology, while the same might be said of the 1890s and the three following decades in the study of nutrition and human and animal metabolism. The reformers' notions about child health were also based on the experience of a middle-class society in which children were larger; better fed; less anemic; freer of rashes, chilblains, and sniffles; less prone to serious diseases – and where birth rates had already begun to decline. These notions also represented a conception of infancy and early childhood as "precious" though "priceless," to use the terms of a sociologist who has studied contemporaneous American assumptions about childhood.[6] Working-class mothers were actually more fulsome in their appreciation of older children who helped at home or earned cash for their families.[7] The new health standards, too, emanated from a middle-class culture that equated physical health with goodness and, indeed, had been obsessed with health since the mid-nineteenth century (Haley, 1978, esp, chap. 1, pp. 3 and 19).

My view of the Infant Welfare years owes a great deal to Anna Martin, a perspicacious suffragist social worker with the nonconformist Bermondsey settlement in Rotherhithe, South London, from 1898 until the 1920s. Martin witnessed the Infant Welfare movement and the changes associated with it from the vantage point of the waterside married women of whom she was a passionate advocate and spokeswoman; she was vividly conscious of the fresh burdens Infant Welfare legislation imposed on women. She referred bitterly to a *political* alliance between organized working-class men and upper-class male legislators to establish elements of a welfare state on the cheap by squeezing more money and work out of the disenfranchised poor wives of Britain. As Martin tells their stories, every one of the ordinary problems the mothers of Rotherhithe faced — sick children, unwanted pregnancies, unemployed husbands — was deepened by national and municipal interference with their longstanding neighborhood-based survival systems — systems that were already all too delicate balances of material and human resources. Taken together, they created a climate that discouraged women from having babies (A. Martin, 1919, pt. 3, p. 961).[8]

While the working-class clients of the new agencies sometimes welcomed and complied with the professionals, they also resisted their advances or reordered them to suit older needs and habits. Styles of opposition ranged from what anthropologist Emily Martin calls "nonaction" (1987, pp. 183–9) to sabotage, outright refusal, or organized acts of rebellion. A model stressing mothers' passive acquiescence and middle-class professionals' unchallenged social control is inappropriate in the context of London's well-established, female-centered neighborhood networks upholding common ideas of mothers' rights and children's place. Linda Gordon's convincing analysis in *Heroes of Their Own Lives* of Boston women's attempts to manipulate volunteer child protection agencies to their own advantage is more applicable to these inner-London households. To be sure, the London mothers, unlike the Boston women whom Gordon surveys, did not have a choice about whether to call in such figures as borough health visitors or sanitary inspectors. Yet even these visits could sometimes be turned to advantage: they might include referral to a clinic, a dinner program, a charity distributing free trusses or eyeglasses, or a training school for a blind son, and even an admonition that another pregnancy was out of the question — professional advice that a woman could pointedly relay to her husband (L. Gordon, 1988).

Despite the welfare orientation of their work, sanitary officers, school personnel, and doctors all nonetheless conspired to put a woman, in Martin's words, "in a state of being continually driven to live beyond her means" physically and financially. These regulations had enormously increased the hours of work a mother had to do to send, for example, three, four, or five tidy, well-shod, and nit-free children to school each day. For wives, the price of noncompliance with this motley but ubiquitous set of laws and regulations could be not only "countless humiliations" but fines, jail sentences, or the loss of child custody. To be a mother in these new circumstances was to be little more than "the unpaid nursemaid of the State" (A. Martin, 1913, pp. 1239–40; 1919, pt. 3, p. 960).[9]

WORKING-CLASS WOMEN AND THEIR CHILDREN

Middle-class women had for several generations been defined, at least in prescriptive literature, around their identity as mothers.[10] But for the bulk of working-class wives (possibly excepting the 10 or 15 percent married to "labour aristocrats"), the effort to ensure household economic survival had a greater claim on their attention than rearing the individual child.[11] Until the late Victorian years or later, working-class mothers, like poor mothers in earlier centuries, saw themselves as *workers* for their husbands and children; productive rather than emotional functions were at the center of female identity.

The economic arrangements in working-class families in most parts of late nineteenth- and early twentieth-century England reflected the mother's central role in the family and the father's institutionalized peripheral relation to his children in particular. Husbands "paid" their wives each week an unvarying sum that was often called the wife's "wage." "Good" husbands paid their wives nearly all that they earned; bad ones paid smaller and more irregular sums. It was the wife's job to run the household on whatever she got from her husband, combined with whatever earnings she and her children could contribute (see Oren, 1973). While in the poorest London districts perhaps a third of wives worked for pay at any given moment,[12] nearly all would have done so during their married lives. The importance of the unpaid work they did in the home was also acknowledged by their community. Preparing decent meals from scanty ingredients; foraging in shops, streets, and charitable organizations for food, clothing, blankets, and fuel; handling the pawnshop assistant, the corner shopkeeper, the landlady, the school board visitor – all were motherly skills and honored as such.

London's poor mothers were attentive to babies' needs for sleep, holding, and feeding, perhaps by way of keeping them quiet in small, crowded homes. The mothers were, however, on the whole, very hard on toddlers whose needs to explore and move about were impossible for them to accommodate; two- and three-year-olds were commonly kept in highchairs or tied into ordinary chairs for hours while their mothers did household chores. After infancy, working-class children shared the rigors of the family economy; few young people seemed to believe in a right to relief from the discomfort of hard work, lack of sleep, scanty food, and chronic health problems (Humphries, 1981).[13] Older children – helpers, allies, and often intimates of their mothers – were exploited by our standards, saddled with onerous babysitting responsibilities, placed in paid jobs before and after school, or enlisted in home manufacturing.

The Infant Welfare movement's proposition that mothers did, if they carefully enough followed the instructions of health visitors or doctors, have full power over child life and death was presented to a female working-class public accustomed to toil and worry over sick children, mourning and regret over dead ones, but not to self-blame. Mothers knew in graphic detail what their children needed to be healthier (fresh milk, fruit, extra house room, medicine for a sickness) and how little they could afford these things. The women were quite clear that it was usually material circumstances and not their own failings that threatened their children's lives and health.

Maternal consciousness about children's health was organized around the possibility of a death or maiming. A child's death was a familiar event in turn-of-the-century London, where the infant mortality rate was about 150 per 1,000. In some of the poorest and densest parts of Lambeth, though, or Kensington, rates were over 400.[14] In a large group of South London patients of the General Lying-In Hospital (whose records I examined for the years 1877 to 1882), nearly two-thirds of those over 35 had experienced two child or infant deaths; the pattern for a group of Guy's Lying-In Charity hospital outpatients in the 1890s was similar.[15] The nearly universal (and much deplored) habit of buying burial insurance for young children on weekly payments of one or two pennies to cover the costs of a funeral speaks of parents' need to consider the possibility of such deaths. Funeral arrangements were a constant subject of neighborhood gossip, as women shared their worries and plans for their own families' funerals or assessed the propriety of others'. Mothers' speech bristled with the consciousness of the nearness of a child's death: "Oh, you'd be better all of you dead"; "It's a blessing the Lord took my other five"; "All alive, thank Gawd."[16]

The heroic mothers who figure in innumerable family histories and contemporary accounts, watching night after night over feverish children ill with typhoid, whooping cough, or scarlet fever, were literally battling against death. The threat of death was the point at which they pawned the contents of their homes for medicines, extra milk, and doctors' fees, the point at which they ruined their own health through constant care.[17] George Acorn's pseudonymous 1911 London autobiography describes the death of a baby brother some decades earlier and his mother's heroic nursing while she simultaneously worked to cover the extra expenses of illness:

She would work like one possessed, her dexterous fingers moulding box after box almost too quickly for the eye to follow....Although her head was bent over her work apparently oblivious of all else, she would start up at the least cry from the ailing child, and rock it to her bosom until she could lay it down, enjoining silence on us all, and then resume her work as if her life depended on it.

Eventually the baby got much worse and a doctor was sent for. "Suddenly a look of fear came into her face. She seemed afraid of something; then, bracing herself as if for some frightful task, inclined her ear to the child's mouth. She gave a piercing scream, and whispered brokenly, 'My God, he's dead!'" (Acorn, 1911, pp. 35–8).

Conditions that brought children only discomfort, even profound discomfort – toothache, itchy skin rashes, or nearsightedness – made little claim for their heroic treatment. By ignoring them themselves, parents taught their children to ignore these unpleasant ailments. Late-Victorian and Edwardian medical people who encountered this lack of attention en masse were astonished at the success of an entire culture in denying the importance of perpetually running noses, squinty eyes, scabies, and impetigo; children afflicted with these conditions ran about cheerfully apparently quite without distress. Their medical problems were not actually neglected; they were, more accurately, simply not seen.

HEALTH VISITING

London was late in establishing health programs aimed at mothers and children, schemes that received no national funding or organization until 1907. Manchester and Salford began a comprehensive system of sanitary inspection and health visiting in the 1860s, and a number of county and municipal authorities instituted home health visiting or milk depots for babies in the 1890s and early 1900s – St. Helens, Liverpool, and Glasgow among them. All of London's health programs began in the twentieth century, however, using mostly volunteers working with enterprising borough medical officers. The London County Council (LCC) agreed in 1901 to partly subsidize the salaries of infant life inspectors. Local initiatives in the capital had national implications: G. F. McCleary, the Fabian medical officer of health from Battersea, and Liberal M. P. John Burns put Battersea on the political map in 1902 with their infant milk depot and babies' clinic (M. Moore, 1977; Dingwall, 1977; Dwork, 1987, pp. 105–7; Rowan, 1985).

The 1907 Notification of Births Act, a permissive law that was immediately adopted in 20 of London's 29 boroughs, made possible the elaborate system of home visits to infants and mothers that in some boroughs took in every child born into a non-middle-class household. A new profession for women, the health visitor, took shape. As Blanche Gardiner, the newly appointed Sanitary Inspector for the Prevention of Infant Mortality in St. Pancras, reported in 1908, the act made it possible for authorities to send an "advice card" to each mother "within a few days" of every birth in the borough, followed by the arrival of a health visitor. Her colleague Dora Bunting put it more vividly in her description of the St. Pancras Mothers' and Infants' Society: "Directly a baby was heard of they pounced down upon it." By 1910 the London medical officer of health, Shirley Murphy, reported only three boroughs (Islington, Camberwell, and Greenwich) where there was no infant visiting. There were ten boroughs, on the other hand, in which 60 percent on more of the homes of newly registered births were visited by a combination of paid sanitary inspectors, professional health visitors, or volunteers. Clinics, schools for mothers, and similar institutions had sprouted by then in all but a handful of the 29 greater London boroughs.[18]

Some health visiting schemes were very extensive. In 1915, when there were about 3,000 births in the borough, Kensington's three women health visitors, two of whom were away for part of the year doing "military work," nonetheless managed to pay well over 5,000 visits, most of which involved giving infant care instruction. The North Islington School for Mothers, founded in 1913, listed, by 1917, a staff of three visiting women doctors, five nurses, and 37 volunteers, the majority of whom acted as visitors. They had even trained seven women as home helps, among the first in the country.[19]

Unlike district nurses, health visitors were generally instructed to do nothing in the homes they visited, not even wash or dress babies. Their job was only to offer advice. Somewhere between one and two weeks after a birth the health visitor was to call, offering instruction on sleeping, feeding, household hygiene, and childhood diseases. The job of health visitors was not only to insert such medical ideas into the home as antisepsis, the value of breastfeeding, the dangers of sharing a bed with infants, and the prevention of rickets, but also to accustom women to seek medical help in routine infant and child care, not just in matters of life and death (Kanthack, 1907, p. 37; see also Cavanagh, 1906, p. 196). Midwife Emilia Kanthack's six 1906 lectures for St. Pancras volunteer health visitors drew attention to many conditions that required a doctor's attention: when pregnant women had swollen extremities, fits, or pelvic deformities; when mothers were bottle-feeding their babies; when babies developed severe diarrhea or had signs of rickets (Kanthack, 1907; pp. 26, 51, 81, 75, 58, 66). The mothers themselves would have defined some of these ailments as occasions for a doctor's visit, others as distinctly not. More significant in the social history of medicine and of motherhood was the visitors' subtext: many things can go wrong with babies, and only the doctor knows for sure what to do when any of these things happens.

Kensington's first salaried health visitor, a Miss Gauntlett, was unhappy with her observer's role in homes where there was so much malnutrition and "distress" crying out for material help.[20] According to a nurse Cunliffe who wrote to Sylvia Pankhurst's journal *Women's Dreadnought* in 1917, health visitors' incessant questioning "frightened" many working-class women, most of whom had something they wanted to hide from authorities. As the nurse wrote, "Health visitors call at the homes and ask the mothers all sorts of questions as to their general affairs, such as 'What rent do you pay?' 'What wages does your husband get?' 'Is he good to you?' I cannot see what good these questions do."[21] As their main function was to teach, even impose, a new set of mothering practices, they were bound to seem, as the nurse put it, "officious."

MEDICAL "DEFECTS" AND THE SCHOOL CARE COMMITTEES

School medical examinations were yet another effort to reshape mothers' assumptions and practices. The 1907 Education (Administrative Provisions) Act required that district education authorities carry out annual medical checkups of all school entrants and leavers. Supported by women's and labor groups as well as the public health establishment, the bill had been opposed by the British Medical Association as a disastrous incursion into the livelihood of private physicians (Ferguson, 1977, pp. 42–4; Thane, 1982, p. 77; Newsholme, 1935, pp. 393–6; Gilbert, 1965, p. 149). For the metropolis, with its three-quarters of a million public school children, the inspection was a truly gargantuan undertaking, and the project got off to a very slow start. But in the years that followed, the school medical staff was augmented. There were 90 LCC school nurses by 1910 and by the summer of 1912, a staff of 34 full-time school medical officers as well (Hirst, 1981, pp. 281–300; LCC *Annual Reports*, 1910, 3:149).

As with earlier, less formal kinds of monitoring of children's health by teachers or visiting nurses,[22] the object of the inspections was as much the mother as the child. Many schools made special efforts through their Care Committees (volunteer social workers attached to each school in poor districts) to get mothers to be present at the examinations, but the numbers who did so varied enormously from school to school. Care Committee members often attended the inspections, making their own claim over the children's bodies often attended the inspections, making their own claim over the children's bodies and over the mothers' caring practices. Even if the examination took literally a minute as Marion Phillips's 1910 pamphlet charged,[23] the inspections were still events at which the child and its mothering were displayed to the authorities. Women scrubbed and dressed up their children for the occasion. The mother in Bow who grabbed the boots from the feet of one of her just-inspected children to bring home for another to wear to the next inspection was amply demonstrating the pressure the inspections imposed on her. So (in a quite different way) was the woman from the notorious Campbell Road in North Islington who, when told by school officials that her son's shirt was too dirty to wear to school, sent the boy the next day in a clear, just washed shirt which was still "wringing wet."[24] Indeed, nurses and doctors rather gleefully reported the maternal failings they uncovered during the inspections in the way of nails, pieces of wire, and pins on clothing in place of buttons, and many of them confiscated the evidence. An East London school doctor, for instance, noted that inspection at one of his schools yielded "quite a collection of wire nails which were used as clothes fastenings."[25] At the Popham Road School in Islington, a nurse fastidiously reported to the Care Committee that a recent inspection had found 180 children who had their clothes pinned together, while 174 were "properly fastened."[26]

School medical inspections are a good example of the sort of welfare measure Anna Martin deplored: seemingly protecting children and providing a service to families, the medical examinations involved a modest state outlay but a heavy charge on mothers. Many of those involved in school-based social work considered that offering diagnoses without easy and inexpensive access to treatment was a real cruelty.[27] The 1907 act mandating medical examinations for schoolchildren provided no school clinics, however, for the ailments discovered by the doctors. Such clinic systems existed in other towns, but proposals for London were opposed by moderates on the LCC Education Committee as too expensive, and Margaret McMillan's privately funded Deptford clinic was the only one in operation in the London schools in the prewar years (Phillips, 1910, p. 19). Instead of clinics, the LCC had worked out a complicated financial and administrative arrangement with a number of private hospitals for treating the children. The hospitals' location mostly in inner London meant long trips into town for children from Kilburn or Tottenham, and mothers complained of this as well as long waits at the hospitals, repeated trips, ineffective medical care and high prices.[28]

In the school year ending July 1912, the doctors uncovered about 60,000 eye, ear, nose, throat, and ringworm cases among the London children. Getting them treated was the job of the Care Committees, which in the "deterioration" years were especially active in the surveillance of childhood, and motherhood. Named Health Sub-Committees of board school managers in the nineteenth century, their title was changed to Relief Sub-Committees in 1900 and to Care Committees after the 1906 Education (Provision of Meals) Act, into which they were written as the main providers of the children's dinners and investigators of their families' means. These ladies and gentlemen, under 5 percent of whom were working class according to an 1884 survey, were at first attached to groups of schools where they were involved in choosing teachers, enforcing attendance, dealing with school fees, organizing school dinners, and screening the applicants (P. Gordon, 1974, pp. 152–66; Spaulding, 1900, p. 112). In the twentieth century, especially after 1906, they did more service work among the schoolchildren; serving meals, getting mothers to seek medical treatment for their children, and badgering parents to find apprenticeships for their school leavers rather than better-paying but dead-end jobs.[29] In 1909 there was 5,500 Care Committee volunteers in London, working from one to four days a week in their schools and districts; by 1914 the figure grew to at least 8,000 (J. Kerr, 1916, p. 4; Summers, 1979, p. 34).

These workers had the capacity to help mothers and their children and, goaded by the parents, they often exercised it. The Bay Street School Committee in central Hackney, for example, managed to locate a Fund for Supplying Spectacles to Poor Children, which paid for three pairs of glasses for local children in 1908; the Poplar district committees decided to supply meals on weekends and to the younger siblings of school-age children during the transport strike that caused such suffering in the area in the summer of 1911.[30]

Like health visitors, Care Committee volunteers, were, from the mothers' vantage point, practically inescapable. While committee members often viewed medical follow-up work as tedious and unrewarding,[31] from the mother's side, the Care Committee visitor, no matter how kindly, was a menacing personage. The visitor could define a mother's refusal to bring a child to hospital as a form of "neglect" and refer the case for investigation by the National Society for the Prevention of Cruelty to Children under Section 12 of the Children Act, a procedure that committees did use occasionally.[32] The Children Act of 1908 also provided a new set of legal protocols under which parents could be compelled to have their children stripped, clipped, and bathed (while their clothes baked in special ovens) at borough "cleansing stations." Care Committee members were often the ones to enforce Education Authority orders to send lousy children to the hated cleansing stations against the furious protests of their mothers.[33] Holborn headmistresses (in 1914) complained of "abusive parents" invading their schools over head-lice issues. In Peckham the problem was that "parents defy nurses' orders and dirty [that is, lice-infested] children remain in school."[34]

If active and well organized, Care Committees could harass parents quite persistently. Thus when Cecilia Osborne's mother, in Shoreditch, refused to have her child medically treated, the mother was visited twice by local committee members, a third time by a special LCC liaison officer. A group of Islington parents whose children were diagnosed as needing eyeglasses were chased down by a local Care Committee, which had also requested that the LCC authorize their sending "worrying letters" to those who had duly got the glasses but had not paid for them.[35] For women with schoolchildren, changing discourses, legislation, and knowledge about health, nutrition, and families appeared most concretely in the form of cheerful but frightening School Care Committee visitors.

"IGNORANT OLD WOMEN" OR "MEDICAL SUPERVISION"?

The Infant Welfare workers frequently spoke of "maternal ignorance," by which they meant that the mothers thought about health, children, and their own duties in the wrong ways and honored the wrong authorities – their relatives and neighbors rather than doctors or health visitors. Infant Welfare specialists all over the country waged an active campaign against "old wives" administering gin and pickles or opiates to babies, "ignorant old women who have buried 10 out of 14 or 15," as one social worker put it (Dyhouse, 1978, p. 262; Blagg, 1910, p. 15). Health visitors, Emilia Kanthack declared in 1907, would have to contend with the fact that the mothers were by and large "pitiably ignorant and superstitious, full of prejudices, and often stuffed with dreadful advice from terrible old gamps and dowagers in their immediate vicinity." What was needed, wrote a commentator in the *Toynbee Record*, were young mothers "who are able to launch out into the experiences of motherhood unchained by superstition and vulgar prejudice" (Kanthack, 1907, p. 4).

The medical approach defined itself as superior to and incompatible with any other theory or practice of child care, giving trained outsiders permission to intrude in an intimate relationship. Even the most welcoming and mother-oriented of Infant Welfare workers jeopardized their carefully forged neighborhood relationships in its name. Social worker Clara Grant, for instance, must have been the scourge of Bow as she went about the streets snatching pacifiers from babies while ingeniously diverting their attention; her proud recital of these rather obnoxious deeds, of course, stemmed from her certainty that she was protecting the babies from the microbe-laden comforters (Grant, 1930, p. 83).

The newly professionalizing fields of nursing and public health that were so central in the Infant Welfare campaign worked to disseminate some pieces of the new body of knowledge in medicine and public health. They taught the superiority of mothers' over cows' milk in its varied commercially available forms, the importance of "proteid matter" in the diet, and methods of preventing the spread of tuberculous bacilli from one infected family member to another. The proponents of a more medical childcare had something substantive to teach, but they were not always right. Margaret McMillan was proud, for example, that her clinic had carried out "over 700 operations" for adenoids and tonsils in one year early in this century; most of them would today be viewed as unnecessary. Thousands of London children in these years had their skulls heavily irradiated, too, as a treatment for a very nonlethal (if disagreeable) condition, ringworm.[36]

Middle-class teaching and teachers were not always welcomed as emissaries from a better world. Said a nursery worker in 1904, "I do not think that my Hoxton mothers would let a lady in if she said: 'I hear that you have got a baby and I want to teach you about it.'" Investigators doing a well-intentioned study of widows on out-relief in Lambeth in the 1900s found a suspiciously high number not at home.[37] The Fabian Women's Group's weekly visitors in Kensington, beginning their study of "the effect on mother and child of sufficient nourishment before and after birth," were painfully aware of the wary courtesy they were being offered (Reeves, 1913, pp. 8, 16). District nurses, probably the most popular of all those who entered the homes of the poor, were not always desired in working-class homes either. Finsbury women admitted them only when the local general practitioner threatened to refuse his services to those who would not allow the nurses in, and there were scattered reports of hostility elsewhere as well. Indeed, one school nurse had to have a police escort, so much hatred had her delousing activities generated.[38]

Medical and public-health knowledge was part of a foreign culture from the point of view of working-class mothers. In the first decades of this century the health ideas of London's poor mothers differed fundamentally from those of the medically educated practitioners they encountered, and this helps to explain patterns of compliance and areas of dispute. The mothers' case histories – long narratives in which illnesses were put in their familial and economic contexts – sidestepped the "elaborated codes" demanded by doctors and nurses.[39] Medical personnel often jokingly complained about cockney loquaciousness, a ready source of amusing (and often quite affectionate) sketches in nursing journals. Popular perceptions of medical procedures and technology – injections, thermometers, surgical procedures, hospitalization – as unnatural and dangerous assaults on bodily integrity led to parents' frequent refusal to let their children enter fever hospitals (for infectious diseases), and to the mass refusal of vaccination in many working-class London districts by the end of the nineteenth century. The medical belief in the efficacy of removing adenoids and tonsils (which lasted into the 1960s) also frightened London mothers, who quite naturally, as Anna Martin repeated, viewed it as a process of "cutting children's throats." Their contemporaries in New York's lower East Side had rioted in 1908 to prevent busses from taking children from their schools for such operations (A. Martin, 1919, pt. 2, p. 559; Ewen, 1985, p. 143).

Mothers and health workers were at loggerheads over the maternal role in children's health care. It was over rashes, head lice, and runny noses that battle lines were drawn between housewives and medical workers. The School Care Committees, which enforced the doctors' prescriptions, were therefore on the front lines of a minor war. As Barbara Drake, a member of one of the Care Committees, dryly put it in 1910, "The type of medical treatment urged by the School Doctor, treatment of eyes, ears, throat, and nose, is the type of treatment for which the average mother sees the least necessity."[40] Perfect health was a state mothers had never imagined. Teeth that did not actively ache were left alone, and were pulled out by dentists or pharmacists when they called attention to themselves by hurting too badly. Baby teeth were certainly ignored. "He never has toothache" and "It isn't as if they was 'is second teeth" the school workers heard repeatedly from parents in defense of their foot dragging to take children to dentists for fillings.[41] The heartbreak of a South London stonemason, devastated by the school doctor's prescription of glasses for his son, suggests, too, that parents might have seen the wearing of eyeglasses as a sign of serious disability.[42]

Prescriptions for eyeglasses and for dental work often required large cash outlays from parents and multiple visits to clinics or hospitals.[43] A Kensington mother whose child needed glasses took literally months to get them paid off at two pence per week (Reeves, 1913, p. 183). Mothers needed to spend their household cash on food, rent, and fuel. Routine well-child health care had a feeble claim on this very scarce money. In the winter of 1910, when a group of more than 50 children from the Popham Road School in Islington were discovered to need glasses, a large minority of parents resisted the Care Committee visitors and refused to provide them. One of the mothers, a Mrs. Stephen, when visited by a committee member, said that she was "unable to pay, and stated that the child did not need the glasses her eyesight being quite good." A Mrs. Hollings also "disputed the necessity of the glasses," according to the Care Committee's minutes. For that committee the balance sheet for the year ending in March 1911 showed a lot of parental foot dragging on glasses or other minor problems: of 29 boys referred for treatment of various sorts, 15 had never been; of 32 girls, a third remained untreated, and at least five of the female cases involved unbought eyeglasses.[44]

The excuses mothers offered for their failure to carry out the doctors' orders outline a distinct system of maternal allegiances very different from those being advanced by school health workers: to wage earning, to the housekeeping budget, and to domestic tasks. For the mothers, too, the care of smaller children had precedence over what they perceived as the relatively minor needs of an older child, a child whom mothers expected would contribute money and work to the household, not drain them away. The mothers complained repeatedly to Care Committees that they could not leave their paid work, or their home duties, to bring a child for medical treatment. As a woman in Rotherhithe who had failed to take her daughter to hospital commented, "If I take Lizzie to the hospital, what with fares, medicine, and someone to mind the others while I'm gone, it will cost me one-and-six. *I don't see the good of taking money off the food to put it on the medicine*" (A. Martin, 1913, p. 1242; 1918, pp. 1100-1). Benjamin Atkins's mother told visitors in West St. Pancras in 1916 that "she is quite unable to leave her other children to take him to Treatment Centre." Among the many Popham Road School parents in Islington who refused to get glasses for their children, some said they could not pay for them, while a Mrs. Bearfield simply said that it was "inconvenient to leave her stall to take the boy to the hospital."[45]

*   *   *

The major legacy of the Infant Welfare era was mothers' (and increasingly, fathers' too) much greater public accountability for the failures and flaws, small and great, physical and moral, of their offspring. After 1904 a long decade of propagandizing about mothers' vital contribution to national efficiency, and emphasis on their skill as the barrier between life and death for their children, coexisted, as it happened, with a massive and distinctly extragovernmental campaign for female suffrage. This unlikely brew may have begun raising the demands and expectations of ordinary working-class women, a situation that the domestic experience of World War I only accelerated. Rather than becoming "unpaid nursemaids of the state," slaving to ensure middle-class comfort for a dozen children on a workingman's wage, working-class women incorporated the Infant Welfare movement's definitions of motherhood into a new sense of their own rights in relation to husbands and even to children. A Rotherhithe workingwoman with whom Martin talked after the war drew her own conclusions about the new maternal regime: "Sometimes I hanker after another baby, but then I say to myself the pleasure of it would only last a year or two, and afterwards *there'd be nothing but worry*" (A. Martin, 1919, pt. 3, pp. 960–61). Women's desperation to avoid the "worry" of an extra child, and their growing determination that care and worry not engulf them entirely, can be seen in the rapidly declining fertility rates of those who married during and after the Infant Welfare era.

NOTES

1   "Investigation and Coordination," *The School Child*, June 1912, p. 9.
2   On the Infant Welfare movement, see Dwork (1987), Lewis (1980), Gilbert (1966), Rose (1985), Dyhouse (1978), Davin (1978), and McCleary (1933).
3   London County Council (LCC), *Annual Reports* (1910), vol. 3, p. 12.
4   School medical officers were to certify which children needed the free food (Thane, 1982, p. 76).
5   In 1915 all stillbirths after 28 weeks of pregnancy also had to be registered with local medical authorities.
6   Karl Pearson was among the first, in the 1890s, to note that birth rates were declining much faster among the prosperous classes (Soloway, 1982b, p. 153); Zelizer (1985).
7   I examine this point in chapter 4 of my forthcoming study, *Love and Labor in Outcast London: Motherhood, 1870–1918*.
8   This is one in a three-article series attacking the Infant Welfare movement.
9   See also A. Martin (1911), pp. 38–44.
10   See Gillis, this volume; also Davidoff and Hall (1987), chaps. 3 and 7; Branca, (1975), chaps. 6 and 7; J. Lewis (1984), chap. 3; J. S. Lewis (1986). M. J. Peterson's study of a large group of upper-middle-class urban women, however, uncovered many who took their motherhood very casually (1989).
11   See E. Roberts (1986) for evidence for this position; also Chinn (1988).
12   On the importance of wives in family economies, see Heather-Bigg (1894). Charles Booth found that a third of East London households relied on the earnings of both spouses (1969 [1902], pp. 37–49, 300–1, 310–11, 322–3).
13   On girls, see Davin (forthcoming).
14   *Report of the MOH for Lambeth*, 1895 and 1905; Borough of Kensington, *Annual Report of the MOH for 1905*, p. 12; Hope (1917), vol. 1, p. 212.
15   There were 256 women in this group. Stillbirths made up only a small proportion of these deaths (General Lying-In Hospital, York Road, Outpatient Registers, July 1877–November 1882, Greater London Record Office [GLRO], HI/GLI/B22/vol. 1). My thanks to R. Murray, unit administrator, Acute Services, St. Thomas's Hospital, for permission to use and cite these records. Guy's Lying-In Charity, [outpatient] Maternity Record, GLRO, H9/GY/B22/vol. 5. Calculations taken from early 1892 through late 1894 (every case; 1,314 in all).

16   As recorded by teacher and social worker Clara Grant (1930), pp. 100, 104.

17   I examine this issue in *Love and Labor*, chap. 3.

18   St. Pancras MOH, *Annual Report for 1908*, pp. 28–9; *Proceedings of the National Conference on Infantile Mortality*, 1908, p. 69; LCC *Annual Reports* (1910), vol. 3. See, however, Winter (1985), 189–203.

19   Borough of Kensington, *Annual Report of the MOH for 1915*, p. 8; Campbell (1917), vol. 2, pp. 87, 90.

20   Borough of Kensington, *Annual Report of the MOH for 1905*, p. 59.

21   E. H. Cunliffe, "Health Visitors: A Nurse's View," *Women's Dreadnought*, Sept. 22, 1917, p. 857.

22   See Davin (forthcoming), chap. 10, on schools and health before the turn of the century.

23   Mothers who did attend, she found, might have waited as long as three hours for the minute-long inspections (M. Phillips, 1910, p. 8). See also Ferguson (1977), p. 43.

24   Grant (1930), p. 76; "Difficulties in a Very Poor District," *The School Child*, February 1912, p. 6.

25   Dr. Lewis Hawkes, a member of the Charity Organisation Society, longtime resident of Finsbury, and general practitioner there, testified at length before the 1903–4 Inter-Departmental Committee on Physical Deterioration. His report to Doctor John Kerr, London's medical officer for education, is in LCC, *Annual Reports* (1910), 3:137.

26   Minutes of the Popham Road School Care Committee, Islington, 1909–11, GLRO, EO/WEL/2/6, Nov. 5, 1909.

27   "The Health of the Children," *Toynbee Record*, January 1909; McMillan (1909); M. Phillips (1910); "Care Committees," *The School Child*, March 1913, p. 1.

28   Hirst (1981), pp. 291–2; M. Phillips (1910); "The Treatment of School Children at Hospitals," *The School Child*, February 1913.

29   See their discussions in the *Toynbee Record* during these years and, after 1910, in *The School Child*, published for the thousands of School Care workers nationwide.

30   Bay Street School Care Committee minutes, March 31, 1908, GLRO, EO/WEL/2/1; on children's meals in Poplar, see LCC *Minutes of Proceedings*, July, 16 1912, p. 267; July, 2 1912, p. 90; July, 23 1912, p. 362.

31   See reports in *The School Child*, July 1910, p. 15, and March 1913, p. 4.

32   An excellent discussion of the legal and social concept of medical neglect in contemporaneous America is found in L. Gordon (1988), pp. 127–30.

33   The story of an attack on lousy children by Care Committee workers at the Wood Close School in Bethnal Green in 1910 is found in the Care Committee minutes for 1909–10, GLRO, EO/WEL/2/10.

34   Central Consultative Committee of Head Masters and Head Mistresses, *Minutes of Miscellaneous Resolutions Subcommittee* (Nov. 1909–June 1921), vol. 2, pp. 14, 44, 77, 88, 96. These records are in the GLRO, EO/GEN/3/2. Based on research notes kindly supplied by Dina Copelman.

35   Popham Road Care Committee minutes, April 8, 1910. The LCC refused the request.

36   McMillan (1919), p. 191; "Medical Treatment of London Children," *Toynbee Record*, January 1912, p. 48.

37   Test, Miss Eves of the Maurice Hostel, *Parliamentary Papers* (PP), 1904, vol. 32, qq. 7763, 7764, 7700; Royal Commission on the Poor Laws and Relief of Distress, *PP*, 1910, vol. 52, appendix II (Report on an Inquiry into Cases of Children Whose Parents Were in Receipt of Outdoor Relief in Lambeth).

38   Test, Lewis Hawkes, *PP* 1904, vol. 32, qq. 12987–9; *The Sanitary Officer*, July 1910, p. 280.

39   On case history taking, see the glosses on Basil Bernstein offered by E. Martin (1987), pp. 195–7. For contemporary accounts of taking case histories, see Berdoe (1891), pp. 560–63; and "A Plaster Party," *The Nursing Record*, March, 21 1889, p. 105.

40 Letter to the Editor, *The School Child*, February 1910, p. 16. Drake was the secretary of the Charing Cross Road School Care Committee.

41 "Medical Treatment of L.C.C. School Children," *Toynbee Record*, October 1912, p. 6; "The Treatment of School Children at Hospitals," *The School Child*, February 1913, p. 12.

42 Eldred (1955), pp. 43–55. On eyeglasses, see Frere (1903), p. 124.

43 "The Medical Treatment of L.C.C. School Children," *Toynbee Record*, October 1912, p. 6; "The Treatment of School Children at Hospitals," *The School Child*, February 1913; Frere (1903), p. 124.

44 Popham Road Care Committee minutes, April 22, 1910; June 16, 1911.

45 North St. Matthews School Care Committee minutes, Jan. 28, 1916; Popham Road Care Committee minutes, April 22, 1911. See also Curtain Road Care Committee minutes, May 6, 1910.

4

Men's "Marital Rights" and Women's "Wifely Duties": Changing Conjugal Relations in the Fertility Decline

Wally Seccombe

Great advances have been made in the study of gender relations in the 1970s and 1980s, but very few of them are reflected in demographic theories of the fertility decline.[1] Sexual desire and conjugal power are absent from the mainstream paradigms of fertility regulation: it is as if demographers believed in the Immaculate Conception – for everyone. The fundamental problem with standard theories is that they are conceived at the level of the reproductive couple taken as a unified subject. They assume, in other words, the perpetual existence of harmonious needs and aligned interests between husbands and wives with regard to childbearing, sex, and contraception. This is unacceptably naive; an adequate theoretical framework must allow for spousal differences in procreative objectives and the means used to achieve them. We need not adopt the obverse premise: that conflict on these matters is universal or invariably of a zero–sum character. But because the costs and benefits of childbearing and childcare are not evenly distributed between spouses, there are valid grounds for expecting that divergent objectives will frequently arise. In this essay I present an account of the fertility decline among selected working–class populations of northwestern Europe – an account centered on spousal relations and specifically on the changing terms and conditions of marital coitus.

The European fertility decline was due almost entirely to the reduction of marital fertility: changes in the age and incidence of marriage – which had been the key regulators of the birth rate in Western Europe in the early modern era – made little or no contribution (Coale and Treadway, 1986, p. 52). Out-of-wedlock births subsided concomitantly, but this trend accounted for less than 10 percent of the aggregate contraction. In most regions, the reduction of marital fertility was achieved entirely by means of "stopping" – the deliberate cessation of childbirth prior to menopause. In the rest, stop-

the bulk of the change (Knodel, 1977a). The fertility
istoric watershed in two respects: the birth rates of entire
w lows, and the stopping mode of fertility regulation was
practice for the first time.

INITIAL MEANS OF STOPPING

How was stopping accomplished? There is evidence that changes in four
practices contributed: (a) a rise in the incidence of induced abortion; (b)
more frequent resort to coitus interruptus; (c) a decline in coital frequency
by deliberate abstention; and (d) increased use of contraceptive devices.
Because this essay concentrates on the last three practices, I will consider the
first briefly.

The incidence of induced abortion (relative to live births) rose substantially around the turn of the century all across northwestern and central
Europe.[2] Rates peaked in the 1920s, with German hospitals reporting two
to three times as many cases as in the prewar years (Woycker, 1984,
p. 126). In Britain, studies by hospital gynecological departments and women's
clinics estimated that roughly 16 to 20 percent of pregnancies were deliberately terminated. The Inter-Departmental Commission on Abortion, issuing
its final report in 1939, confirmed these as reasonable estimates (Gittins,
1982, p. 164). A 1899 report in the Westminster Review maintained that
most abortions in Britain were still obtained by single women (Saver, 1978,
p. 91). Forty years later, the Inter-Departmental Commission concluded that
"the overwhelming majority of abortions occur among married women...
[and] that abortion is relatively more common in the case of mothers in the
higher age groups than in the case of younger mothers" (Gittins, 1982, p.
164). A parallel rise in the proportion of abortions obtained by married
women was detected in Germany (Woycke, 1984, pp. 130–33). Evidently, a
great many abortions conformed to the stopping pattern: they were sought
by married women approaching the end of their childbearing years. It seems
reasonable to conclude that a rise in the abortion rate contributed considerably to the decline of the birth rate prior to the widespread use of contraceptive devices in marriage. But because a great many working-class women
in the nineteenth century had also sought abortions, it is unlikely that rates
would have risen sufficiently in the early twentieth century to account for
most of the fertility decline at that time.

Turning now to the role of coitus interruptus, abstention, and contraceptive devices, we find that changes in any or all of these methods entail
a profound alteration in the conduct of conjugal sex. No explanation of
declining fertility that fails to take account of these changes can be termed
adequate. Given the pace of the decline, daughters and sons were evidently

breaking radically with the sexual mores of their mothers and fathers. What had brought about this far-reaching revolution in reproductive consciousness and coital behavior? To answer this question, let us consider personal testimonies in which working-class women and men from Britain, Germany, and Norway recount their reproductive experiences in the first quarter of the twentieth century.

In the case of Britain, vivid accounts are preserved in two collections of letters. The first was sent to the Women's Co-operative Guild in the years just prior to World War I in response to an inquiry from the guild urging its members to recount their childbearing histories (Davies, 1978 [1915]).[3] Writing about reproductive experiences that had occurred in the 1880–1910 period, guild members were representatives of a largely *prelimiting popu-lation*. A second set of letters was sent in the 1920s to Marie Stopes, the famous campaigner for the dissemination of contraceptives to the public.[4] In the very act of writing to Stopes to solicit birth-control assistance, her correspondents were moving beyond the wish to restrict fertility to the realm of practical action. Consequently, we should regard them as representatives of a *limiting population*, although one that had been largely ineffective thus far.

Ernest Lewis-Faning conducted a survey in 1946 that furnishes a useful check on several themes found in the British correspondence (Lewis-Faning, 1949). His questionnaire was administered to a quasi-random sample of married female patients found in all departments of general hospitals in England and Scotland. Interviewers inquired as to whether respondents had attempted to limit births at any time in their married lives, and if so, what means were used. The strength of the survey for our purposes was that Lewis-Faning divided the sample into three social classes (on the basis of the husband's occupation): class 1, professional and middle class; class 2, skilled manual labor; and class 3, unskilled manual labor. He tabulated respondents' answers by class and longitudinally by cohort on the basis of the year of marriage dating back to 1900.

For Norway, we have a source comparable to the British correspondence, an immense archive of 4,300 letters written by women from all over the country and sent to the Office for Maternal hygiene in Oslo between 1924 and 1929. They have been extensively analyzed by Ida Blom; I am relying entirely on her assessments (Blom, 1980).[5] The German evidence takes a somewhat different form – the results of surveys done by the Berlin doctor and sex researcher Max Marcuse in 1911–13, and by Doctor O. Polano of Würzburg in 1914. In these surveys, roughly two-thirds of the working-class respondents reported using some form of birth control, so I shall treat the majority as exemplary of *first-generation limiters*. Here, I am using James Woycke's dissertation (1988) and R. P. Neuman's (1978, pp. 408–28) analysis of the surveys.[6]

In the early stages of the decline, what means were people using in their efforts to avert conception? In Lewis-Faning's retrospective survey (1949), nine in ten limiters before 1920 had relied on coitus interruptus.[7] More respondents marrying in the 1920s employed contraceptive devices, but the proportion was still less than one-third. The German pattern was very similar. In Marcuse's study, 77 percent of limiters relied on coitus interruptus, and in Polano's, 83 percent did (Woycke, 1988, p. 39). The Stopes correspondence presents a rather different picture. Forty correspondents published in *Mother England* cite abstinence as the method they were currently practicing or had attempted to pursue in the past, while withdrawal is mentioned by only 13 correspondents.[8] This may be due to Stopes's disapproval of the latter method, and also to the correspondents' reticence to be too explicit. Data from maternal clinics in Manchester and Salford indicate that both withdrawal and abstinence were widely practiced by working-class couples, although the former more frequently (Gittins, 1982, pp. 165–9).

In sum, the evidence points strongly to coitus interruptus as the most popular method of birth control in the first phase of the decline.[9] Yet the Stopes correspondence and the clinic data suggest that attempted abstinence was not negligible and may well have been underestimated in the surveys of Marcuse and Lewis-Faning. Historical demographers generally assume that couples trying to limit births before the widespread use of contraceptive devices would naturally practice coitus interruptus as a less stressful method than prolonged celibacy (van de Walle, 1980; Knodel and van de Walle, 1986, p. 403). But withdrawal was much less secure, and this generated another kind of stress – the fear of pregnancy, mentioned by several female correspondents who favored abstinence for this reason. Perhaps most women writing to Stopes failed to mention withdrawal because they did not take it seriously as a birth-control option (Gittins, 1982, p. 162). The technique depends on male commitment and control; it is likely that many women did not have much faith in being able "to push him out of the way when I think it's near" (J. Lewis, 1984, p. 18).

The rhythm method was not available to couples practicing abstinence or withdrawal in these decades. There was an awareness that the chances of conception were unevenly distributed over the menstrual cycle, but the process and timing of ovulation were not understood. Prevailing medical theory had it exactly backwards, postulating that the "safe time" was mid-cycle (McLaren, 1983, p. 51). Couples abandoning a random schedule of intercourse in favor of this advice would have considerably increased their chances of conception. (It is little wonder that the method was dubbed "Vatican roulette.") In any event, the rhythm method was not widely practiced. The implication of such ignorance is clear: abstainers had to avoid intercourse at all times, and withdrawers had to separate every time. Both methods would have been a great deal easier to employ, particularly in obtaining men's full cooperation, if they could have been practiced for a specific week each month and relinquished in favor of normal intercourse the rest of the time.

The determination to "keep right" in an era prior to the general use of contraceptives created an acute dilemma, because the only "proper" (healthy, natural, and moral) avenue for the sex drive was uninterrupted coitus within marriage. Noncoital forms of sex play were clearly beyond the pale for the vast majority of working-class couples, a testament to the rigidity of their sexual socialization. While only a small minority were prepared to experiment, this portion undoubtedly increased as the pressure mounted to avert conception. Woycke detects a rise in oral sex and anal intercourse in Germany in the early twentieth century, citing the independent reports of two physicians who were convinced that such practices were "shockingly frequent" among working-class couples (1988, p. 37). In her introduction to *Mother England*, Stopes noted that "in a very few [letters], one or two sentences too intense for publication have been cut out"; these were probably references to noncoital sex. There is one allusion to sodomy in *Dear Dr Stopes* (Stopes, ed., 1930, p. vi; Hall, ed., 1981, p. 15).

All sources agree that contraceptive devices of any type were infrequently used by working-class couples before 1920. In Lewis-Faning's survey, less than 10 percent of working-class women marrying before 1920 report any use of mechanical means by either partner. The German findings are similar (1949, p. 52; Neuman, 1978, p. 418; Woycke, 1988, pp. 33–9).[10] Given the widespread desire to limit, why were barrier methods and spermicides not used more often? Stopes's correspondents bluntly described their own lamentable ignorance of the most elementary matters of human reproduction and contraception. Most had heard tell of various "remedies," and many had tried devices and drugs promising to "put you right" that were sold by charlatans and quacks. Contraceptives were often confused with abortifacients, an impression that was undoubtedly reinforced by unscrupulous advertisements for various products in the penny press (Stopes, ed., 1930, pp. 19, 75; Hall, ed., 1981, p. 36; Blom, 1980, p. 51). Repeatedly, respondents complained that these commodities were injurious or ineffective, often both (Stopes, ed., 1930, pp. 4, 47, 57, 75, 110, 128, 146, 153, 155, 157, 166; Hall, ed., 1981, p. 29). Furthermore, contraceptives were expensive items on a tight working-class budget. In Germany around the turn of the century, rubber condoms cost about five marks per dozen, roughly a half-day's pay for a skilled worker (Neuman, 1978, p. 419). In Britain as well, contraceptives were expensive and often difficult to obtain in working-class districts (Brookes, 1986, p. 159). Several correspondents complained to Stopes of the expense of contraceptives, and others were unable to figure out where they could be purchased, indicating that in many neighborhoods they were not yet sold over the counter in local shops (Stopes, ed., 1930, pp. 77, 86, 99, 103, 105, 124, 148, 155, 170). Finally, some women who thoroughly disliked sex with their husbands (as many did) feared that the regular use of contraceptives would remove a compelling rationale for refusing sex in the face of their husbands' "lustfulness," Morakvasic concluded. "For such a woman the use of a contraceptive would remove her strongest weapon in the game of sexual politics" (Morokvasic, 1981, pp. 136–7).[11]

People's fear of contraception was based partly on a well-founded suspicion of bogus products but also on misconceptions about the harmful side effects of "preventatives" (Stopes, ed., 1930, pp. 128, 147). The advice of doctors was a major source of such misapprehensions (Woycke, 1988, p. 110). Leaders of the British Medical Association condemned contraceptives as unnatural and warned that all sorts of maladies would befall their users. Advocating semen as a cure-all elixir for women when absorbed through the vaginal wall, many doctors opposed anything that interfered with the intermingling of secretions; similar misconceptions were propounded by German and French doctors (see Soloway, 1982a, pp. 111–12; Woycke, 1988, 110–21; and McLaren, 1983, pp. 44–64). Thus many doctors felt it was their duty to impede the spread of contraceptive knowledge and devices. Thirty-five correspondents in *Mother England* mention that doctors had refused to inform them about contraceptive devices, even as they warned patients of the dangers of further pregnancies: "When the last baby was born the doctor said can't you finish up but when I asked him how…he just laughed. What's the use of saying finish up when they won't tell us poor women how to" (Stopes, ed., 1930, p. 134).[12] For many working people, fears of physical injury and mental disorder were blended with deep moral reservations and aesthetic distaste; they regarded contraceptives as "repulsive and unnatural" (Davies, 1978 [1915], p. 94; Stopes, ed., 1930, pp. 3, 21, 42, 58, 84, 98, 119). Condoms had an unsavory reputation, being associated with prostitution, extramarital liaisons, and the prevention of venereal disease, which *was* the principal context of their use at this time. People's compunction in this regard was buttressed by the major Christian denominations, Catholic and Protestant, that "viewed with alarm the growing practice of the artificial restriction of the family" urging "all Christian people to discountenance [such means]…as demoralizing to character and hostile of national welfare" (Soloway, 1982a, p. 99).[13]

PROCREATIVE RISKS, CONJUGAL POWER, AND SEXUAL RESTRAINT

Insofar as women bear most of the burdens of repeated childbearing and child care, we would expect them to be more highly motivated than men to call a halt. The evidence bears this out. Women's dread of future pregnancies and their fierce determination to bear no more children is an especially prominent theme in the Stopes correspondence: "I have tryed many Pills But Have not seen the desired effect. Please Help me! I have Had my share,… but I am frighten to death, with what I have gone through, My life is only a living Hell, Yours truly" (Stopes, ed., 1930, p. 123). Similar passages could be cited at length: pleas for help – urgent, fearful, on the brink of despair – by women who recount horrendous experiences "in confinement" and whose pain and disabilities were often highlighted by the ominous warnings of attending doctors and midwives that another birth could kill them (Stopes, ed., 1930, pp. 44, 75, 79, 86, 131, 153). The fear of pregnancy under such circumstances can easily be envisioned. Stopes's correspondents describe sleepless nights, worrying themselves sick, moments of terrible anguish when their "courses" were overdue, and bitter regret and recrimination at a "slip in a moment of weakness" after years of total abstinence. The assessments of Angus McLaren and Lenard Berlanstein on working-class couples in France and Woycke's judgment on the German evidence concur with my reading of the British materials: while most men agreed on the need to stop, women were the driving force behind family limitation (Woycke, 1988, p. 88; McLaren, 1983, pp. 132–3; Berlanstein, 1984, p. 144).[14]

When women grew determined to cease childbearing, were they able to alter the sexual conduct of their husbands to lessen the risk of conception? In marriages where husbands adamantly refused to cooperate, wives had very little influence and were forced to submit to their husbands' sexual advances: "I am sorry to say that my husband is one of those who think we ought to let Nature, as he calls it, have its way and that if I have twenty children it is only my duty as a married woman to put up with it. I am always dreading my husband wanting his wishes fulfilled and I am powerless to prevent him"; "My husband who is a Catholic does not believe in stopping life by any means. When I say I do not want any more he gets very nasty with me and won't try to keep me right" (Stopes, ed., 1930, pp. 145, 100). In these circumstances, women often became inured to coital risk, resorting instead to abortions (which they could seek on their own initiative) to deal with the hazards of repeated pregnancies.

Where husbands were not reported to be coercive, most female respondents indicated that they were able to reduce coital frequency through dissuasion, deferral, and evasion. Some developed the habit of "staying up mending," retiring after their husbands had fallen asleep (Burnett, 1984a, p. 260). While they could put off intercourse for a time, the vast majority of female respondents could not steadfastly refuse a cohabiting husband his "conjugal rights." Periodic "connections" were seen as essential in preserving conjugal harmony: "To maintain the domestic peace, I must nevertheless once in a while let my husband 'have his way'"; "I cannot always refuse my husband as it only means living a cat and dog life for both of us" (Blom, 1980, p. 150; Stopes, ed., 1930, p. 83). The sex drive was perceived as an implacable pressure that would continue to mount if not punctually released; sooner or later it had to be satisfied. "I don't think any man and woman that really love each other can resist nature however much they try," thought a woman writing to Stopes; "we have tryed very hard but still the third baby came." A man confessed, "I have seriously tried to hold myself in check but its impossible...yet when I fail to keep myself in control well there's more trouble and it has caused me many a restless night, and bad feelings between the wife and I" (Stopes, ed., 1930, pp. 168, 43).

Many women who had managed to "hold out" for several months realized they could not continue to do so; they wrote to Stopes with urgent requests for contraceptive information: "Since my last baby was born six months ago, my husband and I have not cohabited as I am so afraid of anything happening again....We cannot go on like this any longer as we are both only young....My husband is getting fed up. Think how hard it is in one room" (Stopes, ed., 1930, pp. 83, 105, 147, 162).

Women feared the consequences of marital abstinence, "knowing there is much unfaithfulness on the part of the husband where families are limited." A Norwegian woman explained to the staff of the Oslo clinic, "If you deny your husband his desire, the law gives him a right to go to another and that is something which a wife who loves her husband will avoid. What should I do?" (Blom, 1980, p. 150).

Women who were gratified to gain the active cooperation of their spouses were often worried about the effects of celibacy or withdrawal on their partners' health: "I will tell you something I dare not tell no one else. I have found out that my husband is abusing himself, you know what I mean. It is worrying me terribly because I am afraid to let him have anything to do with me. I am sure he will do himself some harm" (Stopes, ed., 1930, p. 91). Given the perceived imbalance in the sexual appetites of men and women, it is not surprising that most of the concern as to the potentially harmful effects of abstinence was focused on men (Stopes, ed., 1930, pp. 168, 35, 43, 101, 3, 144, 91, 106, 145, 166; Hall, ed., 1981, pp. 15–16).[15]

The way men approached their wives sexually was immensely important to women (Davies, 1978 [1915], p. 171).[16] Selfish or "lustful" men were roundly condemned, even by wives who did not contest their right to intercourse whenever they felt like it. On the other hand, a considerate husband deserved a forthcoming wife. The obligation of reciprocity within an unequal relationship generated self-sacrifice on the part of the subordinate partner, inducing many women to feel that they were treating kind husbands unfairly by denying them their marital dues: "I feel mean in refusing, that which as a married woman I have a right to give, for my husband has been so fine, so patient, kindly and considerate, yet there is always the fear [conception] might happen the first time I agreed." A woman's empathy could be dangerous in this context: "I was so afraid of being caught again that I stopped all intercourse, then my husband fell ill and of course I had to humour him a bit, the result was another baby" (Stopes, ed., 1930, pp. 53, 41; Blom, 1980, p. 150; Stopes, ed., 1930, pp. 120, 59, 161).

Because women feared pregnancy more than men did, the consequence of differential distress for the ratio of sexual desire is apparent. Several women reported that the dread of another pregnancy had destroyed their passion for "connections" with their husbands (Stopes, ed., 1930, pp. 70, 85, 139, 161, 163, 164). The widely held belief that females who became highly aroused during intercourse were much more likely to become pregnant, particularly if they had orgasms, must have dampened many women's ardor (Charles, 1932, p. 26). Some women were frank to admit that they found no pleasure in intercourse but were nevertheless concerned for their husbands: "I have never at any time had a desire to be with a man and even with my Husband I never get any sensation or feeling. My Husband on the other Hand is very Lustful....I would like to satisfy his desires yet I am terrified at the thought [of getting pregnant] and it causes unpleasant scenes in the Home" (Stopes, ed., 1930, p. 11).

For a substantial minority of women, however, their own sexual desires, together with their husbands', made prolonged abstinence untenable. The prevailing view of feminist historians is that working-class women in the past disliked sex and wished for as few encounters with their husbands as possible. Elizabeth Roberts, in her oral history interviews with British working-class women in Preston and Barrow, reported that "sexual intercourse was regarded as necessary for procreation or as an activity indulged in by men for their own pleasure, but it was never discussed in the evidence as something which could give mutual happiness. No hint was ever made that women might have enjoyed sex" (E. Roberts, 1984, p. 84).[17] The Stopes correspondence is not nearly so bleak in this regard. While several correspondents confirm the conventional stereotype, others present a more balanced and mutual picture, with female passion apparent (Stopes, ed., 1930, pp. 2, 21–2, 40, 58, 70, 105, 114–15, 151, 161, 165, 168, 176). These correspondents were all women: "I have a lot of 'Spanish blood' too in my veins which doesn't help any; living as we do is wearing my nerves to pieces"; "When two people are so fond of one another as we are, as I have one of the best, you like to get the best out of life"; "At certain times of the Month we nearly get beyond control...it is strange for us to go four years without proper connections"; "My husband tells me to control and hold myself in check, well I can, but we do without kisses, and oh, lots of other little things that help make life pleasant"; "Its impossible to put passion entirely out of our lives, for its the love I bear my dear husband that makes me yield to him at such times"; "I am very passionate as well as he, and we have been so wonderfully happy and I do so want to make this happiness last" (Stopes, ed., 1930, pp. 114–15, 4, 61, 156, 136, 53).[18]

While for many women sexual consent was motivated by love and affectionate reciprocity, others experienced their "wifely duty" more as a moral obligation. For these women, "living as nature and God intended us to do" was a basic tenet of Christian marriage; to withhold sexual consent was selfish and sinful (Stopes, ed., 1930, p. 40). Perhaps more important than church doctrine in the strict sense was the pervasive conviction that procreation was natural; one dare not interfere with Mother Nature. A north Lancashire woman interviewed by Elizabeth Roberts recalled visiting her doctor and breaking down when he confirmed that she was pregnant.

> He said, "Its no good crying now, its too late!" I felt like saying that it wasn't the woman's fault all the time. You are married and you have got to abide by these things....They don't know what I have gone through to try to avoid it, you know. we never would take anything in them days. God had sent them and they had to be there. I'm not a religious person, but that were my idea. (E. Roberts, 1984, p. 88)

For this woman and many others, the marriage contract entailed "abiding by these things" – remaining open to the risk of conception while doing her conjugal duty. Wrapped in the ideological mists of procreative naturalism lurked the brute force of men exercising their conjugal rights: "I thought, like hundreds of women do today, that it was only natural, and you had to bear it....My husband being some years my senior, I found that he had not a bit of control over his passions....[A] man has such a lot of ways of punishing a woman if she does not give in the him" (Davies, 1978 [1915], pp. 48–9). Under these circumstances, it was extremely difficult for many women to communicate their most basic wishes to their husbands. Many did not even try. A guild member confessed, "I may say here that I did not want any more....Of course, I can see now that I was a good bit to blame, because I thought I was only like other women would be, and kept all to myself." For their part, many men looked the other way. A Berlin journeyman was asked whether his wife practiced any form of birth control. He said he did not know but thought she "probably looks after that herself because she didn't want the last two children" (Davis, 1978 [1915], p. 43; Neuman, 1978, p. 423). Without the active cooperation of husbands, celibacy was out of the question. Even with husbands' consent, abstinence and withdrawal wracked marital relations with tension, bitterness, and alienation: "Our love seems to bring us more suffering than anything else;" "the result is our married life is spoiled and we are gradually drifting apart" (Stopes, ed., 1930, pp. 80, 114).[19]

While women were generally keener to cease childbearing than were their husbands, men were increasingly willing to exercise some self-restraint in the marriage bed. The prevalence of coitus interruptus as the principal form of birth control establishes a prima facie case for male cooperation. Marie Stopes accused working-class men of being more impervious to their wives' wish to avoid conception than "better informed" men. Eleanor Barton of the Women's Co-operative Guild held the same view (Stopes, ed., 1930; p. 40; J. Lewis, 1984, p. 16). Yet in reading *Mother England*, I was impressed with the reported willingness of most husbands to restrain their sexual desires. Ida Blom's reading of the Norwegian correspondence also suggests a very substantial degree of male collaboration. In the British letters, men who are portrayed as being cooperative outnumber uncooperative males two to one, with the former constituting a clear majority even among female correspondents.[20] These men were praised by their spouses as being careful and considerate; they did not "worry" their wives by insistent sexual demands, and they kept themselves "under control": "My husband is very good and for three years has not had a real 'pleasure' in order to keep me right" (Stopes, ed., 1930, p. 20).

Where spouses found themselves in dispute over reproductive priorities, what was the nature of their discord? Hypothetically, conflict might arise for three reasons: (a) couples could differ on the desirability of having another child; (b) they could disagree over coital frequency and other aspects of sexual conduct; or (c) they might have divergent approaches to birth control. The correspondence indicates that the latter two were the primary bones of contention. Simmering tension arose from men's sexual impulsiveness or lack of discipline, based on the reckless assertion of their conjugal prerogatives, rather than from their desire to have more children than their wives wished.[21]

The attitudes among uncooperative men varied.[21] A minority were intensely hostile to the use of contraceptives of any sort and were resigned to accept the number of children that nature, or God, provided. A French-woman reported, "My husband saw that I wanted to cheat nature. He flew into an awful rage; I was afraid that he would kill me; I resigned myself to the ordeal and now I am going to live with the continual fear of a fifth child" (McLaren, 1983, p. 133). Some men were ambivalent or simply indifferent to the prospects of another pregnancy: "My husband doesn't care if we have a dozen, so long as he satisfies his own selfish desires" (Stopes, ed., 1930, p. 121). A third group of uncooperative men shared their wives' desire to avoid conception, often feeling very intensely on the matter, but were adamant that it was a woman's responsibility to look after herself. Evidently feeling that their virility and marital rights were at stake, they refused to alter their sexual conduct in the slightest (Stopes, ed., 1930, p. 72; Neuman, 1978, pp. 421–4): "My Husband is inclined to get angry each time there are signs of another arrival and thinks I ought to take all expense and blame on my shoulders, although I do my level best to keep right" (Stopes, ed., 1930, p. 72); "He was so angry [to discover that I was pregnant] he never came into my room again for two months....[S]ince then he has been very cruel to me because I will not submit to his embrace" (Hall, ed., 1981, p. 15). Eleanor Rathbone, who campaigned for the family allowance, perceived the connection between men's sexual prerogatives and women's economic dependence in marriage. She said that men's physical access was "still enforced on their wives as part of the price they are expected to pay for being kept by them" (Rathbone, 1986 [1924], p. 197).

THE CONVERGENCE OF MEN'S INTERESTS WITH WOMEN'S

To engender family limitation, both spouses must have a strong *desire* to cease childbearing and the *capacity to take effective action* toward that end. The dilemma for a great many working-class couples in the early twentieth century was that the two necessary conditions of deliberate limitation were disjoined. Women were strongly motivated but lacked the power to avoid coitus and the means to avert conception, while men had it in their power to abstain, withdraw, or use condoms but were not sufficiently motivated to restrain their sexuality with any consistency. Until such time as men came to fear the prospect of another child strongly enough to exercise sexual self-discipline, there was bound to be unspoken stress, if not open conflict, between spouses over the terms and conditions of intercourse. The rate of abortion for married women – rising very considerably from the turn of the century – is a measure of this conflict, representing, as it does, women's fierce determination to terminate pregnancies that their husband had not been conscientious enough to prevent. A substantial minority of pregnancies had always been greeted with a sinking heart and feelings of trepidation for the future, but in the first quarter of the twentieth century this proportion was evidently rising.

If married women were already keen to shorten their childbearing careers, what brought husbands around to their way of thinking? A more insistent attitude on the part of women accounts in part for the increased willingness of men to exercise self-restraint. Ethel Elderton noted in 1914 that contraception was fairly widely practiced by working-class couples in the northern textile districts: "The married women have frankly told our correspondent that they make their husbands take precautions to prevent conception, the two methods of prevention in use being the sheath and coitus interruptus" (Elderton, 1914, p. 61). But the major impetus, in my view, was the underlying shift in the family economy, moving men's reproductive interests increasingly into line with those of their spouses (Levine, 1987, pp. 160–76). In the surveys of Lewis-Faning and Polano, the outstanding reason people gave for wishing to cease childbearing was that they could not afford another child. Stopes's correspondents concurred, referring most frequently to the husband's wage or irregular employment, implying that his was the primary and often sole income.[22] As men contemplated the arrival of another child, breadwinner responsibilities weighed heavily on their minds: "I don't want to be the cause of bringing children into this world and not being able to keep them"; "I am only a working man it take all my time to feed and cloth them if there should be any more I doo't know what we should do" (Stopes, ed., 1930, pp. 14, 17).[23]

Proletarian parents had not always regarded additional children as a net cost. In the traditional family wage economy, children worked from a young age, and their contribution was readily apparent to parents. A French miner's wife was asked why she had seven children. "They come naturally," she replied, "and then, when they grow up, they contribute their wages to the family; it helps balance the household budget" (L. Tilly, 1985, p. 404). A Shoreditch matchmaker told Lady Dilke in 1893, "Of course, we cheat the School Board. Its hard on the little ones, but their fingers is so quick – they that has the most of 'em is best off" (Rubinstein, 1969, p. 61). The next generation of parents would arrive at the opposite conclusion. When referring to children in economic terms, they treated them as a net cost (Neuman, 1978, pp. 424–6).

The contrast between the Victorian and Edwardian generations can best be appreciated by looking at the difference in the dependency ratio at that point in the family cycle when the question of stopping first arose: when parents were in their mid- to late thirties and their eldest children were becoming teenagers. Through most of the nineteenth century, working-class youth took paid jobs from age ten or eleven if not earlier, earning more than enough to cover the costs of their own upkeep. As mothers entered the final phase of childbearing, the income of the eldest would ease their families' economic pinch. In the Edwardian era, however, the eldest children were still attending school fairly regularly when a mother reached her mid-thirties and had to determine whether to go on conceiving or to try to call a halt (Caldwell, 1980, pp. 225–55). Parents could not anticipate any substantial income supplementation from children for another two or three years. Furthermore, the tradition of youth remitting their full wages to their parents had weakened by this time, particularly for boys in their late teens; even when they did go out to work, their income was less secure from the parents' standpoint. Older daughters were not as likely to be available to mind the young ones, freeing mothers to seek employment. The delay and dissipation of children's economic contribution was accompanied by higher costs associated with prolonged schooling and regular year-round attendance (Ross, 1983, p. 20). At the same time, the potential supply of surviving children was increasing, as infant and child mortality declined sharply. This development widened the disparity between the desire for smaller families and the old procreative regime. Facing these prospects, the family's primary breadwinner was increasingly inclined to share his wife's view of the need to quit childbearing.

It was not poverty per se but the prospects of a lower living standard that gave proletarian couples pause for thought. The blunt admission by so many that they "could not afford any more" ought to be interpreted in this way – as a matter of relative well-being, not absolute death. In the words of German workingmen: "With children you can't amount to anything these days. We're still young and we want to have life a little better"; "We want to get ahead, and our daughter should have things better than my wife and sister did" (Neuman, 1978, pp. 425–6). It was the upper layers of the working class that first began to limit. In 1907 Sidney Webb noted that the birth rate had declined far more among members of the Hearts of Oak Friendly Society (the largest benefit society in Britain at the time, with 272,000 male members) than among the general proletarian populace. He argued that it "gave proof of thrift and foresight...[among] the artisan and skilled mechanic class," the primary base of the association (Webb, 1907, pp. 6–7). In the twentieth century, taking control of one's fertility became a mark of working-class self-reliance and respectability, while the prolific poor were pitied or ridiculed. Formerly, fecundity had been associated with masculine virility; now uncontrolled childbearing was considered to be reckless imprudence, a self-inflicted source of poverty. As a German father declared, "Four are enough already. We're already laughed at for having four" (Neuman, 1978, p. 425).

Together with underlying shifts in the value of additional children, changes in reproductive consciousness galvanized the fertility decline. What was the nature of this transformation, especially for women? The dominant recollection of the older guild women who had not limited their childbearing was of stoic resignation; they would have liked fewer children but had felt it was beyond their control: "At the time it was much more usual to trust Providence, and if a woman dies it only proved her weakness and unfitness for motherhood"; "In my early motherhood I took for granted that women had to suffer at these times, and that it was best to be brave and not to make a fuss" (Davies, 1978 [1915], pp. 39, 33). In the midst of such resignation, women "got caught," and babies "just came" and kept coming. A consoling faith that the Lord would provide for all those He sent was extremely common among prelimiters (E. Roberts, 1984, pp. 87–8). A Catholic factory worker from the Rhineland, married 20 years with five living and three dead children, hoped that no more would come but comforted himself with the thought that "if there are too many, then the dear Lord, who puts them in this world, will also feed them" (Neuman, 1978, p. 423).

The guild correspondents deeply regretted the prudish reticence of their mothers to provide them with sexual or reproductive information, vowing that this silence would not be repeated with their own daughters (Davies, 1978 [1915], pp. 50, 64, 70, 72, 116, 118, 156): "I was married at twenty-eight in utter ignorance of the things that most vitally affect a wife and mother. My mother, a dear, pious soul, thought ignorance was innocence, and the only thing I remember her saying on the subject of child-birth was 'God never sends a baby without bread to feed it.' Dame Experience long ago knocked the bottom out of that argument for me" (1978 [1915], p. 44). Among the daughters of procreative fatalists, stoicism finally crumbled. They began to take an instrumental attitude toward their health, considering repeated and uncontrolled pregnancy to be a preventable malady. Increasingly, they perceived the relationship of sex to procreation as a matter of probability and risk, rather than blind fate or God's will. Even though mechanical devices were still widely rejected as harmful and repugnant, contraception had finally come "within the calculus of conscious choice" (to use Ansley Coale's [1973] felicitous phrase). What had brought about this transformation in women's, and then men's, consciousness?

The rapid increase in the routine intervention of doctors in working-class pregnancy and birthing in the early twentieth century seems to have been a catalyst. In the second half of the nineteenth century, about 70 percent of all babies born in England were delivered by midwives without doctors in attendance; in the poorer districts the proportion was undoubtedly higher (Wohl, 1983, p. 14). By the interwar years, the pattern had changed dramatically; all but the poorest families could afford their services at confinement. The majority of correspondents who refer to the matter at all indicate that doctors attended their home births.[24] In these same decades (see Ross, in this volume), working-class homes were invaded by a burgeoning army of middle-class charity visitors and state officials. The home visits of public health nurses would have augmented the doctor's influence in turning pregnancy from a natural event into a medical problem (J. Lewis, 1984, pp. 36–7; see also J. Lewis, 1986, p. 101).

While refusing to help women obtain contraceptive devices, doctors did legitimize women's fears concerning abnormal and protracted childbirth. The doctors' solemn advice fills the Stopes correspondence, their most common instruction being to avoid further pregnancy, complete with terrifying warnings of the dire consequences of failing to. Their admonitions must have buttressed many a woman's resolve not to sacrifice her health on the altar of her "wifely duty" to her husband. Medical talk provided working-class women with a vocabulary of scientific authority to better envisage and describe the inner workings of their bodies and to assign terms to their maladies. The letters are full of such borrowed terminology – *prolapses, embolisms, glyosuria, sciatica* (Stopes, ed., 1930, pp. 24, 40, 56, 76, 78, 84, 92, 96, 98, 101–2, 113, 115–6, 160, 163, 167; Hall, ed., 1981, p. 30). Imported into working-class speech, this alien discourse had its uses. It helped erode the mysteries of the female body, which for so long had been shrouded in ignorance, shame, and "mock modesty" (Davies, 1978 [1915], pp. 64, 70, 72). Medical discourse made it increasingly difficult to regard the maladies associated with childbirth as natural, a manifestation of God's will. Certainly infant deaths, formerly regarded as inevitable, were now considered preventable. Perhaps most important, "the doctor's orders" were a powerful tool in convincing husbands that they ought to restrain themselves, or else terrible afflictions (with impressive Latin names) would befall the missus. Several male correspondents reveal the deep impression that a man-to-man talk with the doctor made in persuading them to put concern with their wives' health above their own sexual desires: "The doctor attending my wife 'forbade' any more children"; "I must not forget what the doctor says. My considerations are for my wife and my four children" (Stopes, ed., 1930, pp. 57, 17, 31, 46, 65, 108, 171).

Feminism, predominantly a middle-class movement, also seems to have had a diffuse impact on working-class women, fortifying their resolve to stop having children. Victorian feminists had attacked the notion that a man had the God-given right to have sex with his wife whenever he felt like it, regardless of her wishes. John Stuart Mill denounced the prerogative of spousal rape as a "most disgusting barbarism, to enforce the lowest degradation of a human being, that of being made the instrument of an animal function contrary to her inclinations" (Mill, 1929 [1869], p. 59). This argument seems to have made ideological headway. In the matrimonial law reforms of the late-Victorian era, men's "conjugal rights," traditionally sanctioned through the wedding vows, were tempered and relativized (Holcombe, 1983; Minor, 1979). As the guild women set down their thoughts two decades later, many expressed a feminist position: "The wife's body belongs to herself....[I]ts the men who need to be educated....[N]o animal will submit to [sex on demand]. Why should the woman?" (Davies, 1978 [1915], pp. 27–8). A woman writing to Stopes in 1923 presented a lengthy thought experiment in gender reversal: "To the men who would condemn you, I would like to give one month as a mother in a working man's home.... They would have to feed that family, wash for it, bake for it, clean for it, make a good big dinner...make old clothes into new. This would be fairly hard but 'God Help Them' what would they do if they were handicapped by pregnancy. You wouldn't have one enemy" (Hall, ed., 1981, p. 18). Against the traditional pronatalist morality of the church, several of Stopes's correspondents articulated a feminist counter-morality, anticipating the modern prochoice slogan "every child a wanted child." Taking dead aim at the traditional Christian belief that God would provide for all, they insisted that it was "wicked to bring children into the world to practically starve" (Hall, ed., 1981, pp. 16, 22; Stopes, ed., 1930, pp. 111, 120, 61). They redefined the maternal ideal: "What real mother is going to bring a life into the world to be pushed into drudgery...because of the strain on the family exchequer" (Davies, 1978 [1915], p. 90). Many correspondents argued that it would be unfair to their present children to have any more (Stopes, ed., 1930, pp. 25, 64, 72, 73, 89, 92, 93, 102, 106, 110, 118, 120, 130, 142, 167, 168). Recalling their own reproductive experience prior to family limitation, guild members were generally encouraged that the times were changing: "I now see that a great deal of this agony ought never to have been, with proper attention. It is good to see some of our women waking up to this fact"; "Working-class women are...far more self-respecting and less humble than their predecessors" (Davies, 1978 [1915], pp. 62, 46).

Even if men's determination to stop was not as intense as their spouses, all that was necessary to avoid numerous conceptions was that husbands be willing to accede to their wives' wishes. Spousal cooperation did not make withdrawal and abstinence secure methods; "moments of weakness" and "slips" were commonplace, as the letters attest. But a very considerable reduction in births was nonetheless achieved through a determined application of methods that remained notoriously haphazard on an individual level. To continue the birth decline, reaching the low birth rates that have prevailed in the developed world since the collapse of the postwar baby boom, it has been necessary for the great majority of reproductive couples to replace "natural" methods with the regular use of contraceptives. In the first phase of the transition, however, withdrawal and abstention were sufficient to produce a dramatic reduction in the birth rate. What changed in the first quarter of the twentieth century was not the means of birth control but the realization by masses of women and men that sexual restraint was both possible and necessary. From that time on, the desire to avoid pregnancy took precedence over the desire for unimpeded coitus in increasing numbers of working-class bedrooms.

NOTES

1   A genuine "community of scholars" is an endangered species in modern academia – at least that has been my experience. The group that crafted this collection was one such community. My deepest thanks to all of them for insightful reflections on this essay. The text's remaining deficiencies are stubbornly mine.

2   Sauer (1978), p. 91, has made the case for an increase in Britain, Woyke (1984), pp. 125–6, has done the same for Germany, Blom (1980) finds evidence of an increase after World War I in Norway, Treffers (1967), pp. 299–300, for the Netherlands, and Shorter (1982), pp. 191–7, presents a range of evidence for several regions of northwest Europe.

3   Replies were received from 386 members, covering 400 cases; of these 160 were printed. The book, edited by the guild's general secretary, created an immediate sensation when published in 1915.

4   Written in the 1920s, they are found in a chapter of Hall, ed. (1981), entitled "The Lower Classes," and in a more extensive collection published by Stopes in 1930. Stopes drew some 200 letters from her private files received in 1926 from working-class people with surnames A to H.

5   I am most grateful to Ida Blom for her patient correspondence with me in English and to Kari Delhi for translating key passages of Blom's work.

6   Woyke's text was originally a doctoral dissertation completed at the University of Toronto in 1984, and it is this version that I cite. Thanks to Edward Shorter for drawing my attention to his student's thesis.

7   Lewis-Faning groups all birth-control practices into two categories, "appliance" and "non-appliance" methods. Strictly speaking, abstinence and the rhythm method were included with coitus interruptus in the latter category, but the author reports that the combined incidence of celibacy and cyclical abstinence was negligible, so that "non-appliance methods may be taken throughout to refer to Coitus Interruptus" (1949, p. 8).

8   On abstinence, see Stopes, ed. (1930), pp. 9, 11, 16, 17, 22, 28, 31, 35, 36–7, 39, 40, 41, 43, 47, 52, 54, 58, 59, 63, 66, 68, 70, 74, 91, 104, 113, 114, 117, 120, 124, 130, 138, 139,

147, 153, 159, 161, 164–5, 166, 177; on withdrawal, see pp. 3, 8, 36, 47, 50, 61, 74, 84, 98, 101, 130, 144, 160. In some letters, it is not clear whether references such as "my husband holds himself in check" refer to abstinence or withdrawal, and of course both methods might be tried by the same couple at different times. I have assigned all such references to one or other category on the basis of my best guess as to the primary means used.

9   Many women mention prolonged breastfeeding as a means of limiting fertility (Stopes, ed., 1930, pp. 8, 16, 55, 62, 64, 73, 77, 99, 148, 155, 170). The suggestion was often raised by nurses who were not prepared to recommend contraceptives. Delayed weaning is a spacing technique; it is practically useless to women attempting to stop. Correspondents rejected it outright for their purposes, agreeing with the popular adage "If a woman want from children to be freed, to trust nursing's but a broken weed" (McLaren, 1984, p. 67).

10   The mass distribution of condoms to soldiers during World War I undoubtedly increased their postwar use (Peel, 1963, p. 120). However, insofar as their wartime purpose reinforced the close association of "French Letters" with prostitution and the prevention of venereal disease, it is doubtful that their distribution and use would have had much of an impact on conjugal use right after the war.

11   Many Victorian feminists opposed birth-control devices for the same reason. See Bland (1986), p. 129.

12   See also pp. 5, 17, 20, 24, 49, 63, 68, 69 (2), 79, 80, 83, 94, 100, 101, 108, 111, 113, 115, 124, 125, 131, 132, 134, 137, 141, 142, 150, 153, 154, 157, 170, 171, 172, 173.

13   The Church of England did not condone the use of birth control until the Lambeth Conference of 1930.

14   I found only one instance in *Mother England* where a husband was keener to quit than his wife. In two cases, men wanted to use condoms, but their wives refused for religious or aesthetic reasons; in the latter, the woman is portrayed as being intensely keen to quit (pp. 42, 58). Roberts (1981), p. 91, cites a woman who wanted a large family while her husband had other ideas. A few such cases can be found, but they appear to be extraordinary.

15   It was widely believed that abstinent men were more likely to contract tuberculosis than their sexually active counterparts (McLaren, 1983, pp. 132–3).

16   See also pp. 27, 48, 66, 99, 99–100; and Stopes, ed. (1930), pp. 148, 158.

17   Lewis finds "copious evidence...of women who felt no sexual pleasure because of fear of pregnancy, and there is some indication that working-class women may have internalized middle-class ideas of passionlessness and its correlate: male sensuality" (1978, p. 139). Branca asserts that "there is no sign of sexual pleasure in [working-class] marriage" (1978, p. 139).

18   Because Marie Stopes was widely renowned for her manual *Married Love* (which sold out six editions in it first year of publication), it seems likely that women writing to her were biased toward those who found pleasure in conjugal sex. Even so, the correspondence indicates that at least a substantial minority of working-class women did enjoy sex with their husbands. The picture Roberts presents of universal dislike strikes me as unrepresentative.

19   See also pp. 2, 3, 4, 9, 22, 27, 31, 35, 40, 41, 43, 47, 53, 54, 58, 61, 66, 70, 80, 85, 91, 98, 101, 113, 122, 124, 136, 144, 162, 164–5.

20   Women vouch for the willingness of their husbands to cooperate through abstinence or withdrawal on the following pages of Stopes, ed. (1930): pp. 4, 17, 19, 20, 41, 54, 65, 68, 70, 84, 91, 112, 114, 117, 124, 125, 130, 132, 135, 141, 144, 147, 153, 159, 177. Men declare their willingness to cooperate on pp. 14, 22, 31, 42–3, 47, 58, 74, 161. Because men would not have been writing to Stopes if they were not keenly interested in avoiding conception, they must reflect the more cooperative end of the spectrum. I am not inclined to infer a similar bias in the husbands of female correspondents, because there were compelling reasons for wives who wished to limit, but whose husbands were indifferent or hostile to this objective, to write to Stopes for information concerning female

contraceptives. However, a great many letters came from women who describe themselves as being at risk of conception without ever mentioning their husbands. It is impossible to tell whether these women: (a) were being taken against their will (i.e., raped), (b) felt that it was wrong to refuse to do their "wifely duty," or (c) had strong enough sex drives to rule out abstinence or withdrawal as viable options. If we add some of these correspondents as inferred cases of male uncooperativeness, the correspondence as a whole would be more nearly balanced.

21 Contrary to the standard models of fertility regulation, a difference in the desire to halt childbearing is not necessarily manifest as a divergence on optimal family size. When women and men are asked how many children they would like to have in contemporary surveys, their answers frequently do not differ much (Mason and Taj, 1987, pp. 611–38). My impression from the correspondence is that this would have been the case for working-class women and men in Britain in the first quarter of the twentieth century. But they did differ, often dramatically, in the intensity of their desire to stop. This suggests that the degree of motivation is not a linear reflection of the size of the potential child surplus (a demographic theorists' postulate) for two reasons: because the anticipated costs of the excess will not be evenly borne, and because differences in sexual desire and contraceptive onus have been left out of the equation entirely.

22 In the Lewis-Faning survey, 49 percent of the skilled laborers' wives and 67 percent of the unskilled laborers' wives answered in this fashion (1949, p. 178). In Polano's Würzburg survey, economic constraints were cited by 45 percent of all respondents (Neuman, 1978, p. 424). A full citation of the Stopes, ed. (1930), references would be so copious as to occur on almost every page. The following exemplify the range of issues involved in the correspondents' concern to halt childbearing in order to make ends meet: pp. 8–9, 39, 48, 91, 92, 110, 132. Male unemployment was frequently mentioned: pp. 12, 14, 23, 28, 41, 79, 88, 92, 103, 118, 124, 159, 166.

23 See also pp. 57, 59, 66, 93, 103, 173; Neuman (1978), pp. 424–6.

24 The routine hospitalization of births was a later development. In 1927, 15 percent of all births in Britain occurred in hospitals; by 1946, 54 percent did (Lewis, 1980, p. 120).

5

The Sexual Politics of Reproduction in Britain

Angus McLaren

The two major traumas that dominate the twentieth-century
novel of working-class life are, not the strike, not the factory
accident, but early and unwanted pregnancy and hasty marriage, or the back street abortion.
— Ken Worpole, *Dockers and Detectives* (1983)

In the latter decades of the nineteenth century, Britain experienced the
beginnings of a sustained decline in marital fertility. Couples who married in
1861–9 had on average 6.16 children; those of 1890–99, 4.13 children; and
those of 1920–24, 2.31 children. The crucial first phase of the fertility
decline was clearly a consequence of the methodical use of traditional
methods of birth control – withdrawal and abortion. Later surveys suggested
that only a tiny percentage of couples married before 1910 used mechanical
contraceptives (Wrigley, 1969, p. 197).

The spread of new means of fertility regulation was more a result than a
cause of the initial drop in family size. Ironically enough, many of the early
twentieth-century birth-control advocates in Britain and North America,
facing enormous public hostility, sought to distance themselves from traditional fertility-control methods; indeed, they attempted to advance the
cause of contraception by turning to their own advantage the widespread
bourgeois fear of a perceived abortion "epidemic." They argued that the
question was not *if* family size was to be limited but *by what means*. The use
of modern forms of contraception would, they argued, remake the working-
class family, which would come to resemble its middle-class counterpart
both in its reduced size and in its values.

Birth-control advocates were, more than any other group, responsible for
the notion that a great discontinuity separated the traditional world, in which

limitation of family size was impossible, and the modern, in which it was feasible. In this essay I argue that this was not so; birth-control advocates themselves played an ambivalent role in changing behavior. They sought, on the one hand, to create and respond to a demand for a particular type of family limitation that was appropriate for a particular family form; on the other hand, they attempted to reduce reliance on methods they could not tolerate – methods that spoke to the needs of a different class and culture.

Abortion was widely used by working-class women, although they were obviously concerned by the dangers it posed. If the birth controllers were simply responding to their clients' demands, one could have expected them to have sought to provide safe, legal abortions as well as to distribute contraceptives. In fact, the popularizers of contraception sought to steer women away from inducing miscarriages. "Birth control," wrote Margaret Sanger, "is essentially an education for women" (1923, p. 254). Appropriate family behavior and sex roles were, as the following analysis suggests, central to the curriculum. The first half of this essay establishes the significance of abortion as a means of fertility control. The evidence of doctors – although obviously biased against such practices – necessarily provides the starting point for such an analysis. The second half of the essay examines the responses of the birth controllers to abortion. Notions of "right" and "wrong" ways to control fertility were socially determined. Even in an age heralded by some as the "twilight of parenthood," the use of one form of fertility control (contraception) was perceived to be normal, hence accepted, and that of another (abortion) perverse.

ABORTION

The reader of the leading British medical journals of the 1890s such as the *Lancet* and the *British Medical Journal* is struck by physicians' reluctance to discuss abortion. The medical profession argued that the inducement of miscarriage was both medically and morally wrong as well as a criminal offense; doctors only condoned the termination of a pregnancy if a mother's life was in danger and full medical consultation took place. Many women had to rely on self-induced abortions as a form of fertility control because doctors, though they might advise restriction of family size, failed to provide the information on contraception that would make it safely possible. Earlier in the century doctors might have opposed abortion because of the dangers it posed for women, but by 1900 hospital operations could be performed with relative safety. The profession thus forced women to look for aid elsewhere.

What preoccupied doctors were the many irregular practitioners providing real or purported abortifacients to a large clientele. The medical profession especially scrutinized the work of midwives, pharmacists, and herbalists. In

1892 medical witnesses before the Select Committee on Midwives' Registration testified that unsupervised midwives would "increase criminal abortion."[1] Physicians had always viewed midwives as professional rivals for the control of birthing; now they demanded more stringent regulation of midwifery. Pharmacists also were harshly criticized: "The registration of chemists has not prevented them from selling oceans and tons of medicine each year for the purpose of causing abortion." Similarly, when a Wigan herbalist was convicted of selling abortifacients, the *Lancet* lamented, "What things go on and what crime is practiced in the name of herbalism."[2] When a physician was tried for abortion, however, the *Lancet* did not call for closer government supervision of his profession.[3] Doctors, in short, turned the public concern over abortion to their own purposes – eliminating competing semiprofessional healers.

Physicians were as much concerned by the fact that some abortifacients did work as by the fact that quacks sold some that did not. A woman would first seek to "put herself right" by drinking an infusion of one of the traditional abortifacients such as tansy, quinine, pennyroyal, rue, ergot of rye, savin, or cottonroot. Ergot of rye has long been used by midwives to induce labor.[4] The effectiveness of these home remedies is hard to determine, but doctors believed that some, by sufficient irritation of the lower bowel, could induce expulsion.

If the drugs failed, a woman might try bleedings, hot baths, violent exercises, and large quantities of gin. After that came the riskier step of attempting a dilation of the cervix with slippery elm, a sponge tent, or catheter. The Higgison syringe for a soap and water douche began to be used after World War I. The woman turned to the abortionist as a last resort. The quickening of fetus at about the sixteenth week customarily put an end to any further attempts at miscarrying.

The dangers posed by these drugs may might well have been exaggerated. The general public usually became aware of a woman's attempt at abortion only when something went seriously wrong; a successful inducement of miscarriage would pass unreported. Moreover, it is likely that doctors, opposed to women's attempts at "medical self-help," would seek to frighten them by portraying in lurid terms the risks run. Savin, ergot of rye, diachylon, pennyroyal, and quinine crystals were potentially poisonous and had to be used with great care. Yet several of them, such as ergot, were to be eventually taken over by professional obstetricians. Slippery elm was used to dilate the cervix; a similar technique involving a form of seaweed was used until at least the 1950s in British hospitals (Polson and Tattersall, 1959, pp. 545–59; Polson, 1963, pp. 430–37).

Doctors further recognized that women did not always rely on quacks or pharmacists but could discover for themselves the sorts of medications they needed. The best example of such medical "self-help" in the 1890s was the discovery and expanded use of a lead compound, diachylon, as an abortifacient. Its use came to light when the *Lancet* reported in 1898 on the lead poisoning of a 23-year-old married woman in Sheffield who admitted to "taking stuff" to bring on a miscarriage (Crooke, 1898, pp. 255–6).[5] A few years earlier there had been many incidents of lead poisoning in Sheffield owing to contamination of the town's water supply. Local women were quick to note that those who were pregnant had aborted and so struck on the idea that a small amount of lead could be used to induced miscarriage. Diachylon was readily at hand in every working-class home for use on cuts and sores as a plaster and for drawing milk away after parturition to relieve swollen breasts. Now it was put to a new use (Crooke, 1898, p. 256).[6] What impressed physicians was that this abortifacient was not a patent medicine or a quack cure popularized by handbills or newspaper advertisements but a home remedy passed on by word of mouth. Although its use spread, it spread slowly, "for the women of this class do not travel farther than to and from their nearest market town or centre. The direction of the spread along the northern part of thickly populated manufacturing populations, subject to bad trade or overcrowding" (Hall and Ransom, 1906, p. 511). In 1906 this use of diachylon was still restricted in area. By the time of the 1914 Parliamentary Report on Infant Mortality, it had spread in Lancashire. An investigator reported that diachylon was retailed in pennyworths and made up into pills. One pharmacist admitted to selling 14 pounds (500 pennyworths) – in one year.[7]

Ethel Elderton's survey of fertility trends in the north of England turned up evidence of the same practices. One Yorkshire woman declared, "Six out of ten working women take something, if only paultry stuff....One tells another....[I]t's all done in secrecy. One woman said to me, 'I'd rather swallow the druggist's shop and the man in't than have another kid.'"[8] Quacks all over England also attempted to turn the demand for abortifacients to their own profit. Diachylon was sold as "Mrs. Seagrave's Pills," and a host of other purported cures for "female ills" were offered under female brand names. Even "respectable" medical companies sought to exploit the situation. The 1914 Select Committee on Patent Medicines was told that, "In the instructions headed 'Advice for Females' accompanying 'Beecham's Pills,' women suffering from 'any unusual delay' are recommended to take five pills a day."[9]

Who were the women seeking abortion and how did they view their right to do so? The evidence suggests that they were predominantly from the working-and lower-middle classes, but one has to be cautious in making such a generalization (Knight, 1977, pp. 56–68; McLaren, 1977, pp. 70–81). As contemporary commentators noted, the abortions of middle-class women less often came to the attention of the authorities because they could afford more skilled methods (Engel, 1912, p. 257). Indeed, the law punished not so much the act of abortion as the poverty of women unable to afford a discrete physician.[10]

"I have been told that these abortionists will make from £2,000 to £3,000 a year in Manchester and other large towns," stated Dr. R. Reid Rentoul.[11] His claim that middle-class women were asking their doctors to provide them with abortions was substantiated by an exasperated contributor to the *Lancet*: "There is apparently a good deal of ignorance on the part of some women about the right and wrong of the matter. Not very rarely a women will say that when she and her husband married they agreed that there should be no family...and she will, after the occurrence of two months amenorrhoea has suggested a pregnancy, come to her medical man asking him, as she may euphemistically term it, to help her."[12] Such a woman, continued the writer, believed that, despite the law, there was no crime as long as the child was not alive; and to argue with her was "futile."

Middle-class women's reliance on abortion declined with the increased willingness of their husbands to use contraceptives. The evidence suggests, then, that working-class women provided the main clientele for home remedies and quack cures. Doctors' hostility to contraception was probably of scant importance to working-class women deciding to resort to abortion. They had little contact with physicians and would have had difficulty broaching a delicate subject with someone so obviously of a different station in life (Rice, 1939, p. 44).

Doctors could imagine abortion only as a result of either ignorance or desperation. One should certainly not minimize the physical hazards and the moral anguish faced by working-class women who were led to induce a miscarriage. Few could have viewed abortion as the preferred means of controlling their fertility. Nevertheless, the practice was for a number of reasons a logical form of birth control. Though dangerous, it provided a woman with some control of her own body. It meant that she was not completely helpless if her spouse was opposed to contraception.[13]

To what extent did men share abortion decisions? When in 1917 the National Birth Rate Commission asked whether husbands supported their wives in their use of abortifacients, Sir Thomas Oliver replied, "Yes. I think there must be many cases where the husband does acquiesce in the act done by his wife; but at the same time I am...certain...that [sometimes] the husband was perfectly ignorant of what his wife had taken" (Marchant, 1917, pp. 318–19).[14] In a cooperative household a couple might well agree, should contraception fail, on the necessity of abortion. Nevertheless, some working-men were opposed to contraception and viewed the imposition of fertility control as in some way an attack on their manhood. *The Little Woman in the Little House* (1992) quoted the complaint of a working woman who had nine children in 15 years but could not get her husband to cooperate: "But he said it was his rights, and he'd have consumption if we took precautions." It was no surprise that such women enjoyed the war years: "And you do get your nights to yourself, and no fear of another blooming kid" (Eyles, 1922, pp. 142, 132). For the interwar period, Richard Hoggart still reports that "the husband's shyness and an assumption that this [fertility control] is really her affair often [means]…that he 'can't be bothered with it' " (1971, p. 45).[15] Josephine Klein's findings were similar: "Husbands are not expected to abstain from sexual intercourse, or to use their own methods of contraception, though a 'good' husband is often commended for being 'careful' " (1965, vol. 2, p. 439).[16] Havelock Ellis believed that inducement of miscarriage was "perhaps specially marked among the poor and hard-working classes" (1910, vol. 6, p. 603). Thus for the working class abortion was both a supplement and an alternative to contraception.

A second reason for working-class women's resort to abortion was that, given the difficulty of using contraceptives, it could seem simpler from their point of view to have the desired number of children and then use abortifacients to "stop." Spacing of births was attempted through extended nursing. In contrast, the middle classes, as contemporaries noted, had a more complicated fertility strategy: they used contraceptives to postpone, space, and finally stop births.[17]

A third reason for working-class women's more frequent recourse to abortion mentioned to the National Birth Rate Commission by a member of the Women's Industrial Council was its cheapness. A woman might know about contraception but not be able to afford the syringe, oils, quinine, or condoms or have the privacy and running water that made douching possible. "Methods of prevention are disagreeable and difficult, as well as being expensive," she reported (Marchant, 1917, p. 279).[18] Many women, this witness asserted, thought it much simpler to wait until after conception and then taken diachylon, gin, or salts. The crochet hook, she claimed, could with a bit of midwifery skill be used quite safely. Eyles reported the same sort of stratagems but was less optimistic about the outcome (1922, p. 159).

A fourth reason that working women might view abortion as a "thinkable" option was that, though it posed a serious threat to a mother's health, it could involve the least human cost (Davis and Blake, 1955, p. 235). The working-class couple's postponing the decision of controlling pregnancy to later in the reproductive cycle gave them time to assess whether they could support an additional child. There is no doubt, however, that abortion contributed to the maternal mortality rate. Dame Janet Campbell declared in 1924 that abortion-related deaths were responsible for the particularly high maternal death rate in the industrial and textile centers of Halifax, Blackpool, Bury, Barnsley, and Bradford.[19]

Finally, although many of the women who sought abortion understandably viewed it with fears and regrets, perhaps even as "wrong," they nevertheless considered that it was their right. Middle-class male doctors repeatedly expressed annoyance that working-class women refused to accept the idea of fetal life from the moment of conception. Yet this concept was relatively new. Abortion was not a statutory crime in English law until 1803, and the notion that life did not exist until the woman felt fetal movements

– quickening – was only legally denied in 1837. Only in 1861 did the Offenses against the Person Act make it a crime for a woman to abort herself; earlier prohibitions had all been directed at the abortionist. The idea that the woman less than three months' pregnant who sought to "put herself right" was committing a crime was a product of the late nineteenth century; even in the early twentieth century much of the public did not perceive abortion as a crime.[20]

Such attitudes were revealed every time serious observers questioned working women. Havelock Ellis stated that women felt no regret and could not fathom the legal and medical opposition to abortion (1910, vol. 6, pp. 601–10). The Birkett Committee on abortion later reported, "Many mothers seemed not to understand that self-induced abortion was illegal. They assumed it was legal before the third month, and only outside the law when procured by another person" (Simms, 1974, pp. 114–16). Well into the twentieth century, working-class women took pills not to abort but "to bring on their period." That they did not intend to harm a new life was indicated by their abandonment of such tactics once quickening occurred. An investigator of a Liverpool slum reported that the typical Catholic resident of Ship Street "regards birth control as a sin but abortion before the age of three months a perfectly legitimate measure....[T]he majority have at some time or another tried to bring on an abortion" (M. Kerr, 1958, pp. 137, 174).

Only if all else failed was the abortionist called in. Many abortionists were not the sinister figures portrayed by the medical profession but older, lower middle-class and working-class women. It is likely that the working-class abortionists of the late nineteenth and early twentieth centuries were not all that different from those Moya Woodside interviewed in Holloway Prison in the 1950s. Out of 44, all had been married, all but three had children, 13 were grandmothers, and 22 were over 60. There were few crimes in which one would expect to find so many elderly women involved. These women did not believe their activities "criminal" but elicited by "compassion and feminine solidarity."[21]

CONTRACEPTION AND CLASS

How did the proponents of birth control respond to the abortion issue? The first British organization to defend contraception – the Malthusian League – did so on the basis of the argument that labor could only improve its living conditions by restricting its numbers (Ledbetter, 1976; McLaren, 1978, pp. 107–15). That those members of the working class who were in fact pursuing a family limitation strategy resorted to old-fashioned and frequently dangerous remedies was, the neo-Malthusians believed, due simply to a lack of adequate contraceptives. Nevertheless, the league was slow to respond. Only from 1913 onwards did it begin to interest itself in public meetings;

only then did it fully appreciate working-class women's reliance on abortion. One of the movement's leaders, Bessie Drysdale, spoke of a young girl in Sussex who "told me that she had never heard of preservatives, only of people taking drugs." Another wrote to the *Malthusian*, "We know no preservatives though I have taken pills given me when two months but have always been afraid." A husband asking for information stated, "The wife has been taking a 5s box of capsules to bring on her courses, but it is no good." A "Mrs. S." of Middlesborough reported that the "respectable" had little idea of the extent of illegal operations: "Any working man or woman knows that there is any amount of this business going on, sometimes with terrible results."[22] The league was outraged by the working-class's frequent recourse to abortion. Referring to what he took to be working women's stoical acceptance of the necessity of abortion, a contributor to the *Malthusian* of March 1890 complained, "When they are 'in for it,' they are ready to resort to even criminal means of escaping evils which they would not guard against when they had the power."[23]

The Malthusian League turned its face adamantly against such tactics. Its leader, C. V. Drysdale, expressed the hope that "the greatest care will be taken to avoid any confusion between the results of prevention of conception on the one hand and of abortion or attempted abortion on the other" (Marchant, 1917, p. 95). Indeed, the league's reluctance to establish a birth-control clinic was based on its concern that the public would naturally assume that such an institution would provide abortions (Soloway, 1982a, p. 190). Similarly, in the 1920s doctors still cited as the reason for their refusing to provide contraceptive information that such counseling gave one a reputation that drew "the denizens of the underworld to flock to one's surgery."[24] The league made its stance clear by repeatedly castigating the use of female pills and abortifacients.

It has been estimated that the Malthusian League issued about three million pamphlets and leaflets between 1879 and 1921. Only in 1913 did it finally begin to provide practical information on contraception to supplement its tracts on Malthusian economics. In its long life the league did little more than confirm the suspicion of many within the working class that fertility restriction was a means to protect the interests of the propertied.

Marie Stopes, not the Malthusian League, was responsible for the popularization of the birth-control ideology in England. She discovered birth-control work in her own particular voyage of self-discovery. In 1912, after a year of marriage to a Canadian botanist, it slowly dawned on Stopes that all was not well. The sexual ignorance of some university-educated women of Edwardian England was such that Stopes did not understand that her husband was impotent and that the marriage had not been consummated. Only in 1914 did she start proceedings for an annulment. She then began the serious study of the problems of sexuality and birth control, seeking information from the books of the Reading Room of the British Museum.[25] In the

Society for Constructive Birth Control and Racial Progress that she founded in 1921 and through her writings, Stopes was to popularize a particular type of fertility control used for particular purposes.

Stopes's social preoccupations were made clear in the columns of *Birth Control News* on the racial and national necessity of birth control. Stopes, like the neo-Malthusians, was as concerned to raise the fertility of the upper classes as to lower that of the working classes. She argued that the struggle for survival was being reversed with the "unfit" now outbreeding the fit and the country threatened by "race suicide" and degeneration (Sanger, 1923, pp. 86ff). Contraception, in limiting the numbers of the unskilled and the ignorant, would necessarily improve national health. The working woman had to be taught birth control, Stopes asserted, because "such knowledge is not only essential to her private well-being, but essential to her in the fulfilment of her duties as a citizen" (1928b, p. 207).

Although those who bought Stopes's books were no doubt mainly members of the middle class, her chief preoccupation was the working class. During the 1920s she lectured to countless laboring audiences about rational methods of fertility control used by the wealthy and well-educated.[26] Their adoption would, she believed, improve workers' lives and ease the load of the middle classes, weighed down by "crushing" taxes. "Contraception is obviously indicated," she wrote, "rather than the saddling of the community with children of a very doubtful racial value" (1923a, p. 37). Such sentiments were echoed by the eugenicist C. P. Blacker, who reported that between August 15 and September 15, 1924, a group of Guy's Hospital externs asked 78 new mothers in the district if their babies had been intended or not. The answers received included "This one was a haccident" and "This one was a bit of a slip, 'e was." Thirty-one of the children were wanted and 47 were not. Blacker concluded that if such ignorant and congenitally unhealthy women were permitted to go on breeding they would produce vicious children, the prey of "Communist agitators and Bolsheviks" (1924, pp. 460, 564).[27]

"Soon," Stopes prophesized, "the only class callously and carelessly allowing themselves to hand on bodily defect will be the morons of various grades, sometimes called the 'social problem group'" (1935, p. 116). For those who were unable or refused to use the birth-control devices available to them, she prescribed sterilization. Her repeated references to "the thriftless, unmanageable and the appalling prolific" and "the hopelessly rotten and racially diseased" reveals her total lack of understanding of the life of the lower classes (1928b, pp. 220, 223). Such prejudice also determined the methods of contraception she sought to popularize.

Stopes's first concern was the family – the cornerstone of a stable civilization. Few would have denied that the economic well-being of families was important, but what preoccupied Stopes was their emotional well-being. "The only secure basis for the present-day State," she wrote, "is the wedding of its units in marriage; but there is rottenness and danger at the foundations of the State if many of the marriages are unhappy" (1918a, p. xi). Stopes's goal was the creation of sexually happy couples in which the husband would be sensitive and caring. She believed that women's sensuality was dominated by a "fundamental pulse" that men would have to learn to interpret. In her romantic view, the sex act had to be a "*mutual* affair, not the mere 'indulgence' of a man." She prescribed that her readers seek the goal of achieving mutual orgasm. In unlocking the passions, she promised, one would shift marriage from being "brutalized, and hopeless and sodden" to something "rapturous, spiritual and vital." Her model man and wife were "young, happy, and physically well-conditioned."[28]

Stopes was one of the first to insist that the husband and wife "adore" each other, be "married lovers" constantly "wooing" each other – that is, when not reading up on how it was to be done.[29] In passing she condemned lesbianism and masturbation, not on moral grounds but because they reduced the woman's ability to have a "real union." Stopes thus became one of the chief architects and defenders of twentieth-century notions of hetero-sexuality.[30]

The Malthusian League had supported fertility control on economic grounds (Stopes, 1922). For Stopes, however, birth control was essentially an instrument that, by sparing the woman unwanted pregnancies, would permit the emergence of the happy, sensual family unit in which the woman could delight in motherhood. It followed that the contraceptives Stopes favored would not violate her image of the rational, caring couple. The myth of domesticity conjured up by Stopes must have attracted working-class women; their lives would necessarily have improved if their husbands became more responsible spouses. But Stopes condemned all the contraceptive measures already used by working-class couple. She damned extended nursing, widely used in working-class families to space births, as weakening for the mother (1923b, p. 6). Coitus interruptus was extremely unreliable and a physical and psychological danger, she declared. For women, withdrawal meant not achieving orgasm, being left "up in the air" or, as one of Stopes's correspondents put it, "having to sneeze but not being able to" (1918a, p. 56, 1923b, p. 9). But Stopes asserted that withdrawal also had damaging physiological side effects: "The woman, too, loses the advantage...of the partial absorption of the man's secretions" (1918a, p. 71). Frigidity in women and neurasthenia in men were both attributed by Stopes to with-drawal (1923a, p. 18). Moreover, she asserted, men could be lured into dangerous overindulgence by the simplicity of the withdrawal method. What she ignored was that coitus interruptus, more than any other method of con-traception, required the sort of male cooperation that she claimed to value. She chided the Malthusian League for condoning both coitus interruptus and douching; the sheath she condemned as unromantic and unpleasant (1923a, p. 70).[31]

Stopes's favored methods of contraception were the cervical cap and diaphragm (1918b, passim).[32] For additional safety she recommended a soluble quinine pessary in conjunction with the cap. She consequently argued for clinics in which contraceptives could be fitted. These clinics would both distance birth control from the shady world of rubbergood shops and abortifacients and attract the participation of doctors.[33] The program's inherent flaw was that working-class women were repelled and intimidated by the clinics' male, middle-class, medical aura.

Stopes, like Sanger in the United States, condemned the very contraceptive measures that the working classes found easiest to use and prescribed those that, although the most "effective," were the least often used.[34] Particularly significant in this context was Stopes's continuing preoccupation with abortion. She was aware of and cited statistics to document its prevalence.[35] She asserted that the vast majority of Britons "have babies annually *or* are incessantly bringing on abortions" (1923a, p. 205). She could only imagine abortion as "used by poor and ignorant women denied the necessary contraceptive knowledge" (1923a, p. 54).[36] Abortion, she asserted, would, like prostitution, ultimately disappear as birth control spread.

In her clinic Stopes demanded that staff members swear not to provide any information on abortion (1925). She similarly refused to report the number of women who sought such information because, she explained, the clinic refused to do anything for them. It was impossible, however, to ignore the extent of self-induced miscarriages, and Stopes ultimately produced the book *Mother England*, which consisted of letters sent from women recounting their attempts to end pregnancies. "In three months," she wrote, "I have had as many as 20,000 requests for criminal abortion from women who did not apparently even *know* that it was criminal" (1929, p. 183).[37] A woman wrote in 1922, "When I fell for my last child, a neighbour recommended me to take certain medicines....I have been told of neighbours round about performing monkey tricks on themselves with button hooks and crochet hooks, and although I have lacked the courage for that, I can't help feeling a sort of sympathy."[38] Stopes set out her arguments against such tactics in *A Letter to a Working Woman* (1923). She envisioned the woman "caught" and then, "So you do, or you try to do, a desperate thing; you try to get rid of the baby before it has 'gone too far.'" This, she informed her reader, was "what is called an abortion" and something against both the law and nature. Some might feel the law to be wrong, conceded Stopes: "I know that many thousands of you feel all this is cruel and unjust, but I want to tell you that the law is not cruel, and that it is not unjust" (1923b, pp. 5, 6, 8). In effect, she was saying that the working class would have to change its behavior and adopt a particular form of contraceptive technology – a technology that was not consonant with its preferences.

Stopes, like most birth-control advocates, attacked opponents who tried to confuse abortion with contraception. Her policy – no doubt motivated in part by tactical concerns – was to make a sharp distinction between the two.[39] But the letters of working-class women suggest that they did not agree that the use of one method required the sacrifice of the other; rather, they saw both having a place on a continuum of fertility-control measures.

Working-class women's desire to provide themselves with the greatest possible degree of flexibility in dealing with reproductive decisions was reflected in their language. They rarely used the term *abortion* because it clearly conjured up the image of a doctor carrying out an operation.[40] Working women described themselves as simply wishing to "restore the menses" or "make themselves regular." Likewise, they did not say they had "conceived," which had an irremedial ring to it; they said were "caught," had "fallen," "am that way again," "am a month over my time," "am four months on the way" – all of which implied a *process* that could or could not be terminated.[41] Stopes's standard response rejected the nuances and subtleties of this vocabulary, declaring that such thinking made "it evident that there exists a large amount of ignorance of the law."[42]

Stopes and fellow birth controllers argued that the spread of contraception would eventually lead to the elimination of abortion.[43] Turning the argument around, one might conclude that the failure of the abortion rate to decline in the twentieth century was evidence that many women, particularly working-class women, did not use "rational" contraceptive strategies but went on "taking chances" with abortion (Luker, 1975). What was the incidence of abortion? It is obviously very difficult to assess the incidence of acts that were criminal and therefore hidden.[44] The only *hard* evidence on abortions comes from court or inquest records, usually because of a women's death. These provide a sample of the tragically unsuccessful attempts to induce miscarriage. It is estimated that perhaps one abortion attempt in a thousand resulted in death; even registered mortality from abortion is biased, however, given the family and doctor's interest in hiding the cause of death and the coroner's frequent inability to determine it.[45] Even if one were able to interview nineteenth- and early twentieth-century women, it is unlikely that a more accurate account of abortion could be provided, for many no doubt took an abortifacient in the mistaken belief they were pregnant and were subsequently equally incorrect in thinking they had miscarried.

Taking into account all the difficulties in determining the incidence of abortion, it is nevertheless important to note contemporaries' estimates of the extent of the practice. The editors of the *Malthusian* claimed in 1914 that 100,000 women a year took drugs to induce miscarriage; Stopes referred in 1921 to the "prevalence and horror of the poor and ignorant woman's attempt at early abortion."[46] One of the earliest histories of the birth-control movement in Britain stated in 1930 that "there are few mothers of large families who have not at some time attempted abortion" (Breed and How-Martyn, 1930, p. 18).[47] Dr. Harry Roberts asserted in the *New Statesman and Nation* in 1931 that 25 percent of all women procured or attempted to procure abortion (Simms and Hindell, 1971, p. 67). The British Medical Association suggested that 20 percent of all miscarriages were criminally induced. David Glass estimated that in 1935 that 68,000 abortions were induced (Glass, 1940). The 1939 Birkett Committee on abortion, which reported to the Ministry of Health, concluded that during the previous 100 years the rate had remained relatively stable at somewhere between 15 and 25 percent of all miscarriages.[48]

One way of appreciating the incidence of abortion is to take into account its impact on the maternal mortality rate. At least 500 women died each year in interwar England as a result of bungled abortions. It is difficult to determine the ratio of abortion deaths to the total number of pregnancy-related deaths, but some idea of its impact can be gained by comparing infant and maternal morality rates. The former fell dramatically from 130 deaths per 1,000 live births in 1905 to 55 per 1,000 by 1935, whereas the latter persisted at about 5 per 1,000 in the first decades of the century and indeed began to rise in the 1930s. Childbirth and pregnancy-related death was second only to tuberculosis as the cause of death for women in the 15- to 45-year-old age group and was, as Jane Lewis had reminded us, "the only major couse of death to show an increase during the interwar period." Although women were bearing fewer children, and many of the traditional causes of childbirth-related death were being eliminated, women's mortality rate was kept high by failed abortions. If Dorothy Thurtle was correct in her argument before the Birkett Committee in 1939 that the risks of abortion were no higher than those of giving birth at term, then the 500 or so annual abortion-related deaths would imply the number of abortions to have been close to 125,000 (J. Lewis, 1980, pp. 37–8; Dupâquier, 1986).[49]

Stopes and the birth controllers made only slow headway in their attempts to turn working-class women toward modern methods of contraception. Stopes chose to interpret such intransigence as evidence of "ignorance." What she and historians preoccupied by technological innovations have ignored is that the cultural values that accompanied middle-class methods of contraception deterred their acceptance by the working classes. By 1930 Britain had 16 birth-control clinics and two private consultants, but in nine years these facilities had only dealt with 21,000 patients, about the same number who in a single three-month period wrote Stopes for information about abortion (Soloway, 1982a, p. 277).[50] The vast majority of women relied on traditional methods to limit their fertility. In the poorer household in which the husband and wife used coitus interruptus to limit family size, abortion was often turned to as a "backup method" of birth control. The need for such a safety net is illustrated by the fact that the percentage of working-class couples estimated to use mechanical means of contraception only increased from 1 percent to 28 percent between 1910 and 1930 (Lewis-Faning, 1949, pp. 171, 173; Rowntree and Pierce, 1961; Gittiens, 1982, pp. 162, 170). In households in which the husband did not cooperate with the wife, abortion might well have been the primary method of fertility control. The decision of whether or not to abort was frequently made in the context of female networks to which women turned for advice and assistance.

The importance of abortion as a means of fertility control reveals, first (and contrary to the assumption of women's passivity in relation to their own fertility), the extraordinary risks women would run to control it, and, second, that the working class had its own methods of fertility control long before being exposed to neo-Malthusian exhortations.[51] Birth controllers offered a mixed message: on the one hand, they spoke of more effective contraceptives that many working-class families would no doubt have welcomed; on the other, they offered these contraceptives as part of an "ideological" package. Neo-Malthusians envisioned a model family in which the farsighted and prudent husband would use, or assist his wife in using, mechanical means of contraception for the purposes of ensuring the family's upward economic mobility. The rational mother would not work outside the home but devote herself to her maternal, childrearing duties. For advice on the suitable method of fertility control, the couple would turn to their friendly, progressive physician. He would inform them not only of the efficacy of a medically fitted diaphragm but of the immorality and illegality of abortion.

Abortion was both wrong and dangerous, its opponents declared. The dangers that birth controllers saw in the practice were as much social as physiological. Abortion represented not the harmonious couple but two separate gender cultures in which men demanded their "rights" and women relied on female networks for support; it epitomized not the consumption-oriented, farsighted, rational middle class but the short sighted, risk-taking working class. Stopes and her colleagues sought to remake not only the fertility control decision but the family that made it.[52]

NOTES

1   *Parliamentary Papers*, 14 (1892), p. 25; and see Donnison (1977).
2   *Parliamentary Papers*, 14 (1982), p. 31; *Lancet*, 1 (1989), p. 238; and see also *Lancet*, 1 (1989), p. 468; *British Medical Journal*, 1 (1899), p. 110.
3   *Lancet*, 1 (1898), p. 242. On doctors and abortion, see Mohr (1978); McLaren (1984), pp. 113–44; Smith-Rosenberg (1985), pp. 217–44; Keown (1988).
4   *Lancet*, 2 (1989), pp. 1844–5.
5   See also *Malthusian*, December 1910, p. 48.
6   On reports of plumbism (lead poisoning) as early as 1893 in Leicester, see Scott (1901–2), pp. 148–52.
7   *Parliamentary Papers*, 39 (1914), p. 70. Diachylon was finally placed on the poison list in 1917.
8   *Malthusian*, January 1915, p. 5.
9   *Lancet*, 2 (1914), p. 704. On quackery and abortion, see *Malthusian*, December 1902, p. 89; *Lancet*, 2 (1898), pp. 1651–3.
10 *Malthusian*, September 1883, p. 441.
11 *Parliamentary Papers*, 14 (1892), p. 30.

12 *Lancet*, 1 (1988), p. 235; and see also Banks and Banks (1964), pp. 86–7.

13 On working-class women's difficulties in controlling births, see Reeves (1913), p. 102.

14 On the emotional segregation of the sexes prior to World War I, see Ross (1982), pp. 575–602; Gillis (1985), pp. 248–52.

15 According to Gittens (1982), couples who communicated easily were the most successful in controlling family size.

16 See also Young and Wilmott (1957), p. 6.

17 On nursing, see Eyles (1922), p. 153; on "stopping," see Mrs. Ring's testimony in Marchant (1917), p. 280.

18 On workers access to contraceptives, see also Brookes (1986), pp. 156–63.

19 See also Marchant (1926), p. 96.

20 On the imposition of a new, scientific view of reproduction, see McLaren (1984), pp. 113–44; and Martin (1987).

21 See also Brookes (1983), pp. 165–76.

22 *Malthusian*, January 1911, p. 23; October 1915, p. 76; June 1914, p. 44; April 1916, p. 33.

23 *Malthusian*, March 1890, p. 18.

24 *Birth Control News*, March 1924, p. 2.

25 On Stopes's life, see Hall (1977) and Briant (1972).

26 On working-class responses, see Liddington (1984), pp. 316–25.

27 On his attempt to win his profession's public support for birth control, see Blacker (1926).

28 See also Holtzman (1982), pp. 39–52.

29 To her surprise, Stopes found working-class women wanted to know how to make their husbands *less* rather than more passionate. "The demand for a simple 'pill' or drug to solve such troubles is astonishingly widespread....I am surprised by the prevalence of the rumour that there are drugs which can safely be taken to reduce the man's virility, and that such drugs act directly and only on the sex organs. I think it may not be out of place, even in a book specifically addressed to educated people, to explode this popular fallacy, and warn everyone that *no reliable drug of this nature exists*" (Stopes, 1928a, p. 28).

30 Studies arguing that in the twentieth century women were "conscripted" into heterosexuality have curiously slighted the importance of birth-control advocates like Stopes. See Jackson (1983) and Jeffreys (1985).

31 Stopes also opposed the rhythm method and coitus interruptus.

32 Stopes later accepted the necessity of working women relying on a simpler device such as the sponge; see Stopes (1930).

33 For doctors' response, see *The Practioner*, 111 (July 1923).

34 See Sanger (1928), pp. 294–7. In contrast, early nineteenth-century neo-Malthusians like Francis Place, Charles Knowlton, Richard Carlile, and Robert Dale Owen popularized basic forms of birth control like coitus interruptus.

35 Stopes (1923a), p. 5; *Birth Control News*, November 1923, p. 1.

36 Sanger referred to abortion as the "remedy of utter desperation" (1928, p. 395).

37 See also Hall (1978), pp. 13–46.

38 *Birth Control News*, May 1922, p. 2.

39 For the suggestion that Margaret Sanger opposed abortion as a way of claiming a moral impulse for her work, see Kennedy (1970), pp. 16–17; and Petchesky (1984), pp. 89–95. Such sharp distinctions could only be drawn where birth-control activities were tolerated. Middle-class women in countries like France and Italy where few contraceptives were available in the interwar years would necessarily continue to rely on abortion as a backup method of birth control.

40 Lewis-Faning, in reporting that more women admitted to abortion by drugs (54.1 percent) and douches (25.4 percent) than by instruments (11.5 percent), noted, "Possibly the low position of instruments in the list is due to the fact that those may be more associated in the minds of the women with criminal offence, and so were less frequently admitted" (1949, vol. 1, pp. 162, 170).

41 *Birth Control News*, June 1926, p. 2; October 1923; p. 2; May 1924, p. 2; September 1925, p. 1; February 1927, p. 2; May 1928; p. 2.

42 *Birth Control News*, August 1923, p. 4.

43 *Birth Control News*, November 1924, p. 1.

44 Shorter (1982, p. 196) believes that the late nineteenth-century surge resulted in 25 percent of conceptions being aborted; Mohr (1978, pp. 50–55) places the figure in the United States at between 15 and 20 percent.

45 One German pharmacist claimed to have carried out 11,000 abortions without a single fatality (Leunbach, 1930, p. 64).

46 *Malthusian*, June 1914, p. 42; Stopes (1918b), p. 10.

47 One analysis of 3,296 clinic patients revealed that one-fifth to one-quarter of pregnancies were lost (Himes, 1928, pp. 157–65).

48 Ministry of Health, Home Office, Report of the Inter-Departmental Committee on Abortion, 1939, pp. 8–12. See also Lewis-Faning (1949), pp. 168–72; Jenkins (1940).

49 On Thurtle, see Gebhard (1958), p. 204.

50 Soloway notes that the failure record of Stopes's clients was probably closer to 50 percent than to the 2.5 percent she admitted. It is also questionable whether one could attribute the working classes' slowness in adopting contraception simply to "ignorance" when it was estimated that between 1918 and 1928 15 million books, pamphlets, and tracts on the subject were in circulation (Himes, 1928, p. 163).

51 On Germany, see Neuman (1978) and Woycke (1988).

52 The history of the public defenders of abortion cannot be given here, but it is important to note how they distanced themselves from Stopes's social conservatism. "Any one," wrote F. W. Stella Browne, "who knows the lives and work of the wives and mothers of the working class – or, as I, a Communist would prefer to style it, the exploited class… knows that these women are in no doubt as to the essential righteousness of their claim to control their own maternity. But how? Hardly any of these women…will admit that – often more than once – she has, on finding herself, in the hideously significant phrase they use, 'caught,' had recourse either to drugs or to the most violent internal operative methods in order to bring about a miscarriage" (Browne, 1922, p. 3). The working class needed both simple contraceptives and safe abortions. See Rowbotham (1977), Simms and Hindell (1971), and Brookes (1988).

6

The Contours of Childhood: Demography, Strategy, and Mythology of Childhood in French and German Lower-Class Autobiographies

Mary Jo Maynes

Adelheid Popp, born in 1869 into a family of village weavers in Austria, began her memoirs (published in 1909) with a litany of what she had missed in childhood: "No bright moment, no sunbeam, no hint of a comfortable home where motherly love and care could shape my childhood was ever known to me" (Popp, 1909, p. 1). When Popp's family moved to Vienna when she was ten, it was left to her to complete the residency registration because her mother could not write. She recalled that she left the column labeled "children" blank because she "didn't think of [herself] as child" (1909, pp. 9–10). She recalled, "When I'd rush to work at six o'clock in the morning, other children of my age were still sleeping. And when I hurried home at eight o'clock at night, then the others were going to bed, fed and cared for. While I sat bent over my work, lining up stitch after stitch, they played, went walking or sat in school" (1909, p. 10). At the time, Popp accepted her lot as unquestionable, with the exception of one recurring fantasy: "just once to sleep in." Only later would it strike her that there was injustice in her plight: "In later years I was often overcome by a feeling of boundless bitterness because I had never enjoyed childhood pleasures or youthful happiness" (1909, p. 11).

Two perspectives on her childhood are superimposed in Popp's memories: an account of the remembered events of childhood, including a reconstruction of how she had experienced these events *as a child* and an *adult's* interpretation of those events in the context of an understanding arrived at later in life. As a child, Popp claimed, her fate seemed hard but was unquestioned; as an adult, however, she saw injustice and made an implicit comparison between the suffering child she had been and a vision of what her childhood should have been like.[1] For Popp the adult activist in the Austrian socialist women's movement, her recollections of her childhood crystallized a class experience and bore a political message.

In nearly all of the German memoirs I have read of nineteenth-century working-class childhoods,[2] variants on Popp's theme – how childhood had failed to live up to assumed standards of a proper childhood – recur. Like Popp, many authors describe an idealized childhood only to show how it was denied them. For example, Anna Altmann, another member of the Austrian socialist women's movement, compared her remembered childhood of the 1850s and the imagined childhood of the class enemy:

The garlands woven by the proletariat on the path through life aren't like those of the rich and fortunate, because by the cradle of the proletarian child there stand behind the actual parents a second couple – Father Sorrow and Mother Need – who also claim their rights. Today when I recall...pictures of the past, the first to emerge are the dark shadows of my ruined youth. The golden days that the children of the rich enjoyed under the protection of their guardians were never granted to me. (Altmann, 1912, p. 23)

Franz Lüth, an agricultural day laborer born in Mecklenburg in 1870, put it this way: "The happiest days of a person's life, the golden years of childhood, passed slowly, joylessly and full of despair for small and needy Franz. At home, he was so overloaded with work that not an hour of free time was left. School seemed more like a respite from the treadmill of household work...than intellectual stimulation" (Lüth, 1908, p. 11).

With few exceptions,[3] German workers' childhood accounts tell of deprivation contrasted with an ideal of childhood *not* attained. They brutally contrast the remembered experiences of German working-class children with the dominant ideals defining childhood in other milieux.[4] They also show that this very contrast had become, in the era of working-class formation in the German-speaking world, the basis for a political claim. If, even late in the nineteenth century, "normal" childhood was still denied many working-class children, its elusiveness fed an emergent critique of society and gave some workers an incentive for political activism aimed at least in part at making childhood a possibility for future proletarian generations.

NOT SO BAD, DESPITE EVERYTHING

French working-class autobiographical accounts of childhood tell somewhat different stories. To be sure, there are a few French accounts of childhoods marked by cruelty, neglect, and exploitation,[5] but these tales are notably rare and date from early in the nineteenth century. By the end of the century, stories of sentimental home lives and warm relationships with mothers (and often fathers) predominate even in contexts of material deprivation. For example, Elise Blanc, whose family were tenant farmers in a village near Moulins, recalled the warm rapport of her family life:

I really loved to tease Papa, who returned my teasing. He'd say: "This one deserves to be loved a bit more, because she wasn't nursed long enough." He'd tell [stories]... and I'd laugh with pleasure.
   [If I had a toothache]...I'd seek refuge in my mother's apron, my head on her shoulder and that seemed to bring me comfort.
   We really loved our parents. (Blanc, n.d., p. 255)

Louis Lecoin, born around 1888 as the third of seven children of a day laborer, offers another example from a very different milieu. The family lived from hand to mouth with each of its members contributing in various ways to its survival. Sources of income, Lecoin recalled with apparent pain, included the bread his mother earned by sleeping with the miller. Lecoin nevertheless denied that his childhood was solely a time of suffering: "Am I, despite myself, going to claim to be a child martyr and have you believe that my early years passed in gloom, without horizon, without brightness, with no joy? That would be false! In the first place, my parents never treated me badly" (Lecoin, 1965, p. 17). Lecoin never blamed his parents for their poverty, he claimed, nor did the family's struggle for survival make him sad. Instead, he suggests, it created enormous solidarity among family members and a special appreciation for parents not felt by upper-class children:

In our family we didn't do much hugging, but when my mother rested her hand on my head, I appreciated her gesture as the equal of the most tender caress.
   I have kept from my early childhood, which was very fine despite everything and even though it took place in the blackest poverty, the impression the poor possess one advantage over the rich, in any case a noticeable compensation – I think that the kids of poor folks feel a closer and better affection for their parents – but have I observed well? (1965, p. 13)[6]

Lecoin, writing for a different audience and in a later era than the German accounts cited, felt more compelled to refute the association between material and emotional deprivation than to use childhood suffering to fuel a claim of social injustice.
   One could say the same for Angelina Bardin, a *nourrisson* born around 1901 and who certainly claimed that her mother's abandonment of her at birth later caused her pain. Nevertheless, her foster parents were in her account warm, loving, and supportive. Only when she went to work as a farm servant at the age of 13 did she face abuse in the hands of employers.[7]
   Lecoin and Bardin did not publish their accounts until the middle of the twentieth century (Bardin's was apparently written in the late 1930s).

However, most French autobiographies composed earlier, even those by active socialists and syndicalists, depict childhoods that were "despite everything" not bad. Jean-Baptiste Dumay, half-orphaned before his birth in 1841 by his father's death in a mining accident, lived his early years in difficult conditions. His life story describes his rebellion against the Creusot industrial enterprise. Nevertheless, he writes, he and his mother survived well and he even enjoyed a relatively carefree childhood, supported in part by his mother's widow's pension. The life story of Jeanne Bouvier, born in the Isère in 1865 to the family of a cooper and railway worker, was punctuated by her struggle toward a militant syndicalist consciousness and an arduous self-education, but her economic and intellectual struggle began only when she left home. She recalled her earliest childhood largely in placid terms. Georges Dumoulin also faced severe material deprivation as the child of northern French laborers in the 1880s, but the story of his childhood was dominated by the central role of a loving mother, a warm family life, and success in school. Dumoulin became a militant syndicalist, but his narrative of political evolution did not open with joyless childhood. The French stories, in short, recount injustice but *not* unrelenting suffering as the lot of the proletarian child.

These images of late nineteenth-century lower-class childhood in French and German autobiographies provide a starting point for an exploration of the historical connections between the intimate family history and broader societal transformations. In particular, the accounts of childhood suggest some of the ways in which childhood experiences varied from one proletarian milieu to the other. (It should be noted, however, that in both French and German accounts proletarian childhood was distinguished from dominant norms or practices.)[8] They point to aspects of family life that may well have had ramifications for the evolution of political culture and consciousness. This essay examines the comparative social, demographic, and economic contexts that shaped lower-class childhoods in France and Germany in the late nineteenth century, emphasizing differences in the timing of changes in the conditions of children in these two settings. It also looks at the portrayal of childhood in French and German working-class autobiographies as evidence both of the somewhat different family strategies and the different political meanings that aspects of family life had taken on in the two countries by the turn of the century.

THE DISCOVERY OF PROLETARIAN CHILDHOOD

Historians of childhood have long been concerned with recounting the sociohistorical and cultural process whereby modern notions and institutions of childhood were created. Philippe Ariès marked a new epoch with his pathbreaking *L'Enfant et la vie familiale sous l'Ancien Régime* in 1960. Ariès suggested that childhood as we know it, far from being a universal experience with common characteristics, was created during the early modern epoch. Moreover, this "discovery" of childhood occurred simultaneously with and was connected to the emergence of the modern nuclear and privatized family that became the special preserve of emotion.

Critics have pointed to the limitations of the Ariès thesis. Charles Tilly noted that, despite a certain fuzziness in Ariè's conceptualization of the linkage between demographic change and the emergence of childhood, the demographic prerequisites for the new rationality of childhood – the lowered infant and child mortality that justified both emotional and material investment in children – obtained only in elite populations before the nineteenth century. Morover, as Tilly and others have argued, the evidence on which Ariès relied so heavily – iconographic and memoir literature – was heavily skewed toward upper-class experiences and was other prescriptive rather than descriptive in nature (Tilly, 1973). Linda Pollock (1983) has argued that even the available descriptive literature, largely memoirs, was read by Ariès and many of his followers in an unsystematic and unrepresentative manner. Pollock claims that many of the notions and practices that Ariès associated with the discovery of childhood in the seventeenth century were present earlier in English childhood accounts.

If we take a more circumscribed version of the Ariès thesis – that a particular understanding of childhood and family life and a new set of family practices came to the fore in the culture and practices of the dominant classes of Western Europe in the early modern epoch – as arguable, we are still left with a puzzle. Many of the practices Ariès sees as central to modern notions of childhood simply have little relation to childrearing practices among peasant and plebeian milieux even at the beginning of the twentieth century. When and under what conditions did these practices change?

Research on the history of childhood in more popular milieux suggests several revisions.[9] In the first place, segregation of children from the adult world of work is inconsistent with the family economy that structured family life for peasants and industrial workers. Children worked alongside adults and were central to their economic activities; they left the labor force only between the third quarter of the nineteenth century and the first quarter of the twentieth century at a pace that varied regionally. Proto-industry and the transition to industrial capitalism affected patterns of family work and the demand for child labor, but this demand may have intensified in some areas before it diminished.[10] By the middle of the nineteenth century schools were drawing an increasing proportion of children out of adult activities and into age-segregated groups for at least part of the day. But these changing patterns did not eradicate the persistent view of children as family workers or the persistent need of most families for their children's labor.

Demographic conditions also worked against the emergence of a child-centered family in popular milieux in most of Europe before the late

nineteenth century. The emerging rationality of childhood was most pertinent in a demographic regime of lowered fertility and lowered infant and
child mortality. With the exception of peasant and petit bourgeois France,
where fertility had declined by the early nineteenth century, fertility levels
among the European popular classes remained high until the end of that
century. High levels of infant and child mortality among the poor also
persisted despite the overall mortality decline. In Germany at least, demographic differentials between classes widened before they converged. For
example, in Prussia between 1880 and 1900, mortality rates for the infants of
civil servants dropped from 180 to 153 per 1,000, while during the same two
decades mortality rates for infants whose fathers were unskilled workers rose
from 216 to 237 per 1,000. Even wider differentials were in evidence between
upper- and working-class city neighborhoods (Spree, 1981, pp. 54ff and
69ff).

Although less commonly noted, adult mortality also affected the possibilities for the new patterns of childhood. Parents' likelihood of surviving to their children's maturity affected their nurturing relationships.
For a pattern of childrearing centered on the parent-child (and especially
mother-child) bond to replace the more diffuse supervision of earlier eras,
parents had to survive long enough to raise their children. Demographic
evidence suggests that mothers could expect to survive past their offsprings'
maturation in some areas of Europe by the second quarter of the nineteenth
century. But there were also temporary and regional setbacks in adult life
expectancy, especially where urban and industrial diseases like cholera and
tuberculosis took their toll. Rough estimates from regional life tables suggest
that parental survival to a child's twentieth birthday could not be taken for
granted even in the second half of the nineteenth century.[11] Scattered direct
evidence on parental survival shows dramatic contrasts between the demographic fates of poorer and wealthier populations during the epoch of demographic transition. For example, in the industrial Mulhouse region of
France, in the 1850s, children of artisans and wage earners were three times
more likely than children of *patrons* and white-collar workers to have lost
their fathers by late adolescence. In Germany the mortality rates of younger
adults were especially high in the industrial Grosstädte, and within cities
wide differentials in different neighborhoods marked socioeconomic boundaries. According to Reinhard Spree, social differentials in mortality rates in
Germany only began to converge in the early twentieth century (1981, p.
188; Heywood, 1987, pp. 162–3). What was demographically a common
experience in healthier and better-fed upper-class populations by the eighteenth century – the survival of children to adulthood and of parents to their
children's maturity – was still uncertain for working-class families before the
beginning of the twentieth century.

The eventual withdrawal of children from the labor force, along with the
decline of child and adult mortality throughout Western Europe, permitted

Table 6.1 Occupational sectors of autobiographers' parents

	French	German	Total	%
Father				
Agriculture	7	3	10	17
Industry	7	20	27	47
Tertiary	7	3	10	17
Unknown, other	4	7	11	19
Total	25	33	58	100
Mother				
Agriculture	4	5	9	16
Industry	7	14	21	36
Tertiary	4	6	10	17
Unknown, other	10	8	18	31
Total	25	33	58	100

the diffusion of certain features of middle-class childhood. But its various contours – demographic, emotional, economic, educational, and cultural – moved according to rhythms that varied by region and social class. A variety of norms, expectations, and rationalities coexisted and often clashed. Memories of childhoods lived during this era must be understood in this historical context.

READING AUTOBIOGRAPHIES

The testimony of autobiographers from the popular classes provides evidence about how and when people perceived demographic changes and acted on them, and about the effects of different childhood experiences on adult identity and behavior.

Obviously autobiographies are not representative sources in the usual sense of the word. They are both more selective and more eloquent than the usual demographic-historical sources. Their evidence must always be read with caution and careful placement. I would argue, however, that far from being random or idiosyncratic reflections of their authors' individual trajectories, they are products of collective social, political, and cultural historical processes. We do need to know who wrote autobiographies and what sorts of childhood experiences were especially likely to be connected with the autobiographical urge. Autobiographers emerged from across the occupational spectrum. Table 6.1 summarizes the industrial sectors of the parents of the 58 French- and German-language autobiographers whose life stories are the basis of this analysis. These include not only proletarians of the industrial era (miners, factory workers, railroad workers) but also upwardly or downwardly mobile workers, service workers who proliferated in the growing cities, and agricultural workers. Mothers' as well as fathers' occupations are included, as the great majority of autobiographers described their mothers as having done paid work throughout their childhood. These women's occupations were concentrated in the putting-out and sweated occupations.

Noteworthy as well is the greater presence of factory industrial workers among the parents of the autobiographers in the German sample and the higher proportion of agricultural families in the French. These differences certainly help to account for some of the national contrasts in childhood experiences, but it is important to note that the profiles reflect (although they exaggerate) differences between the labor forces of French- and German-speaking regions in the late nineteenth century that stem from the specific character and pace of industrialization and working-class formation in France and central Europe.[12] Mid-nineteenth-century occupational censuses of France and Prussia show that 52 percent and 55 percent of the respective work forces were still employed in the primary sector. In France the proportion fell only gradually in the second half of the century, standing at 42 percent of the work force in 1901, whereas the Prussian figure had dropped to 34 percent (Kaelble, 1981, p. 120).

Another important feature among the autobiographers is their experience of family instability. The strikingly high proportion of broken homes, especially in the German accounts, is perhaps a signal that autobiographers as a group had somewhat atypical childhoods from this perspective. A comparison with national statistics suggests that although the autobiographers' collective experiences mirror fairly closely what life tables would predict, the German accounts show somewhat more and the French sowewhat less parental loss than would be expected (see table 6.2).[13]

These comparisons between the autobiographies and the broader population of French and German workers help to situate the perspectives they represent. The character of these documents as a particular kind of source with certain generic qualities must also be noted. The recorded experiences were not only filtered by individual memory, and by the selective encouragements that culminated in the texts' writing and publication, but they were also shaped by understandings of the autobiographical form itself – what was and was not appropriate to include, the possible ways in which life stories could be structured – *and* by the author's purpose in writing his or her autobiography. Reading autobiographies as sociohistorical sources requires attention to these qualities and motivations. Rejecting both a transparent reading of memoirs as social data banks and a skeptical dismissal of them as unreliable or unrepresentative, I emphasize the experience-based and culturally constructed character of these sources. I turn now to these

Table 6.2   Parental fate as of autobiographer's fourteenth year compared with hypothetical survival rates indicated by life tables (in %)

	German	French	Total
Assuming abandoning parents as survivors (n = 540)			
Both parents survive	52	70	61
One parent dies	41	24	33
Both parents die	7	4	6
Excluding abandonments (n = 44)			
Both parents survive	48	67	57
One parent dies	43	29	36
Both parents die	9	5	7
Hypothetical calculations (from life tables)			
Both parents survive	62	60	
One parent dies	34	35	
Both parents die	4	5	

texts' salient accounts of childhood in late nineteenth-century working-class milieux, asking what sense adults made of those experiences retrospectively, to see how the broad structural changes were perceived, interpreted, and acted on. The focus here is on various aspects of family strategy regarding children: the portrayal of the demographic regime, child labor, schooling, family size, child care, and emotional attachments between parents and children.

A REGIME OF UNCERTAINTY

Demographic vulnerability had clear implications for the conditions of childhood: the death of or abandonment by a parent was omnipresent in lower-class childhood. The narratives specify the consequences of this demographic regime for the quality of children's lives. The probability of a troubled childhood was far greater in a single-parent household. Often autobiographers point to the moment of parental death or abandonment as the moment when their childhood turned from bright or tolerable to the opposite. For example, Norbert Truquin's mother died when he was six in about 1839. Her death and his father's financial problems and subsequent abandonment of his son signaled the end of Truquin's childhood and his entry into full-time work. Ottilie Baader, born in Frankfurt in 1847, recalled her mother's death when she was seven as the loss of all that was best in her life. For Christian Döbel, a peasant from central Germany born in 1805; Heinrich Dikreiter, born in

Table 6.3 Patterns of child labor

| | Work before age 14 | | | |
	Full time	Part time	Not working	Total
German, born				
Before 1870	8	8	–	16
After 1870	6	7	2	17
Total	14	15	2	31
French, born				
Before 1870	8	2	5	15
After 1870	3	4	3	10
Total	11	6	8	25

Strassburg in 1865; and Heinrich Holek, born in Bohemia in 1885, the loss of the mother signaled the end of all emotional support and happiness or even the end of family life altogether.

Children who lost their father more commonly remembered the loss in terms of its devastation of the family economy. For Lucien Bourgeois (b. 1882), Karl Grüenberg (b. 1891), and Annaliese Rüegg (b. 1879) the father's early death meant precocious entry into the labor force. Parental loss continued to be a major determinant of the quality of childhood for working-class children even in the late nineteenth century. German accounts suggest that the frequency of paternal abandonment in an era of high levels of migration may well have offset the effects of declining mortality.[14]

THE WORK OF CHILDREN

In contrast with the persistence of demographic vulnerability as a feature of working-class childhood even at the end of the nineteenth century, the autobiographies suggest that both patterns of child labor and expectations about it indeed shifted over the course of the century in both French- and German-speaking areas (see table 6.3). A work-free childhood was apparently possible in nineteenth-century French popular milieux. Eight of the 25 French autobiographers reported no significant work before school leaving (here defined as age 14). Of these, several lived on the margins of the petit bourgeoisie and the better-off peasantry. (Victorine Brocher was the daughter of a shoemaker of bourgeois origins; Henri Tricot was raised by grandparents who were shopkeepers; Charlotte Davy was the daughter of a minor railroad employee; Eugène Courmeaux was the son of a *vigneron* and a shop clerk who had become shopkeepers; Frédéric Mistral was the son of the second marriage of a wealthy peasant to a day laborer.) Others who enjoyed work-free childhoods lived unambiguously in the world of manual labor. (Philippe Valette, the son of a rural day laborer and a cook, suggests that he only began to work as a herder at the time of his first Communion; Jean-Baptiste Dumay was the son of a miner killed in an accident before his birth and a seamstress; Angelina Bardin was a foundling.)

In contrast, only two of the 33 German autobiographers reported such exemption from work: Marie Beutelmeyer, the daughter of a downwardly mobile minor official, did not join the ranks of manual laborers until her teens, and Bruno Bürgel was an orphan raised by an artisanal foster family who made few demands on his time. All other German autobiographers report work as an omnipresent and engrossing childhood experience. Heinrich Holek (b. 1885) recalled that he had to help his stepmother at her brickmaking job before and after school. He got up at four to go to the brickyards and prepare the clay for her day's work. After school he returned to help her make bricks and prepare the next day's work. The anonymous author of *Im Kampf ums Dasein* (b. 1880) reported having to make an alloted number of paper bags. Each child had a daily quota of several thousand – more or less according to age. They all had to rise at six o'clock: "Then we would glue until five or six minutes before eight o'clock, in order to be able to get to school by eight....Breaks during school hours were our only recreation and playtime, because at home there wasn't any. In the evening we had to work until our assigned quota was finished" (*Kampf*, 1908, pp. 31–2).

Child labor continued in Germany even as work patterns changed during the nineteenth century. Most late-century memoirists report part-time rather than full-time labor before leaving school – a transition to the disappearance of childhood labor in the twentieth century. Ironically, more schooling along with part-time child labor may have at least temporarily increased the overall pressures on children, especially in those families where sweated labor or family production persisted as the basis of the family economy.

The autobiographers' experiences can also be read as evidence of the association between diminishing reliance on child labor and low fertility strategies. Figures 6.1 and 6.2 summarize the autobiographers' reports concerning the size of their families of origin. Smaller families predominated among the French autobiographers, even those born before 1870.[15] As figure 6.2 suggests, the smaller German families seem to have been the consequence of parental death or abandonment, whereas deliberate fertility control seems more significant in the French pattern. Although several French autobiographers came from the larger proletarian family of five or more children (Lecoin, Léon Jamin, Truquin, Dumoulin, Agricol Perdiguier), it is the less common pattern, as indeed was the case in the French population as a whole.

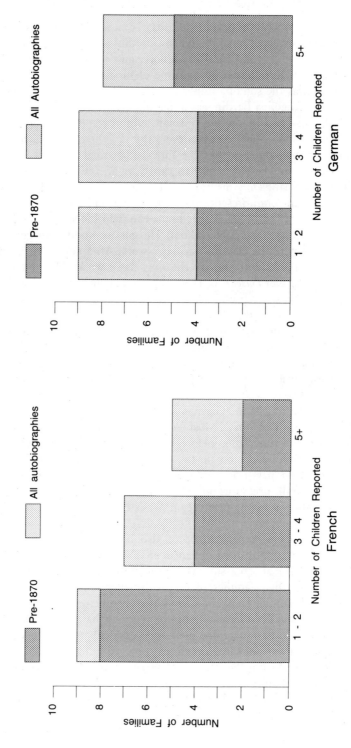

Figure 6.1 Distribution of family size before and after 1870

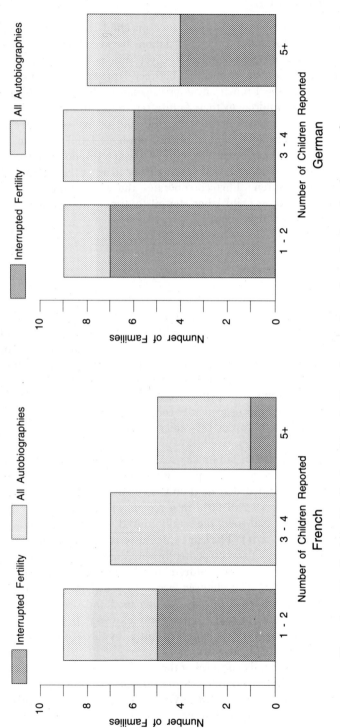

Figure 6.2 Distribution of family size with and without interruption owing to death or abandonment of one spouse

The different national levels of reliance on child labor in these accounts (see table 6.3) substantiate the association between small families and diminished reliance on child labor. Moreover, among the families portrayed in the autobiographies, the connection between large families and child labor was clear for both the French and German narratives. All autobiographers with five or more children in their family reported entering the work force before school-leaving age. Furthermore, four out of five of the French and half of the eight German autobiographers from large families began working full-time before age 14. Conversely, nine of the ten (predominantly French) autobiographers who reported not working prior to age 14 were from families of one or two children. This corroborates the association between high fertility and reliance on child labor central to arguments about family strategy and demographic transition.[16]

CALCULATION OR COPING?

We are still left with the question of the degree of conscious calculation behind these apparently different strategies with respect to numbers of children. If there is an association between large families and the reliance on child labor, can this be read backward as an imputed motive for having many children in the first place? Direct discussions of motives for having children, as opposed to children's treatment once born, are rare; while working-class autobiographers by no means generally considered sexuality or procreation to be taboo subjects, the glimpses they offer into childbearing strategies are at best indirect.

The connection between family survival or prosperity and the availability of older working children was frequently noted. Georges Dumoulin recalled that his father complained that he didn't have enough daughters. His father dreamed of a owning a small farm in a region where daughters might find work, but because he had sons, the family moved to a mining region instead (Dumoulin, 1938, pp. 27ff). The same calculus was evident at the turn of the century to the children of the carpenter Joseph Voisin. He recalled the 1890s as hard years as he raised five children. But by the next decade conditions shifted for the better: "The children began to grow up. The house prospered – we then had a small business selling food and drinks. The mother and daughters took care of that. In 1907, my two sons began to work with me....From this time on, we emerged little by little from our former poverty" (Voisin, 1931, pp. 18–19).

While evidence abounds concerning the awareness of benefits to parents of older working children, and thus of the *ultimate* logic of the large-family strategy, explicit discussions about having children don't make this association. They are governed by different considerations. For example, Marie

Sansgène, a servant from Danzig who had married a literary critic and so had left the working classes by the time she wrote her autobiography, saw the nonchalance of her sister and brother-in-law as characteristic of the class culture she left behind:

They were like the majority of all workers' families – they and their children lived from hand to mouth. When times were good and work was available they did fine and they starved when there was no work. There was never a question of savings.... When we would try to encourage him to try a little harder and improve himself he'd say: "What am I missing? Don't I have a beautiful wife and pretty children? Shouldn't I thank the good Lord?...What do you want, sister-in-law? If I drink a schnapps, that's my business, and if my wife has a kid, that's hers." (Sansgène, 1908, p. 120)

Alwin Ger condemned what he saw as the prevalent irrationality in the mining Saxon families among whom he grew up during the 1860s and whose religiosity, manners, and ignorance he came to deplore as fatalistic:

I often used to hear, when the women would get together in groups and talk, how some among them would raise the question of whether it wouldn't be smarter if the poor had fewer children. But this opinion always brought an angry response. The great majority of the women strongly held the opinion "This little pleasure is the only one we've got left; we're never gonna let them take it from us."
That by this fashion of behaving, with their single bit of pleasure, they make their own lives bleak as well as the lives of their many children – the women never think about this. (Ger, 1918, p. 61)

Both of these writers are discrete concerning their own (presumably different) rationality of limitation. Indeed, in accounts by autobiographers who either came from or themselves produced small families, little is said explicitly about strategy or rationale. The few autobiographers who talk explicitly about their own pregnancies or those of their mates suggest that control over fertility was either unthinkable or unmanageable. Lena Christ, for example, saw her pregnancies as the direct result of her husband's lack of control:

Already after three weeks...my husband once again burned with passion and he overcame with force all the reluctance that a wise nature instills in a mother in such a condition – even among the animals. It was no use to show him the little one who nursed at my breast and say: "Go, don't take the food out of his mouth! Leave me in peace! I am ill!" Once his desire was aroused his reason was silenced....So it happened that after a few months I was expecting again. (Christ, 1921, pp. 290–1)[17]

Max Bromme, who got married in 1895 after his girlfriend got pregnant, did learn something of contraception after his second daughter was born two years later:

One day our foreman brought some Parisian articles along with him to work, which is how I first heard of them. Before this I had not known about contraceptives. The foreman sold me a single pessary for 1.20 Marks. I even bought a second one. After that we'd talk a lot among ourselves about such "protections." Then, you'd hear things that people would never admit in writing. The most sure method was supposed to be "suburban business." "Coitus interruptus" is the technical name for this....Even though I tried the pessaries and even the last-named technique, a year later my son Ernst was born. (Bromme, 1905, pp. 224–5)

Three more children would be born before Bromme brought his narrative to a close in 1905. Despite his explicit association between the augmenting misery of his family and too many and too frequent births, Bromme raised the subject of contraception only to bemoan its ineffectiveness.

In the context of courtship, several autobiographers allude to marriages occasioned by pregnancies, suggesting perhaps that insofar as these pregnancies were strategic at all, they forced a marriage that might not otherwise have occurred.[18] These few glimpses are an inadequate basis for any full understanding of alternative rationales of childbearing. They do suggest that calculating attitudes about the employment of older children could coexist with fatalism about conception. Such fatalism was explicitly condemned in several accounts, but there was a tantalizing silence about strategies among those limiting births (which must have included most of the autobiographers and the parents of the vast majority of the French autobiographers as well). We can conclude little more than that deliberate family limitation was accompanied by discretion concerning its impulse and practices. If having too many children was a fit topic for comment by those who had them, having just the right number apparently was not.[19]

A NOTE ON SCHOOLING

Historians of education have argued that schooling was becoming part of a larger rationality of childhood; they see increasing school attendance as evidence of an increasing tendency on the part of parents to think of their children's schooling as an investment in the future. The comparison between France and Germany in this regard casts some doubt on this straightforward association. Schooling can only make sense as a parental strategy when it doesn't interfere with other demands, especially the need for child labor. Moreover, it serves a strategic end only when the additional years of schooling necessary to open alternative careers for children were available to working-class families. These conditions were rarely filled in the nineteenth century. The pressures inherent in the family economy – its cyclic demand for early entry of children into the labor force and the inaccessibility of higher education – made educational investments impractical for most European working-class families before the turn of the century.[20]

The autobiographical evidence is illuminating about family strategies for schooling. The different timing in France and Germany of the enforcement of mandatory school attendance seems to have held correspondingly different implications for children. Enforcement of obligatory schooling occurred earlier in the German states, long before families ceased to rely on their children for work. The net effect was to intensify demands on children's time. In the competition between school and family economy, children were often the losers. As Margarete Flecken points out in her study of working-class childhood in Germany, "for most children, attending school meant in fact one more responsibility and an additional burden" (1981, p. 132). Schooling's main benefit was that enforced attendance at least set limits on work.

The contrast with the French accounts is again striking. In the early nineteenth century reports of childhoods (Truquin, Perdiguier, Sebastian Commissaire, Claude Genoux), schooling was a marginal part of the child's existence. By the time school attendance was enforced, French children had become more dispensable in the work force. Work and schooling were sometimes presented as alternatives, and the pressures to choose work over schooling could produce wrenching awareness of the injuries of poverty. In the case of Georges Dumoulin, for example, who from the age of eight had to leave school for seven or eight months each year in order to work, this necessity produced in him "a sort of hate against something that appeared to [him] as an injustice" (Dumoulin, 1938, p. 19).

In both France and Germany special dispensations permitted certain children (like Dumoulin, or the more traditional shepherds like Franz Lüth or Heinrich Lange) to be excused from school in cases of hardship, or to leave early. But with the exception of the few children affected by these special provisions, children's time was subject to a competition between work and school that remained intense and relentless in the German accounts. The greater demands of the family economy, coupled with the earlier and more insistent requirement of school attendance in central Europe, meant that for the Germans there was simply no time left for "childhood." In France, where the serious enforcement of school attendance came only at a time when families were not so reliant on child labor, there was more flexibility.

Autobiographical discussions of schooling also suggest that it may have been less critical to family strategy than is often thought. Certainly the Germany autobiographers were more schooled than the French. There is little indication, however, that this greater schooling was regarded in a strategic fashion by their parents. Rather, in most German accounts schooling is recalled more as an obligation that interfered with the child's work than as part of a larger rationality. Only for the few exceptions in which post-primary schooling was a possibility (Holek, Wilhelm Kaisen, Bürgel) is the issue discussed in strategic terms and then the demand for immediate income is found to outweigh other considerations.[21]

While some French autobiographers escaped school entirely or almost entirely (Genoux, Truquin, Jeanne Bouvier) and others left early because of family requirements (Commissaire, Dumoulin), a few continued schooling beyond elementary schooling-leaving age (Charlotte Davy, Henry, Eugène Courmeaux, Mistral, Prosper Delafutry, Lecoin). Delafutry's memoir is especially interesting in this regard because it suggests that this strategic attitude toward schooling could, in late nineteenth-century France, reside even in the milieu of rural day labor from which Delafutry emerged. He was his parents' second child. The first, also named Prosper, had been born in 1844 but died in 1857. The second Prosper, "conceived amid regrets and sorrows of all sorts...was born a year later" (Delafutry, 1886, p. 17). The village mayor later convinced Delafutry's widowed mother to send him to the departmental *école normale*, but the son resisted because he liked farm work better. Eventually Delafutry came to the conclusion that he'd never earn enough to "farm on his own account," so he decided to take his mother's advice and attend the school with support from her and the village (Delafutry, 1886, p. 33ff).

The national comparison again suggests that levels of school attendance alone cannot be read as an indication of a rationality with respect to children who required educational investment. Schooling may indeed have become a component of a new popular rationality earlier in France despite the slower rate there of educational expansion.

PARENTING AND SENTIMENT

A more elusive component of the experience of childhood in the popular classes is the nature of emotional relationships between parents and children. The economic interdependence of family members could feed into mutual appreciation between parents and children (as Lecoin suggested) or to chronic tension over the contributions of various family members. Intergenerational relationships appear more troubled in the German accounts than in the French. In both cases children were more attached to mothers than fathers; portraits of heroic mothers who held families together against the odds were common. Ambivalence toward mother was rarer in the French accounts, and I have found no accounts in French to match the several portraits in German of brutal or abusive mothers and stepmothers remembered chiefly as taskmasters. In the German accounts, moreover, negative or ambivalent recollections of fathers were far more common than in the French and, indeed, were predominant. Many memoirists complain of the violence, neglect, or alcoholic brutality of their fathers.

It is in the autobiographies of two Frenchwomen that "modern" attitudes about motherhood are most clearly formulated. Victorine Brocher devotes long sections of her autobiography to her feelings toward her children. Certainly her ambiguous class location (she was the only child of a shoemaker father who had been born to a bourgeois family) on the margins of the petty bourgeoisie gave her by her own account more freedom to indulge in such sentiments. Indeed, she is fully aware of the luxury of caring for her child herself, even if her somewhat contradictory narrative suggests that even that care was problematic:

I started working, luckily for me I could earn enough money to keep our budget balance, but we did have to go through some really bad times.

How happy I was to be able to take care of my dear child myself! I had to struggle, work very hard, but my dear angel lacked nothing.

That is the only true happiness I have ever known. Mothers who deprive themselves of this happiness don't experience life's greatest pleasure. (Brocher, 1909, p. 67)

Just how Brocher managed to work and care for her child herself only becomes clear later when she mentions that "fortunately, my mother was with me; without her I would not have been able to work and take care of the little one" (1909, p. 68). And even this devotion didn't preclude separation. Brocher continued, "Later, to my great sorrow, I had to separate myself from him. He left for the country with my mother, who adored him. I knew he would be happy" (p. 68). Brocher's hope that her son's poor health would improve in the country was not fulfilled. He died just before his fourth birthday, and her eloquent account of his death's impact on her conveys her maternal sentiments:

I was surprised, altered, I cannot say whether I suffered or not for I had no consciousness of what was going on around me. I couldn't convince myself of the reality of it all.

He who had been my only hope, my only joy, was gone forever. (p. 76)

Brocher's second child was born two years after this death, in January 1868, and Brocher's account of what she experienced at the Paris Commune of 1871 is punctuated by tales of her effort to keep this child alive, an effort that also failed. This early account of motherhood among the poor brings home once again the persistent demographic fragility of the parent-child tie.

Suzanne Voilquin, a haberdasher's daughter who was born in Paris in 1801, tied her decision to marry closely with her desire for children: "Oh! to have children, to concentrate on them this enormous desire to love that tormented my existence, in my view this was the only possible happiness" (Voilquin, 1865, p. 103).

German women autobiographers offer no equivalent paeans to motherhood, even if they reflect maternal concerns. Amalie Poelzer and Amalie
Seidl, for instance, explicitly allude to interrupting their political activities at
certain points in their lives because of their children's needs. Even more
significant, I believe, are the allusions in the German socialist accounts to the
desire to make life better for their children as a motive for political activism.
Thus according to Anna Altmann, "Our whole struggle is aimed only
towards this – to create a better future for our children....The only legacy
that the proletarian can leave behind for his children is to work for better
living conditions" (Altmann, 1912, pp. 60–61). Anna Maier mentioned her
dedication to winning mothers over to socialism "so that the children of the
proletariat will in the future experience more joy in childhood than [she] had
had" (Maier, 1912, p. 109). Even though an ideal childhood still eluded late
nineteenth-century German workers and their children, it was familiar
enough to serve as a model to pursue and even a motive for political action.

CONCLUSIONS

The varying patterns of demography, work, and schooling – and in particular the different relative pace of the processes of industrialization and the
extension of schooling – may go far to explain why late nineteenth-century
accounts of childhood look different in French and German autobiographies.
It would be a mistake, however, to argue that all the interesting differences
between the recollections of childhoods lived in France and Germany have
been explained by the logic of the family economy. The way parents felt
about and treated their children was not simply determined by the family
economic situation. Experiences and memories of childhood were, of course,
always lived and reconstructed in a cultural and political context. If we start
from the family economy model and derive from the constraints affecting
family experiences the sentiments and meanings associated with them, we
run the risk of assuming that what had to be was. It is worth looking
to accounts of childhood for the various visions that could emerge within
similar sets of constraints and for implicit contrasts between what was
remembered and what might or should have been. To what extent did
parental treatment of children seem to follow the only thinkable model and
to what extent were choices purportedly being made? How are we to account
for alternative family images even where the family economies were quite
similar? Louis Lecoin, who described one of the most impoverished of the
French childhoods, nevertheless rejected the title of "child martyr." For
many of the German autobiographers from similar circumstances, it was
precisely to claim this title that they recounted their lives. Their long-held
grievances against parents not infrequently intruded on narratives of child-

hood intended to denounce the economic system. German autobiographers, especially those who wrote as part of the great outpouring of life stories that flowed from the years of socialist growth in the early decades of the twentieth century, had a distinct political motivation for emphasizing the inescapable misery of childhood for working-class children. One could argue that their portraits of their parents reflected this necessity. Still, the undercurrent of bitterness and blame suggests that the authors were not entirely convinced that their parents were nothing more than victims of circumstance. Parents appear simultaneously as victims and as merciless taskmasters and petty tyrants; glimpses outside reveal other families where treatment was not so bad, in contrast with the harshness of their own lives.

These stories suggest that a set of attitudes about children and many family practices associatd with "modern" childhood characterized proletarian milieux in France in the second half of the nineteenth century. This understanding of childhood had apparently become broadly accepted; it was probably fairly independent from the *particular* circumstances in which a family found itself, even if this understanding became possible only because of the particular demographic and economic constraints on family strategy that prevailed in France. These family practices suggest an elaborated and sentimentalized family life, which may well have contributed to the construction of a realm of satisfaction available to ordinary workers. On the other hand, the German accounts of this same era suggest that what had come to be seen as a proper childhood still eluded their authors and that this awareness contributed to the formulation of a social critique.

This question of interpretation with which I close suggests the significance of examining interpretations of social processes. If we wish to make connections between family and demographic history and other streams of historical development, it is necessary to ask if and to what effect changing family experience was reflected in consciousness. The possibility of childhood not only evolved at a different pace for the children of German and French workers, but the relative elusiveness of childhood in Germany took on a particular set of meanings and was transformed into a political claim based on personal experience. In the French accounts, the impact of economic brutality came later in life and was located for the most part outside of the family. Childhood had, already in the second half of the nineteenth century, taken on the glow of paradise so characteristic of dominant models of personality development. In any event, it bears no explicit political edge. In many German workers' accounts, in contrast, missing out on the golden years of childhood became, in the context of an emergent working-class politics, the first step on a life path to rebelliousness.

NOTES

1   Recollections of childhood always reflect both the lived experience of early years as refracted through the prism of memory, and the interpretive framework provided by adult experiences. For a good discussion of the autobiographical perspective, see Lejeune (1971, 1974, 1980).

2   The memoirs on which this chapter are based are drawn from a set of working-class autobiographies I have been collecting for several years. At the time this chapter was written, the set included 58 memoirs of varying lengths first published between 1854 and 1976. Many of the authors' pertinent characteristics are described herein. Among the 33 German-language texts, only five describe childhoods in largely positive terms. The rest dwell on the hardships suffered by the author as a child or describe only exceptional aspects of or periods during childhood in positive terms.

3   See, for example, the autobiograhies of Wilhelm Kaisen (1967) or Heinrich Lange, both of whom were raised by two surviving parents.

4   For discussions of childrearing practices among middle-class Germans in the late eighteenth century, see Schlumbohm (1980, 1983), Weber-Kellermann (1974), and Elschenbroich (1977).

5   Again, the tendency of the autobiographies can be specified more precisely. Only three of the 25 French autobiographers offer narratives of childhood dominated by excessive work and neglect. The greater number alternate between discussions of work demands and other pastimes, discipline and affection.

6   It is important to note one German example, the memoir of Wilhelm Kaisen, who makes arguments similar to those of Lecoin. Kaisen's account is one of the handful of positive accounts of German childhood.

7   Bardin's account no doubt reflects a relatively good fostering situation. The account of Gabriel Jacques, published to reveal the plight of the foundling, shows the opposite extreme. Nancy Fitch (1986) has explored the contours of the foundling experience in the Allier region and suggests some plausible reasons for the quite varying experiences of foundlings.

8   I have included memoirs of people whose families of origin lived by manual labor in either agriculture or industry, or who themselves did so. In part, the scope is deliberately large because of the frequency within individual lives of occupational changes, as well as the salience at this historical moment of transitions, for example, between agriculture and industry or between artisanal and factory industrial settings. The memoirs are drawn from all over French- and German-speaking Europe. See Watkins (1991) for a full discussion of the changing relationship between demographic and political boundaries in the nineteenth and twentieth centuries.

9   For discussions of the literature on the history of childhood in France and Central Europe, see Heywood (1987) and Maynes and Taylor (1990).

10 See especially Kriedte et al. (1981) and Heywood (1987).

11 These are crude estimates from life tables. They equal the proportion of adults alive at the mean age at maternity and paternity who survived 15 years later, as indicated in life tables corresponding to regions and approximate mortality levels. Ages at maternity and paternity were estimated from evidence in Festy (1979), pp. 28–33, and Coale and Demeny (1966).

12 For a useful summary of differences in the character of working-class formation in France and Germany, see Katznelson and Zolberg, eds. (1986).

13 Heywood found that in Mulhouse 21 percent of children who died in the 1850s between the ages of 15 and 19 had fathers who were already dead or missing (1987, p. 163).

14 Poorer children were more likely than wealthier ones to lose a parent through death, and the impact of a parental loss on family on a marginal budget was more likely to be disastrous.

15 For comparable data for the whole French population at mid-century, see Festy (1979), p. 77.

16 For a good discussion of the connections between fertility and child labor strategies, see Levine (1987).

17 The sort of desperation Christ recounts, and her presentation of herself as a victim of her husband's sexual appetites, echoes the reports of British working-class women concerning their pregnancies cited in Wally Seccombe in this volume. In different contexts, this claim could lead to protest or despair (as for Christ).

18 Angelina Bardin, for example, described falling in love with the son of a wealthy peasant family. Because the boy's mother opposed the match, Bardin had no hope. Her friends advised her to sleep with the boy in order to get pregnant, but she refused this advice. Two German autobiographers, Max Bromme and Franz Rehbein, got married when their girlfriends announced they were pregnant. A strategic pregnancy could force a marriage, of course, but there was a risk that it would prompt the father's desertion or his wish to simply continue cohabitation. Discussions on forms of working-class marriage in the nineteenth century include Tilly et al. (1976), Berlanstein (1980), Lynch (1988), Phayer (1977), Gestrich (1986), and Knodel (1968).

19 Part of the explanation for this silence may lie in the political sensitivity of the issue of contraception around the turn of the century. Good discussions of this in the French and German contexts, respectively, can be found in McLaren (1983) and Niggemann (1981). Workers' movements disagreed among themselves about contraception, and some politicized workers saw Malthusian campaigns as counter-revolutionary.

20 For a discussion of aspects of educational change, class formation, and family strategy in nineteenth-century France and Germany, see Maynes (1985b), Müller et al. (1987), and Frijhoff, ed. (1983).

21 For example, Wilhelm Kaisen attended a school designed to facilitate the transfer of *Volksschule* pupils into the *Gymansium*, but he soon became discouraged by his relative backwardness and entered apprenticeship instead. Heinrich Holek attended a secondary school at municipal expense for a brief time, but his studies were continually interrupted by work demands and family moves, leading him to drop out as well. Bruno Bürgel wished, and his teacher encouraged him, to pursue secondary schooling, but his foster father objected that "there was no future in that for a poor devil like him." Not only was his stepfather unable to give him even the money for clothes and supplies, but "he and the foster mother had on the contrary figured that [Bruno] would now begin to support them" (Bürgel, 1919, pp. 36–9).

AUTOBIOGRAPHIES

Altmann, Anna. 1912. "Blätter und Blüten," in A. Popp, ed., *Gedenkbuch*. Vienna.
Anonymous (Popp, Adelheid). 1909. *Die Jugendgeschichte einer Arbeiterin*. Munich.
Anonymous. 1908. *Im Kampf ums Dasein*. Stuttgart.
B (rocher), Victorine. [1909]. *Souvenirs d'une morte vivante*. Paris.
Baader, Ottilie. 1921. *Ein Steiniger Weg*. Berlin.
Bardin, Angelina. 1956. *Angelina. Une fille des champs*. Paris.
Beutelmeyer, Marie. 1912. "Aus Oberösterreich," in A. Popp, ed., *Gedenkbuch*. Vienna.
Blanc, Elise. n.d. "Madame Elise Blanc. L'Ombre court," in E. Guillaumin, ed., *Paysans par eux-memes*. Paris.
Bourgeois, Lucien. 1925. *L'Ascension*. Paris.
Bouvier, Jeanne. 1936. *Mes mémoires ou 59 années d'activité industrielle, sociale et intellectuelle d'une ouvrier*. Poitiers.
Bromme, Max. 1905. *Lebensgeschichte eines modernen Fabrikarbeiters*. Jena.

Bürgel, Bruno. 1919. *Vom Arbeiter zum Astronomen.* Berlin.

Christ, Lena. 1921. *Erinnerungen.* Munich.

Commissaire, Sebastian. [1888]. *Mémoires et souvenirs du Sebastien Commissaire.* Lyon, Paris.

Courmeaux, Eugène. 1891. *Notes, souvenirs et impressions d'un vieux Remois.* Reims.

Davy, Charlotte, 1927. *Une femme....* Paris.

Delafutry, Prosper, 1886. *Les Mémoirs d'un travailleur.* Paris.

Dikreiter, Heinrich, 1914. *Vom Waisenhaus zur Fabrik.* Berlin.

Döbel, Christian. n.d. *Ein deutscher Handwerksbursch der Biedermeierzeit.* Stuttgart.

Dumay, Jean-Baptiste. 1976. *Mémoires d'un militant ouvrier du Creusot.* Grenoble.

Dumoulin, Georges, 1938. *Carnets de route.* Lille.

Genoux, Claude, 1870. *Mémoires d'un enfant de la Savoie.* Paris.

Ger (isch), Alwin. 1918. *Erzgebirgisches Volk. Erinnerung von A. Ger.* Berlin.

Grünberg, Karl. 1969. *Episoden. Sechs Jahrzehnten Kampf um den Sozialismus.* Berlin.

Henrey, Mrs. Robert. 1953. *The Little Madeleine.* New York.

Holek, Heinrich. 1927. *Unterwegs. Eine Selbstbiographie.* Vienna.

Jacques, Gabriel. 1958. *Moi, Jacques sans nom.* Paris.

Jamin, Léon. 1912. *Petit-Pierre.* Paris.

Kaisen, Wilhelm. 1967. *Meine Arbeit. Mein Leben.* Munich.

Lange, Heinrich. n.d. *Aus einer alten Handwerksburschen Mappe.* Leipzig.

Lecoin, Louis. 1965. *Le Cours d'une vie.* Paris.

Lüth, Franz. 1908. *Aus der Jugendzeit eines Tagelöhners.* Berlin.

Maier, Anna. 1912. "Wie ich reif wurde," in A. Popp, ed., *Gedenkbuch.* Vienna.

Mistral, Frédéric. 1906. *Mes origins, mémoirs et récits.* Paris.

Perdiguier, Agricol. 1854. *Mémoirs d'un compagnon.* Moulins.

Poelzer, Amalie. 1912. "Erinnerungen," in A. Popp, ed., *Gedenkbuch.* Vienna.

Rehbein, Franz. [1911]. *Das Leben eines Landarbeiters.* Jena.

Rüegg, Annaliese. 1914. *Erlebnisse einer Serviertochter.* Zurich.

Sansgène, Marie (Anna Hill). [1908]. *Jugenderinnerungem eines armen Dienstmädchen.* Bremen.

Seidl. Amalie. 1912. "Der erste Arbeiterinnenstreik," in A. Popp, ed., *Gedenkbuch.* Vienna.

Tricot, Henri. 1998. *Confessions d'un anarchist.* Lyon.

Truquin, Norbert. [1888]. *Mémoirs et aventures d'un proletaire à travers la revolution.* Paris.

Valette, Philippe. 1947. *Mon village. Récit.* Paris.

Voilquin, Suzanne. [1865]. *Souvenirs d'une fille du peuple, ou, La Saint-simonienne en Egypt.* Paris.

Voisin, Joseph. 1931. *Histoire de ma vie et 55 ans de compagnonnage.* Tours.

III

Community and Class

7

Population Change, Labor Markets, and Working-Class Militancy: The Regions around Birmingham and Saint-Etienne, 1840–1880

Michael Hanagan

Labor shortage is one of the less obvious effects of population decline. This essay explores the link between labor supply and worker militancy in cross-national comparative perspective. The forces that influenced labor supply, both the size of the labor force and the regularity of its participation in industry, are seen as particularly important influences in the shaping of worker militancy. Insofar as they influenced the character of migration from the countryside, a major source of unskilled labor, the availability and nature of domestic industry, the condition of land tenure, and population increase molded the nature of unskilled labor markets in both England and France. In turn, labor-market factors shaped and interacted with national politics in important ways. Although a product of several factors, labor shortage in nineteenth-century France was, in part at least, due to the falling fertility rate. Thus employer policies and worker responses to them may be seen as a partial consequence of the fertility decline with which this collection is concerned.

To examine the influence of rural migration and of delining rates of natural increase, this essay compares one region in England and one region in France. Because increased demand for unskilled full-time workers was particularly acute in large-scale industry and because the nature of factory-worker militancy has long been a focus of special historical interest, it is useful to compare two industrializing centers, keeping in mind that factory industry was much more typical of England than France. We will look at the economic and social background within which large-scale industry developed and at this background's influence on management policies and working-class responses.

To pursue these issues, I have selected to observe roughly similar industrial regions in France – the region around the city of Saint-Etienne, the Stéphanois – and England – the region around Birmingham, including the Black Country. By 1800 both regions were longtime coal-mining centers. Both had a long history of rural and urban domestic production, and both were early centers of metallurgy and of machine construction (see Court, 1938, and Gras, 1904).

Most important for our analysis, urbanization and industrial growth advanced with extraordinary speed in both regions between 1800 and 1880. Birmingham, of course, was one of the pioneer cities of the Industrial Revolution; its population increased by about five and one half times between 1801 and 1881, from 71,000 to 400,774. Although Saint-Etienne was only one third the size of Birmingham, its population increased about five times between 1799 and 1881, from 24,342 to 123,813.[1] Both regions depended heavily on migrants for their industrial growth. Between 1830 and 1880 the rural areas that furnished migrants for the industrial regions reflected national population trends in their respective countries – falling French fertility and continued high English fertility (see figure 7.1). A look at total fertility in the regions contributing most heavily to Saint-Etienne's population shows a long-term decline over almost the whole of the period. In regions contributing most heavily to Birmingham's growth, the decline in total fertility did not begin until after 1880.[2]

To assess the influence of fertility trends on labor-force formation in the industrial towns and cities in the two regions, I first look at economic and social conditions in the rural areas where migrants originated. In an age of extensive short-distance migration, demographic developments in nearby sending areas were of considerable importance to the evolution of industrial labor. The presence of smallholdings and the specific character of domestic industry allowed a mixed farming and domestic industrial economy to survive in the Stéphanois countryside when it was disappearing in the region around Birmingham. Participants in the Stéphanois mixed economy could be easily persuaded to migrate to the industrial city on a temporary, not a permanent, basis. Next I examine the character of migration and of those welfare institutions that strongly shaped migration patterns. Labor shortage in the Stéphanois countryside forced employers to do all they could to build a permanent work force from a population inclined to seasonality and temporary work. In contrast, the relative abundance of unskilled labor in the Birmingham region, willing to work on a long-term basis, posed a different set of problems for urban industrial elites and government administrators: What to do when the business cycle brought unemployment to workers totally dependent on wage work? Finally, I analyze the influence of rural supply and migration patterns on the development of the urban labor force.

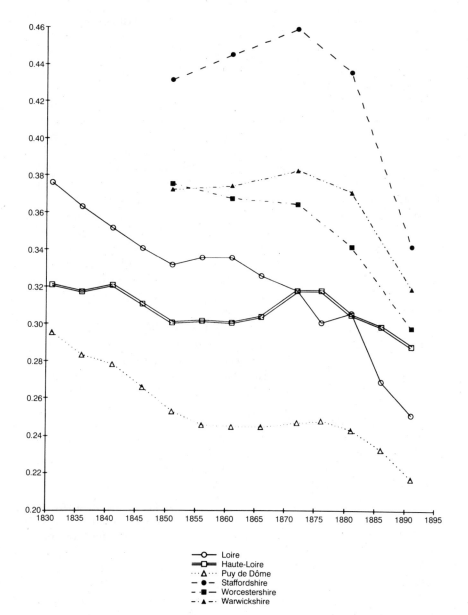

Figure 7.1   Index of overall regional fertility, 1830–90

THE RURAL HINTERLANDS OF INDUSTRIAL REGIONS

Between 1800 and 1880 short-distance migration was an important factor in
the growth of the regions around both Saint-Etienne and Birmingham. In
the region around Birmingham, short-distance migration existed side by side
with rhythmic emigration and return migration and the growth of interurban
migration; emigration was of no consequence in the Stéphanois, but there
too interurban migration was increasing, (see Baines, 1985). A look at conditions in these short-distance sending areas that supplied the majority of
migrants to the industrial city shows one key way in which labor supply
shaped economic development. In the Stéphanois the combination of slow
population growth and the expansion of peasant landholdings allowed the
survival of domestic industry, which in turn permitted many rural residents
to continue to reside in the countryside or to migrate to the city on a temporary basis. In the Birmingham region, in contrast, rapid population growth
and the proletarianization of the rural population led workers to concentrate
permanently in the city, but the plentiful rural proletarian work force also
weakened the bargaining position of industrial proletarians in the city;
domestic industry survived in the countryside only among an ever more
desperate and impoverished work force – people whose livelihood depended
on increasingly marginalized economic activity.

A look at conditions in the countryside surrounding both regions can offer
insight into the character and circumstances of migratory flows. Birmingham
is in the northwestern corner of Warwickshire, adjacent to Staffordshire and
Worcestershire. The coal-mining region of the Black Country, which contributed heavily to Birmingham's growth, is in south Staffordshire. Migration
to the Birmingham industrial region was heavily from Warwickshire,
south Staffordshire, Worcestershire, and Shropshire (Lawton, 1958, pp.
164–77).[3] Saint-Etienne is in the southern third of the department of the
Loire, adjacent to the department of the Haute-Loire. Most migration to the
Stéphanois industrial cities came from the arrondissement of Saint-Etienne,
the arrondissement that contains the Stéphanois coal basin, the arrondissement of Yssingeaux in the Haute-Loire, and the arrondissement of Ambert
in the nearby Puy de Dôme.[4]

At the beginning of the period under study, in the late eighteenth and
early nineteenth centuries, the major similarities between the rural worlds
surrounding Saint-Etienne and Birmingham were the spread of domestic
industry and the presence of a large, mobile population. The Stéphanois
region and the rural areas to its west and northwest are wet, cold, and
subject to great fluctuations in temperature; rye was the dominant crop,
although grazing and dairying were beginning to spread at the beginning of
the century (see Merley, 1974; Garrier, 1973; Gachon, 1933). The Birmingham region is on a plateau but is not as rugged as the Stéphanois; the climate

is more temperate, and, especially on its peripheries, the soil is more suited to grain growing. By the end of the eighteenth century wheat was the region's dominant crop. Warwickshire, Staffordshire, and Worcestershire contain rich grain-growing regions, although the immediate Black Country region is not as well endowed agriculturally as the surrounding territories and divided between arable and grazing regions (Pelham, 1952, pp. 89–106).

Long before the end of the eighteenth century, the spread of rural industries – hardware manufacture in the two areas, silk weaving in the Stéphanois alone – had created a part-time industrial proletariat throughout both regions. Already at the beginning of the nineteenth century the arron-dissement of Ambert in the Puy de Dôme was a center of seasonal industry, many of its inhabitants leaving part of the year to work as day laborers, sawyers, and rag pickers in Paris, Lyon, and smaller but closer cities (Mauco, 1932, pp. 56–7). In both regions the decline of hardware manufacture, a result of industrialization, and the restructuring of arable farming in the Birmingham region released a large number of rural inhabitants for work in urban industry at the beginning of the nineteenth century (Large, 1985, pp. 169–89).

Less consequential at the beginning of the nineteenth century but assuming crucial significance by mid-century was the character of land tenure. At the beginning of the century the Birmingham countryside was dominated by large landholders who leased land to farmers. In the seventeenth century the growth of urban regions nearby increased the demand for grain, which encouraged landowners to enclose land in Warwickshire and Staffordshire (Currie, 1979, pp. 106–16). The controversy over the effects of enclosure on labor supply continues almost unabated. The effects of enclosure depended greatly on the structure of the local rural economy and on whether effects are considered over the long haul or the short term. In the Midlands and the North, rising wages were probably more of a factor in migration than enclos-ure, but even here there is conflicting evidence (Snell, 1985, p. 212; see also Armstrong, 1989, pp. 641–70). The expansion of coal mines led also to enclosures, and many miners may have come from the land as the mines were developed (Raybould, 1984, pp. 59–86; Sturgess, 1971, pp. 173–204). Except for the poor land lying immediately around Birmingham and the Black Country, both Staffordshire and Warwickshire were dominated by a handful of landowning families.[5] In contrast, smallholding loomed large in the Stéphanois countryside and in the rye-growing region that surrounded it to the west and northwest. Except for the rich but unhealthy and thinly populated Forézien plain, a class of large landowners hardly existed in these departments.[6]

To understand the evolution of the regions surrounding the cities, it is necessary to take into account not only the interplay between domestic industry and agriculture but also the effect of urban labor markets on the rural economy. Increasingly, the rural economy of domestic industry and agriculture was transformed by a voracious urban demand for labor. As ruined domestic workers and many day laborers found work in urban industry, the cost of agricultural labor rose in both regions. As D. E. C. Eversley notes, "It is clear enough what brought people swarming into the towns, with or without certificates under the Settlement acts. The wage differentials compared with the agricultural districts is striking" (1964, p. 109).

In the departments surrounding the Stéphanois industrial region, agricultural employers also lamented the high cost of day laborers. In 1866 a landowner from the arrondissement of Ambert, a region that contributed many migrants to the Stéphanois, testified that "one of the great evils of agriculture is the lack of laborers which is due to emigration: and upon returning, the emigrants demoralize those who remain."[7]

The rising cost of labor and the expanding demand for rural products only led to a reinforcement of the differences in landholding patterns that already existed at the beginning of the nineteenth century. In the Stéphanois the relatively poor quality of the land, the high cost of day laborers, and the willingness of workers returning from the cities to buy land at high prices led to an increasing "peasantization" of those portions of the department of the Loire, Haute-Loire, and Puy de Dôme adjacent to the Stéphanois. Between 1820 and 1870 smallholdings shook free from tenancy and sharecropping and came to predominate overwhelmingly in the region (Merley, 1974, 1:358–9).[8] P. M. Jones has show that this expansion of peasant landholdings characterized most of the region of the southern Massif Central during the century after the Revolution (1985, pp. 38–9).

In contrast, in the Birmingham region the better quality of the land, extensive ownership by large landlords, and the new demand for grain products caused by rapid urbanization allowed largeholders to tighten their grip on the land. In Staffordshire large holders, trying to round out their possessions, often bid the price of land up beyond any straightforward economic justification. In 1873 eight families, headed by six peers and two commoners, owned 31 percent of all land in Staffordshire, another 26 families owned an additional 17 percent (Currie, 1979, p. 119). Here proletarianization continued its pace throughout the first half of the century.

Property relations and the character of the land only reinforced the trends of labor supply, tying rural dwellers to the land in the Stéphanois, where birth rates were declining, and breaking these people's ties to the land in the region around Birmingham, where birth rates were high. But property relations and birth rates may have interacted together in a manner that further widened the labor-supply differences between the two regions. E. A. Wrigley's argument that the decline of French fertility occurred as a stage process with different mechanisms motivating the separate stages may very well apply to the Stéphanois (Wrigley, 1985). Declining mortality, however, is not strongly indicated for the departments of the Stéphanois region between 1840 and 1880.

The overall relationship between fertility trends and economic changes in the Stéphanois lends plausibility to David Weir's argument that the French fertility decline and the peasantization of the economy are related (1982). Weir argues that the diffusion and enforcement of private property rights and the evolution of a more reliable wage market, characteristic features of a peasant economy, promoted the adoption of family limitation by peasant families and those wage laborers striving to be peasants. Also, the relationship between fertility trends and economic change in the Birmingham region is consistent with Keith Snell's and David Levine's analyses of high English fertility as attributable to the behavior of agricultural day laborers and workers in domestic industry. Snell argues that the decrease of female work in agriculture and cottage industries resulting from enclosure encouraged unemployed women to marry earlier. At the same time, a decreased demand for male domestic servants, also a product of enclosure, and the disappearance of the commons diminished both opportunities and stimulus for male workers to postpone marriage in order to accumulate money to establish themselves on the land (Snell, 1985, p. 211). Levine has shown how cottage industry, by encouraging early marriage, could also increase fertility in the countryside (1987).

Of considerable importance in defining the character of the industrial labor force, the expansion of peasant holding in the Stéphanois region and its surrounding hinterland also made possible the survival of rural industry within this region. But the rural industry that survived had very different demographic implications than early nineteenth-century rural industry. The association of the spread of peasant holdings with continued participation in domestic industry may seem paradoxical to these accustomed to seeing domestic industry as undermining peasant agriculture through a fertility increase and subsequent redivision of already inadequate landholdings. But between 1820 and 1850 the economic context of domestic industry changed decisively. In the early part of the century and before, rural industry developed in response to agricultural stagnation; it represented a move in the direction of proletarianization. But at mid-century in the Stéphanois, as James Lehning has shown, a large component of rural silk weavers were female family members who lived with smallholders involved in agriculture. In this context, rural industry contributed toward the expansion of peasant holdings (Lehning, 1983, p. 5). Silk weaving was a heavily cyclical fashion industry dependent on orders from Paris that came in early spring and the beginning of winter. Thus rural industry also reinforced the seasonal rhythm of so much Stéphanois industrial life.

Given an initial capital that often came from urban industry, rural silk weaving served to supplement the incomes of families struggling to establish themselves in local agriculture. It enabled families to combat agricultural underemployment and to earn hard cash. The increase of smallholding in the Stéphanois during the first two thirds of the nineteenth century kept many families in the countryside from being forced to join their kin and neighbors in the city. The region's cold winters also meant that many members of small-holding families were available for domestic industry or seasonal migration at a time when both were disappearing in the Birmingham region. In the Stéphanois domestic silk weaving survived vigorously among peasants and a tattered contingent of rural proletarians. In the arrondissement of Saint-Etienne 18.9 percent of the population was involved in ribbon weaving, a predominantly domestic industry, in 1828, only a bit higher than the 16.9 percent involved in 1847 or the 16.7 percent in 1872 (see Hanagan, 1989a, p. 36).

In contrast, around Birmingham domestic industry was fading, remaining alive only among proletarianized and pauperized villagers. In the eighteenth century nail making had been a major source of regional employment, although it was even then the least skilled of the hardware trades.[9] Nail making was year-round work, and the lack of small landholdings meant that those who were engaged in it must live in extreme poverty. The development of mechanized nail making relegated local domestic nail making to a sweated and oppressed place in the local economy, although it remained the major employer in domestic industry. In 1843 a reporter to a government commission, discussing a local nail-making community, began "Lower Gornal is... I imagine, the dirtiest and most uncivilized village in the world."[10] In the 1860s an American who toured the Black Country and visited a nail-making village observed, "It is almost painful to see how patient human labor clings to a sinking industry, as drowning men to the last rope and plank of a wrecked ship" (Burritt, 1869, pp. 211, 217).

PATTERNS OF MIGRATION

The expansion of peasant landholdings in the Stéphanois region and the decline of rural domestic industry in the Birmingham region had considerable impact on the pattern of migration. In Saint-Etienne many unskilled migrants were present in the city on a seasonal or temporary basis; when work was unavailable in the city, these workers typically returned to their rural homes. In Birmingham unskilled proletarians frequently remained in the city on a year-round basis, and the city of Birmingham found it necessary to extensively expand such institutions as the workhouse, which provided shelter to unemployed proletarians.

Migration was of dominant importance in the growth of the urban labor force in both regions, but its structure differed according to region. In the Stéphanois seasonal and temporary migration played a more central role in the recruitment of less skilled workers than in the Birmingham region. In the Stéphanois seasonal and temporary migration connected an urban economy in need of migrants' labor with a rural economy to which the migrant retained kin ties and to which he hoped to permanently return as peasant proprietor. In the Birmingham region the chances that urban savings could be used to establish a position in agriculture were smaller, and the attraction of the homeward tie was proportionately weakened. The few weeks an urban worker might spend harvesting in the countryside was not seasonal migration in the Stéphanois manner. The weaker support found in England's sending area helps to explain why institutions such as the workhouse were so much more important in structuring migration in the Birmingham region than in the Stéphanois.

In the Stéphanois seasonal migration and then temporary migration remained major elements in labor recruitment throughout the first half of the century. The Stéphanois was astride one of the major routes of seasonal migration from the Massif Central toward urban industrial centers, and, in boom times, it was able to attract workers who might have intended originally to travel to Lyon or Paris (Poitrineau, 1983, p. 76). In the late eighteenth and early nineteenth centuries, urban demand for workers often coincided with agricultural surplus, and seasonal migration was the course pursued by the majority of migrants. Water was long the major source of industrial power in the Stéphanois, and canals were the chief transportation routes for coal. The drying up of streams in the July and August heat, which shut factories and slowed transportation, coincided with the harvest season when the demand for rural labor was at its height (Devun, 1944, p. 5).

In the 1820s and 1830s the slow penetration of steam power into the Stéphanois and, in the 1830s and 1840s, the establishment of the first railroad system in France, originally intended to haul coal, routinized production and made possible the growth of year-round employment. As a result, mines, metalworks, and textile factories no longer encouraged the return of their workers for the harvest. Adapting to the new conditions of work, migrants tended to lengthen their stay in the city, spending several years there and accumulating savings for a return to the countryside. Most male migrants working in industry spent their time in the city in boarding houses or boarding with working-class families. Most female migrants were housed in dormitories maintained by the textile plants (see Hanagan, 1989b, pp. 90–91).

To look at the small towns and villages in the Stéphanois countryside that sent migrants to the industrial city is to view a radically truncated population structure. In 1856 the manuscript census for the commune of Saint-Amant-Roche-Savine, which sent many migrants to the Stéphanois industrial city of Saint-Chamond, specifically identified seasonally absent migrants to be counted as part of the commune's population. In 1856, 32.4 percent of the total male population aged 20–29 and 19.4 percent of all household heads were listed as seasonally absent.[11]

These seasonal migrants returning from proletarian labor in the industrial city became landowning peasants. Concerning the dire effects of returning migrants on local agriculture, a landowner from Saint-Amant-Roche-Savine testified to an 1866 government committee, "Ten years from now there will be only small proprietors. Upon the death of the father of the family, the children sell everything piecemeal in order to situate themselves in the industrial regions.... They return with their earnings and buy a small piece of land but do not improve it.[12] Of course, not all migrants to the industrial city returned to the countryside to become peasants, but the large numbers of Stéphanois workers who did were following a course of action largely unavailable to their counterparts in Birmingham.

In the Stéphanois the seasonal migrant generally held ties to a specific community that served to anchor his movements to urban job markets. In the Birmingham region migrants generally lacked close ties to one specific rural community. In this region, the first in the world to see the introduction of the steam engine into industry, the harmony between seasonal labor in agriculture and industry had been disrupted several decades earlier than in the Stéphanois, and the disruption had come as much from changes in agriculture as from changes in industry. Workhouse figures show that seasonal employment in Warwickshire had increased in agriculture during the eighteenth century, probably owing to enclosure, which deprived rural laborers of rights to the commons and hence of cow pasture, fuel source, and garden that might formerly have carried them through the winter (see Pelham, 1963; Snell, 1985, pp. 149−50).

The relative absence of this kind of seasonal or temporary migration is not meant to suggest that kinship or social ties did not shape migration patterns among proletarians in the Birmingham region. It seems likely that many migrants in the 1830s and 1840s exhibited patterns of movement similar to the south Staffordshire worker Emmanuel Lovekin. Going to work at seven and a half, Lovekin moved around Staffordshire and Shropshire, including the Black Country and Birmingham, working as a miner and navy. In 1843 he married, and much of the rest of his life was spent working as a mining "butty," a subcontractor. Most of his many jobs were contracted through kin, his brother or his father-in-law, or through friends, but there was no regular pattern of return, no obvious plan of returning to any specific geographic destination.[13] In both the regions around Birmingham and Saint-Etienne, many workers who had lost hope of returning to regional agriculture displayed such patterns of movement.

Because of the proletarians' loose ties with agriculture and of the rapidly expanding demands of local industry, the Birmingham labor market was particularly mobile and unconstrained, but the underpinning of labor mobility was a compulsory institution, the Poor Law. The relief system, of which the Poor Law was a key element, was indispensable in regulating labor supply in nineteenth-century England. In 1805 it was said that "Birmingham regards not the narrow policy of our laws of settlement, nor does she anxiously trouble herself with who are or are not likely to become chargeable" (Elrington, 1964, 7:323). Indeed, industrial communities such as the rapidly growing Black Country coal-mining towns could hardly afford to pay much attention to the settlement laws. But such a policy could lead to trouble in bad times when work was unavailable in industry or agriculture. In the Stéphanois bad times led seasonal and temporary laborers to return to their rural homes where they might hope to survive by claims on landowning families or by selling whatever claims to land they possessed. For Birmingham's unemployed proletarians, unable to obtain assistance from kin and quickly exhausting any meager assistance provided by friendly societies, there was only the workhouse.

After traveling through England, including Birmingham, in 1833, Alexis de Tocqueville commented,

When one crosses the various countries of Europe, one is struck by an extraordinary and apparently inexplicable sight. The countries appearing to be the most impoverished are those which in reality account for the fewest indigents, and among the peoples most admired for their opulence, one part of the population is obliged to rely on the gifts of the other in order to live....England is therefore the country where the agricultural laborer is most forcefully attracted toward industrial labor and finds himself most exposed to the vicissitudes of fortune....Thus pauperism was bound to grow more quickly in England than in countries whose civilization might have been equal to that of the English. (1983, p. 110)

Although eighteenth- and nineteenth-century French commentators complained bitterly about begging and vagabondism, both crimes were often committed by seasonal migrants on their way to and from their different destinations. Alain Cottereau has claimed that "the agricultural sector and its rural environment...constituted, so to speak, the French proletarian's unemployment compensation, his hospital, and his poorhouse" (1986, p. 142). In the Stéphanois the demands of local middle-class reformers for the creation of a *dépôt de mendicité*, the nearest French equivalent of a workhouse, never secured the support of enough powerful backers for enactment (P. L., 1841, p. 134). In contrast, the course of English migration was complicated by relief laws that restricted, sometimes severely, the right of settlement. But the willingness of mining companies to hire miners for long periods gave these workers rights to local relief and encouraged labor mobility to mining regions.

Certainly, in size and scope, the workhouse in the Birmingham region was an institution that had no analogue in the Stéphanois or even in the nearby Lyonnais. In Birmingham 10,707 paupers were given indoor relief in the workhouse in 1820 and 7,143 in 1830. The number had fallen to 5,446 in 1839, but some of this decline may have been due to the repressive effects of the 1834 Poor Law act.[14] Even though most of the paupers given indoor relief in Birmingham passed through the system fairly quickly, institutions for dealing with the homeless, aged, or beggar populations were incomparably less developed in the Stéphanois. In the 1840s the *hôpital de la charité* of Saint-Etienne had room for only a couple of hundred residents, and charity institutions in the other cities never housed more than 25 or so residents each, although some cities had an additional orphanage or old-age home with room for another 30 residents. Many who resided in these Stéphanois institutions were permanently disabled or handicapped and remained in these facilities for a long period (see Faure, 1986; Pralong and Delomier, 1983).

URBAN PROLETARIAN LABOR MARKETS

Differences in the availability of proletarian laborers in the Birmingham and Stéphanois regions also had an important influence on the structure of work and on the character of industrial administration in the two areas. Even in the prosperous 1850s contemporaries in the Birmingham region recognized that a condition of labor surplus for unskilled workers obtained. In 1857 a speaker addressing the National Association for the Promotion of Social Science meeting in Birmingham noted that "in all departments of unskilled labor there was a tendency to surplus."[15] During this same decade when English contemporaries felt that unskilled workers were too plentiful, Stéphanois mining companies were lamenting the scarcity of unskilled workers. Mine owners noted that, because of the expansion of jobs in construction and railway building in the early 1850s, they were forced to send agents to the Corrèze and the Val d'Aosta to replace workers from the Puy de Dôme and Haute-Loire who had come to work in the mines but were now refusing these jobs for jobs in Baron Haussmann's rebuilding of Paris and in the great expansion of the French railway (Guillaume, 1966, p. 139).

The relative abundance of unskilled labor in the Birmingham region meant that industries employing large numbers of unskilled workers, such as coal mining, could exploit their workers ruthlessly. Coal mining presents an excellent point of comparison for analyzing the position of unskilled labor in the two regions because coal mining was a very important employer of unskilled workers in both and because of the basic similarities in the two regions' coal industry. Both south Staffordshire and the Stéphanois region were old, established coal-mining areas. Pit size was small in both areas, with 40 or 50 workers the average group per pit. Thick coal seams characterized both regions, and there was little need for child labor that was deemed so vital in areas of both England and France where coal seams were thinner (see Raybould, 1973; Flinn, 1984, vol. 2; Gras, 1922).

The availability of local men in south Staffordshire willing to work under harsh discipline was a basic assumption of the ruthless and exploitative "butty system" that prevailed in mining. The "butty" was a subcontractor who worked the mine himself, supplying the horses and tools and hiring the workers, while agreeing to provide coal at a certain price per ton to the owner of the coal concession (see A. J. Taylor, 1960). A reporter to the 1843 mining commission added,

The very name of butty is most odious to the ears of the lower orders in South Staffordshire...and the very general unpopularity which this class of men have brought upon themselves is strikingly evidenced by the impromptu answers of persons (whether miners or not) when unexpectedly asked opinions of butties.... "Butties want hanging by the hundreds; it's the most rascalliest thing that ever was in the world."[16]

The evils of the butty system were compounded when the butty was associated with a drinking establishment, pressuring workers to spend their wages at his establishment. The "truck system," which entailed payment in goods, often inferior goods, was also prevalent in south Staffordshire.[17] The system of coal mining in the Black Country did not depend heavily on incentives. Once the pit had been opened, only the skilled pikemen were paid by the amount of coal that they dug; the rest of the workers, even those who worked at the coal face, were paid by the day.[18]

In contrast to the Birmingham region and its butty system, early Stéphanois miners worked in a much less coercive environment. As in the Black Country, employers trying to attract new workers to expanding mines did not seek to challenge the autonomous labor organization in local coal mining. But the shortage of labor in the Stéphanois deprived subcontractors of the fearsome disciplinary power they possessed in the Black Country; subcontractors in France acted first among equals. Until the 1840s (and in some Ripagérien pits until the 1850s) miners functioned in teams with elected leaders, and these mining teams dug coal and themselves decided how their pay would be allocated among team members (Guillaume, 1966, p. 145). Beginning in the 1840s this system was replaced by a new, more bureaucratic one introduced by the giant company that had come to dominate mining in the region, the compagnies des mines de la Loire, which put professional engineers in charge of the pits. These engineers were charged with hiring, but an incentive system was still extended to all those who worked at the coal face. Their pay depended on how much coal they dug, but this was now determined on an individual, not a collective, basis.[19] The new organization of work depended far less on driving and more on incentive than the butty system of south Staffordshire.

The organization of work and differences in labor supply also had profound repercussions on the nature of the industrial paternalism that prevailed in both regions.[20] In the Black Country mines paternalism essentially occurred on the periphery of the workplace, operating outside the industrial establishment. It was directed toward the community in which workers lived or expressed by providing charity to the poor, who, to be sure, included elements of the mining population. To cite just one example, the fourth Earl of Dartmouth, known to the local poor as "Billy-my-Lord," made annual donations of bedding and clothes to the poor in West Bromwich. Dartmouth supported local Anglican schools, built the first public baths, opened his estate to recreational activities, and enlarged the endowment of the parish church (Trainor, 1982).

Most of the aid channeled directly to miners' families came not from the company or the great families but through the Poor Law, and miners had a real interest in the character of its administration. The injury or death of a miner at work was compensated according to a customary, and manifestly inadequate, rate that could by invoked by local magistrates. Unless their husbands had belonged to one or another of the voluntary worker-run insurance societies, miners' widows, whether old or burdened with young children, invariably ended up on the relief rolls.[21] Butties were often accused of deliberate recklessness with the lives of miners, but in 1843 there was not a single hospital in all of the Black Country with the exception of the Wolverhampton Dispensary, which received a few indoor patients (Page, 1908, 1:302).

In the Stéphanois paternalism centered on these employed at the workplace and was concerned with tying workers to the individual industrial establishment. Coal companies usually provided free coal to the parish priests of mining communities, but almost all the rest of their aid went to their miners and their families. In the process of assembling a labor force, the miner's employers were forced to take into account miners' concerns about accidents and old-age compensation. Good medical care also lessened the time that miners spent off the job with illness. The coal monopoly's medical and accident services surpassed the legal requirements, and, after mid-century, the mining companies began to provide for pensions on better terms than those provided by law (Guillaume, 1966). The medical services offered by the Stéphanois coal mines easily surpassed anything available to south Staffordshire miners. Between 1846 and 1848 the mining monopoly erected three hospitals; by 1853 these hospitals were staffed by eight doctors and 34 nun nurses. The hospitals provided medical care and free prescriptions to all miners employed by the company and to their families (Gras, 1982, 2:533–6).

In south Staffordshire the operation of the labor market was unaffected by the operation of paternalism, except insofar as gifts to parish paupers helped encourage migration. In contrast, in the Stéphanois employer paternalism was designed to discourage miners' mobility and to attract new recruits. In the case of both the accident insurance policies created in the 1840s and the retirement pensions created in the 1850s and 1860s, company programs rewarded the worker who stayed continuously on the job and punished those who left. Pensions were given only to workers who had spent 25 to 30 years with the same company, and a worker who quit work at the mines lost forever all claim for a pension and did not received a refund of even the percentage of his own wages that had been placed in the insurance fund.[22]

THE DEVELOPMENT OF THE LABOR MOVEMENT

The influence of labor supply, the organization of industrial work, and paternal administration on the development of the labor movement in the Birmingham and Stéphanois regions can be seen in the coal-mining strikes that occurred in both regions between 1842 and 1844. In May 1842 a miners' strike began in south Staffordshire that spread extensively throughout English mining. In April 1844 a miners' strike started in Rive-de-Gier in the Stéphanois attracted national attention because of its size and hard-fought character.

The proximate cause of both strikes was the same. The early 1840s was an economically troubled period, and coal-mining companies, faced with surpluses, attempted to maintain profits by cutting wages (Challinor and Ripley, 1968, Tarle, 1936).[23] But neither strike remained long confined to a protest against wage cuts. In both regions striking miners soon expanded their demands to include the reform of those aspects of local coal mining that they found most objectionable. Because of the nature of French employer paternalism, grievances there were directed against the centralized employer; in England, with a different pattern of paternalism and public rather than private welfare institutions, grievances did not converge so neatly.

Although mining militancy in both regions followed a similar timetable and began over the same central issue, the strike movements differed significantly in evolution. These differences stemmed in part from the national-level political issues being debated in England and France, but the character of local industrial administrations also influenced miners' participation in these debates. English management policies made it difficult for workers to ally politically with any section of the middle classes to diffuse their resentment against large-scale employers. In France management policies united workers with sections of the middle classes and focused their attention on gaining control at the workplace.

In the Birmingham region Chartists found some sympathy among local miners. The favorable hearing that many south Staffordshire miners gave to Chartism stemmed from its emphasis on the political elements of worker oppression. In the Birmingham region employers assumed little responsibility for their workers' welfare, and impoverished miners and their families were dependent on the publicly administered Poor Law. The Poor Law was an important concern of the south Staffordshire miners, and their concern led them to listen carefully to the Chartists who had established a center in Bilston.[24]

The miners' strike was prefaced by a series of middle-class challenges to local industrial paternalism – challenges that created a receptive climate for the spread of Chartism in the mining basin. The 1834 New Poor Law, championed so enthusiastically by the newly enfranchised middle classes, was alleged to have diminished the number of recipients of relief in Birmingham (Page, 1908, 1:300). The strengthened political position of the local middle classes and their use of this new power helped to drive home the significance of franchise extension to everyone in the Black Country. The growth of middle-class political organizations in the Black Country strengthened the influence of Liberal nonconformity, which championed low poor rates, implementing the New Poor Law principle of "less eligibility'" but was unwilling even to allocate the money for the law's full funding. Both the Earl of Dartmouth in Wolverhampton and the Ward family in Dudley were advocates of relief against a growing middle class that opposed a too-generous Poor Law administration (Trainor, 1982).

Middle-class support for the repressive principles of the new Poor Law and their refusal to provide financial support on the levels required by the law outraged industrial proletarians. Although the extent of Chartist involvement with the south Staffordshire strike is a matter of considerable debate, it seems clear that Chartist opposition to the Poor Law had special resonance among miners. In a speech given by a Chartist to north Staffordshire miners during the 1842 strike – a speech labeled by Raymond Challinor and Brian Ripley "the most memorable speech of the general strike" (1968) – the speaker found a very receptive audience when he asserted that the passage of the Poor Law was one of a series of laws that violated the principle "thou shalt not murder" (Tholfsen, 1977, p. 78).

The organization of work in mining also influenced the evolution of miners' social and political views. The abusive practices employed by butties caused miners to concentrate on narrowing their employers' role to a wage relationship. The character of butty exploitation led south Staffordshire miners to demand the limitation of employer intervention into working-class life. A demand for the end of payment in kind was one of the principal demands added in the course of the strike, and there was much denunciation of ties between butties and drinking establishments.[25]

Considered in isolation, workers' struggles against reduced allocations for relief and their opposition to important aspects of the butty system – issues that brought workers into conflict with the local middle classes – were a viable negotiating position for the labor movement. To win concessions, however, miners' leaders were forced to moderate their demands and appeal to paternalists for support. Because it created intermediaries between workers and employers, the institution of subcontracting enabled workers to appeal to the alleged benevolence of the owners against the exploitation of the subcontractors, thus invoking the aid of large property against the smaller, more directly exploitative butties. Abolition of the truck system and the system of working men half-days for no pay when carts were not available were striker demands that evoked public sympathy from the aristocratic families. Ironically, of course, it was those families' constant pressure on the butties that were a primary cause of the system's ruthlessness. In 1842 the Earl of Dartmouth's effort to arbitrate the strike was supported enthusiastically by the workers, but it failed because of the subcontractors' and small owners' lack of cooperation (Trainor, 1982).

The miners' strike of 1844 in Rive-de-Gier, like that of south Staffordshire, began as a protest against a wage cut but soon moved in a quite different direction. In the Stéphanois in 1844, employer paternalism at the workplace helped to focus workers' attention on their employers and on the workplace as the locus for reform. The combination of an enlarged concept of the social responsibilities of employers with still-fresh traditions of workplace autonomy and democratic work structure proved an especially explosive combination, and it helped promote the spread of republicanism and socialist doctrines among the miners.

A major issue of the miners' strike was the demand for control over the system of accident insurance created by the coal company. The miners demanded the right to elect representatives who would administer the fund to which they were forced to contribute (Tarle, 1936, p. 262). Such a demand put the miners in direct confrontation with the coal monopoly, but their demand for democratic participation was an outgrowth of the same paternalism that defined the workplace as the unit responsible for medical aid and accident insurance. The workers' demand to participate in such a structure flowed logically from employers' premises.

Workers' identification of sickness and accident insurance as workplace issues greatly facilitated workers' conversion to those republican doctrines that were spreading among professional men, shopkeepers, and artisans in the Stéphanois in the 1840s. Secret societies of Lyonnais republicans channeled aid to the striking miners.[26] Opposition to the coal-mining company as a "monopoly" served to unite a broad republican coalition that came quickly to the fore in 1848 in the Stéphanois (D. Gordon, 1985, p. 46). In that revolutionary year the loyalty of the large coal-mining monopoly to the government added yet another to the already long list of grievances that pitted company against worker.

The miners' continuing battle for democratic election of representatives to the insurance society and control over a company institution led with time to the blending of older traditions of miner autonomy and independence with the newer republican doctrines. In this climate the collectivist doctrines of Cabet, Leroux, and Fourier found support among many miners (Hanagan, 1989a, chap. 1). In 1848, in the days following the overthrow of Louis-Philippe, the miners of Rive-de-Gier announced that, consonant with republican principles, they would henceforth elect their own supervisor at the mines (Blanqui, 1849, pp. 162–3). In September of 1848 the miners of

Rive-de-Gier and other towns met to respond to a government inquiry on the conditions of labor. The report called for miners' control over insurance funds, for the miners' right to elect their own team leaders, and for the republic's help in organizing work in the mines to protect workers from their employers.[27]

In conclusion, population increase, the character of domestic industry, and the nature of rural social structure influenced the character of workplace relations, which in turn helped shape workers' militancy and political goals. If this essay has examined the effect of population decline on labor militancy, it has left unexplored the issue of whether militancy, in turn, influence workers' fertility over the course of the nineteenth century. Was workers' militancy an effort to circumvent the pressures for family restriction, and so an alternative to fertility decline? By winning workers job security and old-age provisions, did militancy enable them to restrict their fertility? These aspects of the European fertility decline need still to be addressed by demographers and labor historians.

NOTES

1   Norman Pounds has noted of the Stéphanois region in the early nineteenth century that "the whole region from Rive-de-Gier to Le Chambon was transformed into one of the busiest and fastest developing industrial regions in Europe. Indeed its only rival was central Belgium" (1985, p. 417).

2   The fertility estimates are Ansley Coale's Index of Overall Fertility compiled for regions in France from van de Walle (1974); for England, see Teitelbaum (1984).

3   Analyzing census material from the mining town of Dudley in the Black Country for 1851, Davies and Hyde note that "75 percent of the adults living in the area had been born elsewhere but very few had come from more than a few miles away" (Davies and Hyde [1970], p. 19).

4   See Merley (1977), pp. 261–75. My own analysis of marriage records for 1856 for the coal-mining and metalworking town of Rive-de-Gier in the Stéphanois basin shows that about 60 percent of brides and grooms were non-natives but that over half of all non-natives originated within 16 miles of the city.

5   For a survey, see D. Smith (1982) pp. 26–35.

6   For the Forézien plain, see Tomas (1963), pp. 131–61.

7   Ministère de l'agriculture, 1867, vol. 9, p. 315.

8   On agricultural change in France, see Hohenberg (1972 and 1974) and Price (1975).

9   On eighteenth-century nailmaking, see Rowlands (1975).

10   Midland Mining Commission, 1843, p. vi.

11   Analysis of the manuscript census of Saint-Amant-Roche-Savine, Archives départmentales du Puy de Dôme, 1856.

12   Ibid., p. 320.

13   See "Emmanuel Lovekin, Mining Butty," in Burnett (1984b), pp. 289–96.

14   Royal Statistical Society, 1840, pp. 434–41.

15   National Association for the Promotion of Social Science, 1858, pp. 544–5.

16   Midland Mining Commission, 1843, p. xxxiv.

17   Ibid., pp. xxxv, xliii, xci, 10.

18   Ibid., pp. xxviii–viii.

19 Archives nationales, BB18/1506.
20 On English paternalism, see the important book by D. Roberts (1979).
21 Midland Mining Commission, 1843, p. lviii.
22 In the department of the Gard, for instance, the mines did refund such funds (Rapport A. Girard, chambre des députés, n. 2760, Séance de 6 Décembre, 699).
23 For a debate on Chartism in the Black Country, see comments by Barnsby (1971) and Griffin (1971).
24 Mindland Mining Commission, 1843.
25 Midland Mining Commission, 1843, p. 10.
26 Archive nationales, BB18/1420.
27 "Enquête de Rive-de-Gier – mineurs de Rive-de-Gier," Archives nationales, c/956.

8

Going Forward in Reverse Gear: Culture, Economy, and Political Economy in the Demographic Transitions of a Rural Sicilian Town

Jane Schneider and Peter Schneider

INTRODUCTION

Theorists of modern population change often adopt a dichotomous paradigm to reconstruct the "transition" from high to low fertility among married women. An early example was Louis Henry's contrast between "natural fertility" before transition and purposive, controlled fertility after, the latter intended to achieve a "target" family size (1961). Too easily confused with a biological determinacy (which was not Henry's intention), the concept of natural fertility gave way to an equally polarizing language of "social" versus "individual" regulation. According to this set of contrasts, births in pretransition populations are structured indirectly through latent customs such as parental monitoring of age at marriage, taboos on extramarital sex, and rules for the appropriate age to cease childbearing or commence inter-course after childbirth. In contrast, the procreating couples of post-transition populations self-consciously limit the number of children they have through "rational" choice. As Charles Tilly has phrased it, "We go from a society in which well-defined collective needs explain group-to-group variations in fertility while individual differences are matters of chance, impulse, and inclination to a society in which collective needs set few constraints on fertility but individual calculation governs it very closely" (1978a, p. 44).

Consistent with the dichotomous categories of collective-versus-individual and customary-versus-rational behavior has been a tendency among some demographers to characterize the transition to low fertility as a cultural transformation. Here as above only two patterns matter – the "traditional" and the "modern." Associated with the small family is the cultural repertoire of industrial and bourgeois Protestant society – individual achievement, a secularized "rational" point of view, and the "liberation" of women from lifelong reproduction. Glossed as "Western values," this presumably integrated bundle of traits is assumed to confront its mirror image in populations that do not practice contraception. Massimo Livi-Bacci (1977), for example, cites traditional culture as the main reason why the Italian South "lagged" behind the North in its fertility decline:

What seems to be at work is the force of residual factors, which we cannot measure statistically. Attachment to traditions; a more extended and tightly knit family system; the stronger weight of social control; the lack of women's emancipation; the weight of the often very conservative teaching of the Church – these are some of the manifold factors of Southern culture [which] affect, in a degree not appreciably different, all sectors of the population without regard to income, profession, or residence. (1977, p. 244)

In 1977–8 and during three subsequent summers we studied the transition to low fertility of people in a single community of southern Italy – a rural Sicilian town that we call Villamaura which had a population of more than 11,000 in the 1920s but only around 7,500 by the 1960s. Our story begins with the overall growth of the Sicilian population in the decades after Sicily's unification with Italy in 1860. Rather than attribute this growth simply to declining mortality and other demographic indices, we seek to locate its motivation in the broader context of a changing political economy. Since the late 1860s investment capital, channeled by state policy, stimulated the development of certain of the island's agricultural and mineral resources, and with this came a simultaneous increase in fertility and fall in death rates. Capital investment had multiple and varied consequences for class formation. In addition, it exhibited the restless dynamism of capitalism's booms and busts. Attending to both the differentiating and the roller-coaster effects of capital, we set the stage for comparing the differential timing and experience of fertility decline among Villamaura's named and socially marked *ceti* (social groups): a rural bourgeois or gentry class, a variously privileged artisanry, a group of relatively affluent landed peasants called *burgisi*, and a large mass (by far the majority) of landless or land-poor peasants, the *braccianti*.

Members of the gentry initiated their transition to low fertility around the turn of the century in a context of collapsing markets for Sicily's agricultural wealth. Artisans began to limit family size between the two world wars, a period that coincided with the Great Depression. The fertility decline of the peasantry also began in the interwar years but did not implicate a majority of either rich or poor peasants until the decades of land reform and improved opportunities for laborers in the 1950s and 1960s. (Villamaura's landed peasants were neither different enough from the landless peasants in the timing of their transition nor large enough in number to warrant full treatment here.)

In examining the links between political economy and culture, we emphasize the following points: (a) No single model of "traditional culture" will explain the fact that southern Italy underwent its demographic transition later than northern Italy, or that landless peasants were the last to be affected, later than the gentry and artisans; (b) Although "Western values" have indeed spread in twentieth-century Sicily, they are a correlate to and consequence of fertility decline, and not its cause; and (c) Rather than breaking with tradition, Sicilian peasants organized the transition to smaller families to realize previously unattainable values of dignity and respectability as defined by their culture.

THE ONSET OF A BOOM

Nineteenth-century Sicily saw the development of a new form of land-holding, new and more intensive uses of land, and new class relations in agriculture and mining, but with marked unevenness over time. Here we seek to identify with some precision a period in which the pace of change on all of these fronts quickened – a period that, as we will see, coincided with a distinctively high rate of population growth. The conjuncture in question lasted from 1868 to the early 1890s when, as it were, the bubble burst.

Why 1868? In the years after the unification of Italy in 1860, a liberal regime with its center of gravity in the Po Valley and Piedmont viewed the South and islands as assets to exploit. Heavy taxes, the most onerous of which were the reinstated tax on milled flour, a tax on animals, and a property tax, were accompanied by the abrupt elimination of tariff barriers, subjecting textile crops such as cotton and linen and manufactured textiles to heavy Italian and foreign competition. Increasing the burden on southern society were a prohibition on the cultivation of tobacco and manufacture of cigars, the mobilization of savings for investment in northern industries through a postal savings system and a newly created national bank, and a military draft (De Stefano and Oddo, 1963, pp. 139–40).

In Sicily public disorders spread from Palermo in 1866 to engulf the rural interior in a full-scale "brigand war" in 1868. Between October 1866 and August 1867, moreover, 53,000 people died in a cholera epidemic. When public security officers were killed at the gates of a few interior towns because people feared they would spread disease, a worried regime in the North felt compelled to switch direction (Brancato, 1977, pp. 136–7). The switch was manifest in inquests and plans that crystallized in the program of General Giacomo Medici, sent to take over the prefecture of Palermo and military command of the island in June 1868.

A supporter of industrial and commercial development, Medici governed Sicily until 1873. The five years of his term constituted what Francesco

Brancato called a "true reversal" (1977). In addition to the promotion of railroads and mass education, he threw his official weight behind the Palermo Chamber of Commerce, whose members spawned a navigation company in 1869, with 13 medium-sized ships by 1873. He instigated the construction of commodity warehouses in Palermo and improved the port until it became one of Italy's most important, with a tonnage increase of 20,000 in the four years after 1869. In addition, Medici presided over the 1868 expropriation and sale of ecclesiastical domain, with the intention of promoting agricultural improvement, and over the conversion of church buildings to state use as schools, police stations, and jails.

Most important, the strong impulse to capitalist development characteristic of the Medici years included the reorganization of finance. In competition with the postal savings system and the Italian national bank, both of which had siphoned funds *from* the island, the Bank of Sicily and other Sicilian financial institutions received autonomous status and legal authorization to mobilize indigenous deposits and savings together with foreign loans to sponsor numerous entrepreneurial and productive activities at home. For the first time Sicily had a banking and credit system that went beyond the limited and traditional areas of public finance, depositor protection, and short-term loans. Instead of these often corrupt salvage operations, the new system nourished the economy, stimulated currency circulation, and spearheaded progress as it constituted funds and made them bear fruit (Brancato, 1977; Giuffrida, 1973, 1980; Pillitteri, 1981).

The reorganization of credit under Medici reversed the currents of money that flowed through the island. Between 1870 and 1895 the Bank of Sicily made 927 loans for a total of 43 million lira, a cooperative was formed to advance credit for planting vineyards, and the Banca Sicula e del Popolo made loans against warehoused agricultural products (De Stefano and Oddo, 1963, pp. 157ff).[1]

Of all the sectors to "take off" with the nourishment of capital, two stand out: the sulfur mines of south-central Sicily and the vineyards of the westernmost province of Trapani. Although small in scale, there were 500 active sulfur mines by 1896, making Sicily responsible for nearly 80 percent of world sulfur production (Caruso-Rasa, 1966; Giura, 1973, 1977; Giuffrida, 1977). Wine-grape production increased most notably during the late 1870s as the phylloxera disease spread through French vineyards, creating a new French demand. In Sicily four times as many hectoliters of wine grapes were produced annually than in 1860, and the extension of land in vineyards, once 120,000 to 130,000 hectares, climbed to more than 300,000, or 12.3 percent of the territory, at the height of the boom (Giarrizzo, 1976, pp. 38–42; Scrofani, 1977). Meanwhile, zones of orchard and citrus groves attracted capital too. In 1862 Sicily exported 500,000 quintals of fruit; by 1887 this figure approached 2.3 million quintals (Scrofani, 1977).

Somewhat different conditions prevailed in the grain-producing interior, where agrarian credit remained scarce or usurious (see Giuffrida, 1980, p. 45) and where exports had actually declined in relation to previous centuries when Sicily had been a prime source of surplus wheat. Nevertheless, demand increased, occasioned by the growth of the specialized mining and vineyard sectors and by a growing population. Indeed, grain prices climbed steadily, along with the prices for land, animal products, and the rent of arable land and pastures (De Stefano and Oddo, 1963, p. 106; Giuffrida, 1969). As if in preparation for this stimulus, Sicilian agrarian economists had visited France, England, and the Low Countries in the early 1800s and returned to fire up a pamphlet literature in favor of "improvement" (Giuffrida, 1980; Pillitteri, 1981; Scrofani, 1977, pp. 87–9). Their efforts, variously reinforced by legislation, were not entirely in vain, for although the arid summers of Sicily's Mediterranean climate inhibited the cultivation of fodder crops and stall feeding of animals, and although there were never enough funds for irrigation projects, extensively cultivated baronies and commons nevertheless gave way to holdings on which wheat and vineyards spread at the expense of pastures, long fallows, and waste.

At the beginning of the century the ratio of pastures to cereals was probably three to two; at the end it was two to three (De Stefano and Oddo, 1963, pp. 103–6; Giarrizzo, 1976, pp. 33–6; Schneider and Schneider, 1976, pp. 114–20; Scrofani, 1962, pp. 217–29, 1977). Except for a temporary dislocation in the mid 1870s, the economic health of interior Sicily seemed adequate to overcome the threat of competition from new granaries in the Balkans, the Ukraine, Egypt, Turkey, and eventually Argentina and North America.

THE SYNCHRONIZATION OF CAPITAL AND POPULATION

We have gone to some lengths to identify the onset of capital formation and investment in Sicily, charting its consequences for the development of the island's productive resources, because this rhythm corresponds rather precisely to the rhythm of population growth. Between 1814 and 1861 population grew by 19 percent, from a little more than 2 million to about 2.4 million. In the next 40 years, the golden age of expanding sulfur and wine production, it grew by almost 50 percent, reaching over 3.5 million by 1901 and exhibiting a rate of growth higher than any other region in Italy at that time (Giarrizzo, 1976). During this period the density of population rose from 93 persons per square kilometer in 1861 to 137 in 1901, with the 1870s and 1880s showing a particular dynamism. Both periods were characterized by slight mortality drops over the previous ten years and a natality increase. As a result, birth rates exceeded death rates by as many as 14 each year, and the overall population grew by 12.5 percent in ten years, compared with only

7.72 percent in the decade 1862–71 (Arceri, 1973, pp. 42–4; Somogyi, 1974, p. 37; SVIMEZ, 1964, p. 62).

To analyze the correspondence of investment activity and demographic expansion, it is first of all necessary to sketch the class-formation processes that developed in the late nineteenth century. In the luxury-crop zones of the coast, small to medium-sized holdings worked by owner-cultivators using mainly family labor prevailed. Mining, at least initially, was a quasi-artisanal activity: miners owned their own equipment and were paid at piece rates for the mineral they extracted. In the interior grain-producing zone, a rural bourgeoisie or gentry class, known as the *ceto civile*, emerged alongside the old feudal aristocracy that it emulated and infiltrated through marriage. The estates that it acquired in the course of the century were leased out under short-term arrangements to rentiers, known as *gabellotti*, who sublet quotas under one-year contracts to sharecroppers or tenants and also worked the land with hired day laborers. Unlike the previous aristocracy that had resided in Palermo and other court cities, the new gentry lived in the rural towns where their holdings were located. Their attempts to replicate court life in these local settings underwrote the expansion of Sicily's remarkable artisanry: tailors, cobblers, stonecutters, masons, blacksmiths, and cabinet-makers manufactured urban luxuries as well as the tools and furnishings of peasant life.

As a rural town of the grain-producing interior, Villamaura exemplifies the demographic and class-formation processes that characterized the zone, its population expanding from 9,000 to 11,000 between 1850 and 1920. A flourishing local gentry inhabited approximately 100 *case civile* (gentry houses), each the locus of continual hospitality, life-cycle celebrations, and the comings and goings of friends, clients, and kin. Although the grand pianos that graced these houses arrived by mule-drawn sledge from the port of Palermo and the fine silks were also imported, local artisans produced most of the fashionable clothing, cabinetry, gunstocks, boots, and wrought-iron balconies that marked *civile* life.

Sicily's emergent *civile* class benefited from the auction of ecclesiast-ical property in 1868. Government architects of the sale envisioned the partition of Church estates into small and medium-sized holdings, each protected from creditors and tax collectors until its new peasant owner could make improvements. In fact, however, only those with capital and con-nections were in a position to bid at auction or to ride out the years between an initial investment and its eventual return.[2] Concentration increased through land seizures against unpaid debts or taxes, through peasants' inability to buy back land they had sold under contracts guarantee-ing repurchase, and through failures to plant or harvest because expenses could not be met. The peasants' vulnerability to land concentration was greater to the extent that they lost their access to pastures, earlier an impor-tant margin of security (De Stefano and Oddo, 1963, p. 100).

Several changes, all more or less related to the processes of class formation just outlined, converged to induce the unusual excess of births over deaths in the 1870s and 1880s. Agricultural improvement, receiving a particular boost from the expropriation and sale of Church lands, was one. In Villamaura deliberations of the town council indicate no problems in local food supply until the 1890s and document the eagerness of town authorities to promote state-sponsored regional fairs devoted to the spread of new agricultural techniques. The resulting consequences for nutrition perhaps contributed to the decline of the annual mortality rate, which for Sicily averaged 32 per 1,000 between 1862 and 1871, 29.2 per 1,000 in the 1870s, and 28.4 per 1,000 in the 1880s. (It was 23.8 in 1902–11, 16.7 in 1922–31, and 13.1 in 1942–51.)

Two public health measures associated with Medici – the construction of cemeteries and systems for piped water in the rural towns – could also have played a role, although data for Villamaura suggest that these measures were not fully operational until after the turn of the century. What did occur on an impressive scale after 1868 was a gentry-instigated architectural renewal in the rural towns. Old piazzas and streets were widened, new ones cut out of crowded neighborhoods, and walls and gates torn down. In Villamaura, as in other towns, the gentry sponsored a public garden, a theater, and a few hundred meters of cobblestone street. According to Leonardo Sciascia and Rosario La Duca, such amenities carried with them the idea of "opening up" dense and unhealthy settlements to clean air and light, lessening the vulnerability of their inhabitants to cholera and tuberculosis (1974, pp. 119ff).

In addition to mortality decline, the Medici years showed a rise in fertility, traceable in part to an increase in the rate of marriage. Averaging 6.89 per 1,000 in the 1860s, the annual marriage rate was 8.11, then 7.85, in the 1870s and 1880s, respectively (Somogyi, 1974, p. 31). Peasants' waning access to land perhaps contributed to this trend, parents having formerly regulated the timing of their children's marriages through their control over a heritable patrimony (see Tilly, 1978a). In Villamaura peasant women with property had a mean age of marriage below that of land-poor peasants in 1860–61 and 1870–71, but in 1880–81 these positions were reversed. Where sulfur mining held out alternatives to landholding, marriage ages were especially low. In the sulfur town of Cianciana (also a component of our study), for example, 55 percent of miners' daughters, 75 percent of peasants' daughters (many of whom married miners), and 68 percent of the daughters of others wed in their teens in the 1890s – these figures all 20 to 30 percent higher than they were in the 1850s. Caltanissetta, the province with the greatest sulfur-mining activity, had the third highest marriage rate in the 1870s, surpassed only by Enna, another province with mines, and by Trapani, where vineyards expanded (Perricone, 1975). For the centers of both sulfur and wine production, the high rates of marriage reflected not only the early ages at which matrimony occurred but the in-migration of young people from towns of the latifundium zone whose families may well have lost their capacity to endow their male children with land (see Renda, 1963).

Also implicated in rising fertility was a decrease in birth spacing. For a sample of marriage cohorts in Villamaura, we examined all of the intervals between the first two children when the first child of the pair was a survivor. Between the cohorts of 1851 and 1881, the average interval between the first and second births fell from 30.7 to 27.6 months. Similarly, the number of birth intervals that would maximize fertility because they were under two years in length (notwithstanding the first child's survival) increased as a proportion of total intervals from 10 to 16 percent during the same period (Schneider and Schneider, 1984, pp. 252–3).

According to the demographic literature, continuous and exclusive infant suckling uninterrupted by supplementary food and long nocturnal separations constitutes a "natural" contraceptive because suckling stimulates hormonal activity that suppresses ovulation (P. Anderson, 1983, pp. 30–32; Bongaarts, 1980; Mosley, ed., 1978, pp. 88–9; Wray, 1978). Once suckling becomes less exclusive owing to the introduction of supplementary foods and less continuous owing to maternal separation, the protective shield disappears, and conceptions follow more closely on prior births. To some demographers (i.e., Short, 1976), a change in breastfeeding, with the associated loss of "natural" contraception, is the most powerful force in modern population growth.

In Villamaura a localized dairy industry based on goats' milk emerged in the late nineteenth century, goats being alone among domesticates in Sicily to increase rather than decrease in number after 1860 (Lorenzoni, 1910, pp. 120–32; Schneider and Schneider, 1976; pp. 141–4). The resulting availability of a supplementary food for infants – it was mixed with sweetened semolina and served as a "pap" – helped to underwrite the shortened birth intervals that our data show. So did the Medici-induced processes of class formation. Members of the rising gentry and those of the more affluent landed peasantry and artisanry who emulated them devalued breastfeeding as a less-than-civilized activity, suitable only for animals and poor peasants. By employing the *baglia* (wet nurse) they increased the probability of conceiving their offspring in quick succession. Dispossessed peasant women, meanwhile, worked at tasks that were incompatible with nursing – gathering wild vegetables in the countryside, gleaning stalks of grain after the harvest, picking olives and grapes for wages, and serving in the houses of the gentry. At home they milled grain by hand to avoid paying the grist tax and manufactured such cottage-industry items as brooms and rope. They most probably gave over their infants to sibling caretakers who fed them supplementary foods, much as poor women did within the living memory of contemporary informants. In this class, too, births succeeded each other quickly, although not until the turn of the century did the infant and child mortality of landless peasant families fall below 40 to 50 percent of live births.

A final explanation for the fertility increase of the 1870s and 1880s is less tangible, but nonetheless intriguing. In has to do with how people may have thought about children in a time of accelerated development. Gino Luzzatto, characterizing Italy as a whole, suggests that, with the construction of the Suez Canal in the 1860s and of the first trans-Alpine tunnel, foreign investors in the Italian economy shifted from a position of pessimism to one of optimism, anticipating links between England and its empire through Italy. "Politicians, scholars, and journalists of the time gave the impression," he wrote, "that the days of the maritime republics were about to be reborn" (1968, p. 73). Moreover, because Brindisi, in the heel of the Italian boot, was to be the port most specialized in linking Europe with the Orient, the buoyancy spread to southern Italy as well. Perhaps in Sicily the new ruling class of incipient bourgeois and landed gentry participated in this optimism by, among other ways, generating and celebrating large families.

In our family reconstitution study gentry families of Villamaura, when compared with families of the other social classes, had a lower incidence of infant mortality and, thanks to the use of wet nurses, closer intervals between surviving children. In addition, several of them called attention to their reproductive success by choosing the names Settimo and Ottavio for a seventh or eighth child, respectively. The famed novelist of Villamaura, Emanuele Navarro della Miraglia, describes a young *civile* protagonist in *La Nana* as follows: he would "grow a pot belly and a beard...practice some honest usury and then, at seventy years, be...laden with rheumatisms and offspring" (1963, p. 35). To the extent that large families spelled dominion in the local status hierarchy, this gentry model may have been hegemonic, with modest, if immeasurable, consequences for population growth.

BUST AND REORGANIZATION

At the same time that indigenously organized capital investments augmented by loans from Italy and the Continent were developing the Sicilian economy, American capital and capitalists, true victors of the American Civil War, mushroomed beside their British forerunners to make good on several decades' worth of railroad building and agricultural improvement in the vast and cornucopic New World. As economic historians have concluded, American economic power played a central role in the capitalist crisis of late nineteenth-century Europe (see Bairoch, 1976).

Trouble began with the arrival by steamship in European ports of cheap, machine-produced American grain, causing the collapse of grain prices by the mid 1880s. The Italian government responded with a tariff that also included protection for the recently expanded factories of the North. The tariff on manufactures led France, whose industries enjoyed an Italian market and whose stock exchange was also faltering, to withdraw capital from Italy and create a retaliatory barrier against Italian products, among them Sicilian fruits and wine.

Until the end of the 1880s, investors in Sicilian vineyards felt sufficiently good about the prospects for wine sales that they financed smallholders to replant as the phylloxera blight began its sweep through the island. The tariff war changed their mood, especially as it became more difficult to borrow in Italy and abroad. This shift cast a shadow on the ground, as land planted in vineyards shrank by almost 200,000 hectares in the 1890s, by 230,000 in 1904. Creditors seized mortgaged holdings that they could sell only at a loss, and thousands of Sicilians emigrated to America. Such was, in Giuseppe Giarrizzo's words, the "desperate epilogue" to an all too brief success story (1976, pp. 38–44).[3] As with the parallel decline of citrus groves and orchards, it left Sicily vulnerable to California's later entry into the luxury-crop market.

The crisis was general, affecting all of the recently expanded sectors and leaving virtually nothing to fall back on. Nevertheless, people associated with the different sectors experienced it in different ways. In contrast to the vineyard zone, where a sudden dessication of credit affected smallholders directly, leading to their precipitous out-migration, the sulfur zone witnessed the reorganization of credit through government intervention in 1896 and the delay of substantial migration by several decades (Caruso-Rasa, 1966; Giura, 1973, 1977, pp. 15–37). In the interior, where grain latifundia dominated both the landscape and the processes of class formation, a different outcome took shape. Here the rapid expansion of the previous decades had increased the ecological fragility of a deforested and eroded landscape, sacrificing the animal patrimony to grain, whose cultivation was pushed into marginal lands where yields were increasingly low. Although the number of planted hectares did not decrease immediately, there were harvest failures in 1892, 1893, 1895, and 1897 in which production was almost halved.

Whereas in the vineyard zone the most vulnerable to crisis were owner-cultivators, in the latifundium interior members of the landed class staved off their own decline by shifting the costs of contraction of the wine industry onto their sharecroppers and agricultural laborers. In addition to the protective tariff, which their national political connections enabled them to get through parliament (and despite the opposition of wine interests), they used local political power to retain a regressive tax structure even in the face of mounting opposition and the peasants' inability to pay. As bosses of the towns, moreover, they called on mafiosi and other strongmen to enforce agricultural contracts and break organized peasant resistance. Records of the town council of Villamaura in the early 1890s indicate that many citizens could not pay their taxes, that the annual religious festival was deeply in debt, and that the town had to loan money to peasants for their daughters' dowries. Bread riots were a threat while, as the notarial archives for the same years show, peasants regularly borrowed seed or money from the gentry at usurious rates of interest (Schneider and Schneider, 1976, p. 123). Similar conditions throughout western Sicily contributed to the revolt of the Sicilian Fasci, in which peasants, artisans, and sulfur miners, inspired by international socialism, organized demonstrations and strikes. Severely suppressed by government troops in the early 1890s, the Fasci mobilization and uprising were followed by migration from the latifundium zone. Thanks to legislation in support of the exodus, a little over a million people left Sicily between 1900 and 1914.

Capital flight and associated out-migration precipitated the transition to low fertility of Villamaura's gentry. Paradoxically, however, the new political and economic context enhanced opportunities for artisans and peasants, encouraging large families among them. Again the reasons were multiple. Returned migrants with savings, plus emigrants' remittances sent back to kinfolk, enabled many peasants to build a second story on their one- or two-room house, with attendant multiplier effects on local crafts and commerce. Remittances also underwrote the purchase of small plots of land whose products were sometimes sold on the new export market created by emigrants abroad. As emigration and landholding absorbed landless laborers, labor contracts improved. In addition, Socialist and Catholic-populist reformers organized cooperatives that advanced credit for the purchase of fertilizers and transport animals and rented latifundia for sublet to peasant sharecroppers. With fertilizers peasants could include legumes, especially fava, in the rotation cycle, thereby improving the soil and gaining a cheap source of fodder.[4] If developments such as these did not motivate couples to want large families, neither did they compel changes to the contrary even though the gentry had, by this time, embarked on a different course.

Around the turn of the century a cemetery was constructed outside of Villamaura and aqueducts for water delivery were finally installed, both projects having been delayed by local quarrels over favoritism in letting the contracts. Meanwhile, intensified crop rotation and livestock acquisition improved the diet of peasants as their somewhat larger houses improved their health. Infant mortality claimed the lives of between 45 and 50 percent of *bracciante* children in the latter half of the nineteenth century, but *bracciante* parents who married in 1899 lost 23 percent, those who married in 1910 lost 24 percent, and those who married in 1920 lost 21 percent (Schneider and Schneider, 1984, p. 256).

The respite, however, was short-lived. Following World War I the United States closed its doors to the migration stream in which Sicilians had participated so heavily, while a Fascist regime in Rome took steps to reverse the encroachment that peasant cultivators had made on large estates. Ostensibly promoting the mechanization of reaping and threshing, the new land policy also furthered the goal of class vengeance, especially as the revaluation of the lira in 1926–9 and subsequent Great Depression "forced many new smallholders into bankruptcy" (Mack Smith, 1968, p. 516). Meanwhile, Fascist laws of 1931 and 1939 restricted the internal migration of rural workers to industrial towns and cities within Italy (Zariski, 1972, p. 41). Notwithstanding a small colonization effort in North Africa and some clandestine migration to America, the interwar years were plagued by the underemployment and pauperization of a labor reserve, trapped until the renewal of out-migration after World War II. As we will show, the artisans of Villamaura responded to the crisis of the interwar years by drastically reducing family size, but on the whole the peasant population did not. A little more than half of the land-poor laborers who married in 1920, and who were not childless, had families of five to 13 living offspring.

VILLAMAURA'S FERTILITY DECLINE

In Villamaura today, the contraceptive pill is readily available in local pharmacies and is purchased without prescription. According to the pharmacists and others, young women, almost all married, are the major source of demand. Among older persons, however, the principal form of birth control continues to depend upon coitus interruptus. Indeed, older men and women express contempt for the pill. "We had to sacrifice," they say, "The pill makes it all too easy and lets them have sex outside of marriage."

A frequently heard euphemism for coitus interruptus is *marcia in dietro* ("reverse gear"). Parallel to the French colloquialism, the label evokes what was once the exclusively male domain of motor vehicles. As one old man proudly explained, "The train can go forward, the train can go backward. I practiced reverse gear for 18 years." Also common, especially among women, is to call the practice *fare sacrifici* ("making sacrifices") or simply, *sacrifici*. Although we conducted interviews with men and women of every social stratum on the subject of birth control, we found no variation in these designations, with the exception that a few artisan women also volunteered a culinary metaphor: "If nothing is in the pan, nothing will cook."

But how was coitus interruptus organized and experienced? Our study compared relations of production and reproduction among Villamaura's main groups during the periods of their respective transitions to low fertility – whether at the turn of the century for the gentry, between the wars for the artisans, or after World War II for the majority of peasants. In each case, we explored connections between major shifts in the group's political and economic circumstances and its adoption of both the values and the practices of family limitation. For the first two groups whose transitions were in the less accessible past, we supplemented the recollections of "veterans" with material culture surveys directed at reconstructing past living standards, and with the "reconstitution" of a sample of marriage cohorts from 1850 to

1940, using a combination of household and vital records. For the peasantry, whose demographic transition was recent, we interviewed a sample of 30 couples who had married between 1950 and 1969, selected at random from a list of households in three neighborhoods known to be predominantly occupied by land-poor peasant families. Although based on different sources, the data enabled us to compare the dynamics of contraception in the three classes.

Where possible in the course of the interviews with laborers, and during the oral histories with older gentry and artisans, we identified people who seemed willing to talk at greater length about their family and fertility experience, and whom we subsequently approached by gender – Peter Schneider talking to men and Jane Schneider to women. This smaller group of about 20 people could not be chosen at random, nor did we ask all possible questions about sexual behavior. The extended interviews, however, did help convince us that people of all three class groups in Villamaura thought of coitus interruptus as a sacrifice of sexual pleasure, but a necessary sacrifice if couples were to enjoy a comfortable and respectable way of life as defined by their local culture.

The Gentry Transition

As we have seen, large-scale emigration from Sicily encouraged peasants and artisans of the early twentieth century to continue to accept as many children "as God sent," notwithstanding an ever-declining incidence of infant and child mortality. Rather different was the situation of the gentry, who did not contribute to the out-migration stream despite the general crisis (Gabaccia, 1984, pp. 61–2). It is true that some of the descendants of this class migrated to large cities in Italy, but this required a costly education at a time when the land no longer yielded generous revenues and the labor force was depleted. Conjuring up an image of "overpopulation," Gaetano Mosca described how teachers at the University of Palermo were subjected to pressure, even intimidation, because too many sons of the gentry were sent there for law degrees (Mosca, 1949, p. 191; Mack Smith, 1959, p. 261).

No doubt a perception of overpopulation within a once privileged group was what led the relatives of one of our informants, a senior citizen of gentry background, to quote such proverbs as "more family, more hunger" (*più famiglia, più fame*), and "one child is nothing, two are precious little [*pica*], three are just right, four are a lot, and five plus the mother are six devils against the father." Unfortunately for our informant, his father, who married in 1899, did not follow the proverbial advice and had nine children, eight of whom survived. Like a Malthusian berating the poor, the son to this day claims that his father should have been able to assess the meaning of a depression in agriculture for a class that lived from landed revenues and plan accordingly. Instead, he squandered a fortune on self-indulgent travel, high living, and incontinent sex and shamefully displayed pride in doing so by naming his eighth child Ottavio.

According to elderly informants of diverse backgrounds, couples in the gentry were the first in Villamaura to experiment with family limitation, and the records show a marked decline in gentry family size around the turn of the century. By all reports, coitus interruptus was the contraceptive of preference. The "little sacks that keep his blood from mixing with hers," namely condoms, were unknown, we were told, until soldiers learned of them during World War I. But coitus interruptus was also viewed with some disdain by the gentry magnates, accustomed as they were to a way of life that rewarded immoderate indulgence with admiration. Descendants of the first contracepting cohort emphasize the access of its men to other alternatives: they exploited their domestic servants and other women of the peasant class sexually (an outlet confirmed by a rising rate of illegitimacy in Villamaura coincident with the gentry transition), and they could also arrange relatively safe clinical abortions for their wives in Palermo. Retrospective accounts also emphasize the legendary martyrdom of gentry wives who are reported to have closed their eyes to their husbands' philandering as well as resigning themselves to long periods of sexual abstinence (see Schneider and Schneider, 1984).

The Artisan Transition

During the interwar years Sicily's population continued to grow, although probably not because of the populationist measures taken by the Fascist government in support of its autarchic and bellicose posture in the world community of nations. Already in 1924 Mussolini had reversed his earlier support for a neo-Malthusian movement that had begun to distribute birth control propaganda in Italy. In 1926 he promoted a national commission to protect "the family" from such propaganda and instituted a tax on bachelors. The tax was increased in 1928 with benefits added for fathers of seven or more children if they worked for the state, ten or more children if they worked in the private sector (Glass, 1967). There is virtually no evidence that people in Villamaura took these measures seriously, and it is more likely that a continued decline of mortality, plus return migration, account for most of the growth. Especially important to people's recollections of the interwar years was an increasingly visible and acknowledged association between large families and poverty – a reverse of the previous pattern when large families bespoke wealth. Contributing to this perception, at the time, was the initiative of local artisans to practice family limitation – with a commitment that, as we will see, was more thorough, ideological, and respectful of women than the gentry model.

According to the elderly veterans of the artisan transition, men perceived coitus interruptus as a learned skill. This is not to confirm, however, the widely held assumption among demographers that withdrawal, in E. Anthony Wrigley's words, "makes the decision to employ contraception and limit family size...a male prerogative" (1969, p. 200). Most artisan men we interviewed seemed to care that their wives experience orgasm and characterized their birth-control effort as requiring a high level of communication and cooperation between spouses – a characterization seconded by women. Reflecting this emphasis on skill and cooperation was the speed and thoroughness of fertility decline among artisans. Two hundred and six families of this class have been archived in Villamaura's *foglie di famiglia*, a file of household records. Although the file is not complete, it does contain a large proportion of the families formed in each of the nine decades between 1860 and 1950. A decade by decade comparison reveals that, until the 1920s, the great majority of artisan couples had between five and 13 living children; from the 1920s on, and particularly after 1930, the great majority had two or, at most, three.

Several aspects of the artisans' way of life (different from both peasants and gentry) contributed to this success. Literate since the late nineteenth century, skilled craftsmen were a vanguard for the transmission of international socialism into the rural towns of the Sicilian interior (P. Schneider, 1986; also Gabaccia, 1988, pp. 44–9). In Villamaura a strong contingent of them formed the backbone of the fledgling Communist party that broke away from its Socialist forerunner in 1922. Persecuted under fascism, this group nevertheless continued to receive international publications, and to hide them, read them, and debate them in their shops. It is said that, unlike other men in Villamaura, if artisans attended church it was not to pray but to listen and criticize. Although we were told by priests that the local clergy had never considered contraception a priority for pastoral counseling or pursued it as a moral issue in confession, Catholic dogma nevertheless held that reproduction was up to God, not men and women. The artisans' workshop conversations challenged this view, even satirizing clerics who preached against the "incomplete act." ("The priest told Tizio that it would be a sin to spill his seed on the ground, so he dumped it in a sack.")

Through conversations in their shops and in the *Circolo degli Operai* (Worker's Circle) that had been founded by about 70 craftsmen in 1907, Villamaura's artisans also raised each other's consciousness about "the French" – a people they had become familiar with through the Ditta Ducrò, a French firm in Palermo that employed cabinetmakers and carpenters from the interior alongside French artisans. Their discourse characterized the French as *più evoluto* (more evolved) than Sicilians, in part for having small families while the mother was still young. These people, it was said, "can pick up a glass of water, drink half of it and put it down again, in contrast to Sicilians who can't stop before the glass is empty." But among Sicilians, artisans were the "most advanced," for although they had little land, they could read. Literacy, plus the urban origins of their respective crafts, linked them to a wider world. We were also told that the workshop conversations included recounting dreams with sexual content – a sort of amateur psychoanalysis for those who were having trouble "reversing gears."

By the 1920s artisans were strongly motivated to redefine family ideals. Accustomed to marrying within their class, they apprenticed their male offspring to succeed them. Shoemakers gave rise to shoemakers, carpenters to carpenters, and so on. Unless working at home, apprenticed boys earned neither room and board nor income – only a token gift on festival days. If the apprenticeship required sojourns to Palermo, there were fees to pay. In addition, artisans aimed for their children to obtain some schooling. Once migration to America ceased to be an option, outlays for apprenticeships became an increasing burden, the more so as the world depression and revaluations of the lira made it ever more difficult for clients to pay their bills.

In addition to their secular worldliness and strong motivation, the artisans' "skillful" exercise of withdrawal was probably enhanced by the already existing companionate structure of their marriages. Shoemakers, cabinet-makers, blacksmiths, and tailors pursued their crafts close to home, in a *bottega* (shop) on the ground floor of their two-storey dwelling. They ate their main meal at midday, seated at table with wife and children. Continuous with these household arrangements, the conjugal pair was likely to cooperate in the work itself. Thus a shoemaker's wife might use her Singer sewing machine to stitch the uppers of shoes whose soles were made by her husband, or the seamstress wife of a cabinetmaker might ask him to critique her designs. Many artisans' wives were also artisans, or ran small shops, and most helped out in the training and discipline of apprentices. As such they participated in their husbands' daytime activities to a far greater degree than did the wives of the agricultural classes, including the gentry (see Wrigley, 1969, p. 200).

Finally, artisans enjoyed a unique pattern of leisure. Known for putting together evenings of dance and song in each other's houses, they also set aside Mondays – the day that neither blacksmiths nor barbers worked – for convivial gatherings in the country. Situated in one of the small rustic houses that some of them owned on the outskirts of the town, such occasions engaged men in political discussions punctuated by music, for artisans were knowledgeable about opera and often played tambourines, whistles, horns, or violins. More or less limited to a single afternoon and evening of the week, these exclusively male gatherings were less a contradiction to the partnership marriage than were the leisure activities of men in the other classes – further support for the gender-balanced quality of the artisans' fertility decline.

The "Late" Bracciante Transition and Sicilian Culture

Until the late nineteenth century in Italy, population and wealth expanded together, landed families having more resources than the peasantry to bring children to adulthood. In the late nineteenth century, however, this relationship was reversed. As shown by Massimo Livi-Bacci's aggregate measures, it was the well-to-do, better educated, and urbanized populations that initiated the decline of fertility, with peasants and laborers coming last (1977).[5] Whereas in Villamaura, the gentry class began to limit family size around the turn of the century and artisans between the world wars, among landless peasants the small family did not become the rule until the 1950s and 1960s, notwithstanding the fall since 1900 of infant and child mortality within this group.

In assessing the lateness of fertility decline among Villamaura's landless peasants, whether in relation to the town's other classes or to the improved survival rate of children, explanations based on "residual" cultural elements are very tempting. For one thing, *bracciante* men and women spontaneously attribute the high fertility of the prewar period to one of two causes – the will of God (*la voghiu di Dio*) or ignorance. The expression *Ogni bimbo, providenza di Dio*, ("every baby is the providence of God") suggests precisely the religious fatalism that demographers often assume to be causal, as does the often repeated claim that in those days people had children with *occhi chiusi* – with their "eyes closed."

Class relations reinforced the perceived absence of "individual controls" among the *braccianti*. One politically conscious wife of a landless laborer recalled thinking how the rich were governed by "brains, culture, civilization" whereas the poor were governed by "instincts." The rich, she thought, were pleased with that arrangement and purposely kept their knowledge of family limitation to themselves. Like *le bestie* (animals), the poor reproduced for the benefit of the rich. Elderly members of the privileged classes volunteered stock phrases like "sexual embrace is the festival of the poor" (*l'amplesso sessuale e la festa del povero*) and "the poorer they were, the more children they had" (*i più poveri che erano, i più figli che avevano*). According to an older artisan, peasants who asked how he managed to have so few children were incredulous at his description of withdrawal during coitus. "But that is why I married her," responded one peasant.

Culturally, the *braccianti* also partook of the pan-Mediterranean value system of patriarchal honor and shame – a system with marked continuity in western Sicily. According to its values, women tolerated in their husbands and appreciated in their sons a certain degree of irresponsible and carefree roving outside the home (Saunders, 1981, pp. 442–4). Correspondingly, the conjugal bond was not traditionally a source of pronounced affection or intimacy. Although it involved cooperation, marriage competed with the ties of affection that united a mother and her children (especially sons), a mother and her family of origin, and the male peer group (see A. Parsons, 1969). Peer groups of adult males gave space to obscene and sacriligious joking – a welcome escape from the constraining, Madonna-like image of women in the home. Until recently the converse of men's freedom to flaunt domestic and religious authority was women's subjugation. Father and brother chaperoned girls before they married, guarding their reputation for chastity. Mother and mother-in-law would inspect the bridal sheets for blood stains after the wedding night. Upon marriage, a husband gave his bride a black dress for her to wear when she became his widow and remained jealous of her chastity until that day.

Whether in fact men dominated women as culturally prescribed is of course an open question, but as George R. Saunders has argued, "since the male version of culture is publicly dominant,...[women] are socialized from childhood to accept the male view of reality" (1981, pp. 448–9). Although women may have harbored cynical doubts, their public acceptance of a role that devalued their intelligence probably also eroded their respect for each other and aspirations for themselves (Saunders, 1981).[6] To Livi-Bacci, such subordination of women, reinforced by religious teachings, was among the most important obstacles to fertility decline in southern Italy. The following description of family life among landless peasants suggests a more complex reality.

Bracciante Family Life

In Villamaura landed peasants (*burgisi*), artisans, and gentry had, by the twentieth century, entered the fashion system of Western capitalism. Most had wardrobes covering at least four categories of wear: work and festival clothes for summer and winter seasons. Women in these classes expected to have a seamstress make them new items of clothing for the patron saint's festival each year. The *braccianti*, however, wore patched clothes, handed down to them by the rich or sent in packets from America. They did not apprentice their daughters to the local seamstresses (in their turn trained to cut patterns in Palermo) and did not have sewing machines at home. *Burgisi* and artisan women prepared their own trousseau of elaborately embroidered or lace-enhanced sheets and bed covers, while gentry women often commissioned this work to the local monastery. But marrying earlier and with far fewer resources, women of the *bracciante* class had neither the time nor the money to assemble more than three beds' worth of simple, appliquéd cottons – "the minimum required for marriage," it was said (see J. Schneider, 1980).

The *braccianti* lived in humble dwellings. Some had a one- or two-room second storey over a combined stall and kitchen on the street level. As late as the 1961 census, however, the majority of Villamaura's landless laborers still occupied rented houses with three or fewer rooms, some that had earlier been stalls or storerooms in gentry houses or that lacked water, a latrine, electricity, or gas. In interviews, both *braccianti* and others stressed that large families in substandard housing could not conform to the rules of modesty that in other classes symbolized respect – especially the rules that humans live separately from their mule or donkey and boy and girl children sleep in separate alcoves, if not in separate rooms. "Men with men and women with women, or God cries and the Devil laughs," was the proverbial expression for this concern.

Eating meat no more than once or twice a year, the *braccianti* were malnourished. They subsisted on thin soups sometimes enriched by vegetables that women gleaned in the mountains, and on *pitirru*, a porridge of grains ground by hand to avoid the tax on milling. Whereas *burgisi* women kept rabbits or hens, *bracciante* women prepared eggplant to simulate meat. Infant nutrition was a special problem. *Bracciante* women collected wild capers or asparagus for barter or sale; they collected other vegetables for the evening soup and worked as laundresses or servants for the gentry. Perhaps in the very early morning they also made brooms for a local merchant. Whatever the activity, it often meant leaving infants in the care of older siblings, who fed them paps. In poor families children had an uphill struggle against respiratory and stomach ailments, even if they did not die. As draft records show, *bracciante* children had lower body weight and smaller stature than children in the other classes, growing up about a head shorter as adults (see Omran, 1981).

Poverty created many other humiliations. Landlords in Villamaura gave out coins and sometimes soup on Sundays; aging *braccianti*, their children too poor to care for them, sometimes begged. Landlords built elaborate mausoleums in the new cemetery and transported their dead in a glass-enclosed, gold-painted (and eventually motorized) hearse. The *braccianti* bore their dead in a rustic, mule-drawn wagon and buried them in underground graves marked only by a cross. Having little or no education in the local elementary school (first established in the late 1860s), peasants in general spoke only the Sicilian dialect and required the intervention of others who were literate in Italian to engage in any transaction with government officials.

The greatest humiliations, however, grew out of the dispersal of the family as a working group. Men aimed for a combination of annual sharecropping and day-labor contracts, but unless they found supplementary work preparing and hauling construction materials they were typically unemployed for about 100 days of each year (see Blok, 1966; Rochefort, 1961). Adult women, as we have seen, combined the care of their own hearths and families with gleaning, broom making, and, to their shame, work as domestic servants. Occasionally they worked for the *burgisi*, washing floors, preparing feed for the animals, and baking bread. More often it was the gentry who employed them as one of their four or five full-time servants. Engaging peasant men for sharecropping, *civile* men often claimed the domestic labor of the formers' wives and daughters as a condition of employment.

The *bracciante* family also dispersed its children in the labor force. Young girls, by the age of nine, learned to bake bread and make pasta on their own, but their main activity in their mother's absence was swaddling, feeding, and taking care of younger siblings. As teenagers, girls found employment in domestic service, their work being remunerated with combinations of room and board, gifts of food, and a monetary wage. Earnings were earmarked for the preparation of a trousseau of bed linens, necessary for their marriage, unless the family was desperate, in which case these earnings went directly to the mother's kitty for food, clothing, festivals, and illness. Such constraints often led mothers to ignore assaults on a daughter's honor by an employer or his son, hiding the fact from the girl's father to ensure her continuous employment.

Boys worked outside the home – at seven or eight alongside their father or grandfather, and then from nine or ten minding sheep for landowners. Memories of child labor are harsh, but, as with girls, desperate parents tried to disregard abuses, sometimes even urging an employer to discipline a homesick child. In landed-peasant families sons' earnings from casual labor were managed by the father for the eventual purchase of land and houses, but in poor families boys either gave their earnings to their mothers to purchase food or, at their father's invitation, put something aside to pay for their own simple wedding and the few pieces of furniture they would need to create a new household. A boy's earnings might also help purchase the bed linens for a sister's dowry.

Among *bracciante* women, breast milk circulated from haves to have-nots in a relatively noncommoditized system of favors and generosity. A woman with plenty of milk might offer her breasts to the fretting infant of a neighbor whose milk was "broken." *Padroni*, in contrast, paid women, some of them *braccianti*, to nurse their babies but expected the relationship to include neighborlike qualities of loyalty and affection. It was preferred, for example, that the wet nurse live-in and favor the employer's child over her own.

Interclass sexual relations were similarly corrosive of the *bracciante* family. Although landlords did not necessarily sleep with the women who served them, it was assumed that they did, so much so that to raise the topic of *servitù* with older *braccianti* in Villamaura today is to evoke diagnostic stories about fallen honor. Especially indicative, because it brings out the element of parasitism in gentry-*bracciante* relations, is the often repeated story of a married servant who, trying to escape the advances of her employer, fell backwards down a staircase, ending up disabled to the point that she could no longer care for her own husband and children.

Among the infants abandoned as foundlings in Villamaura, some unknown number were the legitimate children of parents too poor to raise them. Others, though, were born of brief unions between a gentry father and peasant mother. Town officials, all of gentry status, registered these babies with tell-tale disparaging names of their own invention such as Fortunate Pilgrim, Clear Telegraph, and Giullietta Romeo. The presence of these foundlings in a small community was a constant reminder that the rich exploited the poor in lieu of their own women, their truncated birth parities and "quality" children being won at the price of a population of *creati* – illegitimate children who would also become servants if they survived. As we have already seen, a few *braccianti* recalled thinking that the gentry went out of their way to withhold knowledge of contraception from the peasants, the *civile* way of life being sustained by the "profligacy of the poor."

In effect, servile relations drained energy from one group of families to add it to another. Like wolves, said an old peasant man, the rich "sucked the blood of the poor." *Bracciante* men in general resented the expectation of the gentry that "we give up our lives as well as our labor" to be *sempre spostata* – always at their disposition. This meant sacrificing the needs of one's own family to care for another man's – for example, lending manpower to the seasonal migration of entire gentry households from town dwellings to country villas and back again. As if to symbolize the incorporation of the *braccianti* into their families, landowners addressed them with the intimate *tu* form of the pronoun "you" but exacted terms of address like *Signore* and *baccio la mano* ("I kiss your hand") in exchange. In local memory landlords' patronizing gifts to servants of hand-me-down clothes and leftover food hardly compensated for the flow of family services the other way.

The result was an interdependent demography between the two classes: *bracciante* milk nurtured gentry infants and *bracciante* mothers cared for them, and, as gentry couples reduced their fertility, the *braccianti* increased theirs. In the cohort who married in Villamaura in 1920, peasant women showed an average birth interval of 28 months, against 31 months for artisans and 30 months for the gentry – a difference that reflected the disruption of lactation for peasant women. The busier a mother, the more likely she was to wean her babies early and calm their cries with rocking instead of suckling, with the result that she lost the protection of lactational amenorrhea against new pregnancies. Informants report introducing supplementary foods and mobilizing sibling caretakers as early as three months, then discovering that their breast milk was losing its substance, turning to colostra or becoming spoiled (*guasto*) because they were pregnant again. In such cases the first signs of pregnancy were not the familiar ones of nausea and "cravings" but evidence that the suckling baby had stomach disorders caused by the declining quality of the mother's milk.

More than emigration, demographic interdependence, with its underlying relations of *servitù*, gave *bracciante* families the quality of dispersal or drained energy that distinguished them from landed-peasant families, whose fertility was also high. Having land and livestock, a *burgisi* father mobilized his children to maintain and enhance the family patrimony, putting his sons to work for him or claiming their earnings if they worked for others. As such he could establish a fund for the daughters' dowry and the sons' marriage settlements and insist that the sons remain single and work with him until their sisters were settled. A single household fund underwrote the preparation of trousseaux for these girls, and in hard times both they and their brothers delayed their marriages for years. Hence the mean ages at first marriage of both men and women in the *burgisi* class, evident in the marriage records, fluctuated, rising as high as 28.8 for women and 32.8 for men. For *bracciante* women the mean age at marriage in the interwar years was around 23, for men around 26. According to our interview data, most *braccianti* married with debts and lived, initially, in rented housing. In this respect they fell short of another symbol of respectability – the parents' ability to provide newlyweds with housing of their own (see Gabaccia, 1984, pp. 46–54).

Unlike the *burgisi*, the *braccianti* today do not reminisce nostalgically about large families. Children survived, earned their keep, even earned enough to marry, and cost their parents almost nothing, but neither did they add much to the family patrimony. Many were lost through migration. As for children's contributions to household labor, this took mainly the form of older daughters caring for younger siblings. Of course, today's *braccianti* have lived through the 1950s and 1960s, when their class undertook the transition to low fertility. As a result they too participate in the labeling and shaming of the few remaining nonconformists – poor families with more than five children. One cannot discount the likelihood that today's outlook colors their memory of the past. Yet we were struck by how rarely an image of the large family as interdependent and pulling together emerged in our conversations with them, compared with the other classes. More characteristic were recollections of overworked mothers, colds, and diarrhea and proverbs such as, "If nothing is enough for two, it will do for ten." So much is this the case that members of the first generation of *braccianti* in Villamaura to make a serious effort at family limitation – men as well as women – report having received their mothers' (and mothers'-in-law) approval and encouragement to practice contraception.

For the *bracciante* men life consisted of alternate rhythms: days of intense physical exertion from sunup to sundown and days with virtually no employment at all. Often they spent their idle hours at one of the local taverns, called *bettole*, playing cards and enjoying the repartee of the male peer group. In interviews, aging *braccianti* described how, in this context, the announcement of a wife's pregnancy was celebrated as evidence of her husband's sexual competence. Yet such displays of machismo could hardly compensate for the fact that *bracciante* wives were alienated from husbands and children through obligations of service to the upper class. This situation did not induce a reaction formation so much as it led to resignation – the resignation of what Sicilians call the *cornutu bastonatu*, "the beaten-down cuckold" (see also Davis, 1969). Given the wider cultural context of honor and shame, men felt shame tinged with rage that they could not effectively retain their wives and daughters at home, or even provide separate sleeping places for their male and female children. As we will see, family limitation not only helped *bracciante* women to domesticate men but enabled men to claim the respectability and authority over their households that they had lacked before.

The Bracciante Transition to Low Fertility

Some peasants joined the artisans of the interwar years in limiting family size. Among the 52 landless families in the marriage cohort of 1920, as well as in the household records for marriages of the 1920s and 1930s, about half had between five and 13 living children, discounting childless couples. In almost half of the remaining cases, child mortality, the death of a spouse, or out-migration was implicated, leaving roughly 25 percent of all *bracciante* marriages in which we can suppose that some form of family limitation may have been practiced. Yet statistical and qualitative evidence suggests that a widespread movement for birth control did not occur among peasants until the 1950s and 1960s, when the proportion of *bracciante* families with five to 13 living children fell first to 8 and then to 2 percent. The movement was associated with a substantial change in the circumstances of these families.

First to affect them after the war was a drastic increase in the cost of living associated with severe food shortages. This plus overall economic instability was reflected in a wave of abortions throughout Sicily (Borruso, 1966). Whereas women seeking the occasional abortion had earlier gone to an informal "midwife" of her neighborhood who administered herbal remedies, after the war metal instruments such as knitting needles came into use. Performed by women described retrospectively as "older and widowed," some of whom were local and some itinerant, these abortions often caused hemorrhaging or infection, requiring the (illegal, hence costly) involvement of state-licensed midwives or doctors. Every interviewee on this subject remembered a woman who had died or almost died as the consequence of an abortion and claimed (at least in retrospect) that most women would rather have more children than rely on abortion as a means of birth control. *Meglio figli che malattie* ("better children than sickness"), they claimed.

As far as we can tell, the rapid fertility decline of the peasantry depended on coitus interruptus as in the other classes, although the context for adopting this means was one of increased opportunities rather than a bust-cycle crisis. After the Allied liberation of Sicily in 1945, Socialist and Communist parties regrouped in a renewed struggle for land reform. A 1946 law, passed during a brief center-left government, acknowledged peasant occupations of large estates. Subsequent governments, although more conservative, legislated a 200-hectare limit on the size of holdings, a 60 percent entitlement to the harvest for sharecroppers, and a provision for the expropriation of properties that were left, unimproved, in pasture. A land-reform agency (ERAS) was set up to administer the expropriations and divisions. In 1947, 1 percent of proprietors in Sicily owned half of the arable land; in 1962 the same percent owned about a third (INEA, 1947; Parisi, 1966, pp. 4–5). ERAS meanwhile assigned 76,000 hectares to land-hungry peasants and helped others to purchase 147,000 hectares. The gentry, tempted to shift their investments to urban real estate, were in many cases willing to sell, and smallholders bought about as much again on their own (Rochefort, 1961, p. 162; Schneider and Schneider, 1976, pp. 130–31).

In Villamaura land redistribution in the 1950s was accompanied by two well-remembered public works projects: reforestation in the mountains above the town and the construction of an artificial lake and dam for hydroelectric energy and irrigation. The former was managed by the forestry service of the Italian government, the latter by a private contractor based in Milan. Both provided work to unemployed day laborers, in rotation, at relatively high wages. Several of the men in our sample of laborers who married in the 1950s and 1960s worked for one or both of the new projects and spoke of them in glowing terms. Not only were the wages higher than those paid on the latifundia, but they were actually "family wages" – high enough that a man could liberate his wife from earning an income outside the home and accompanied by fringe benefits that ensured against accident and illness. Most important, the employer signed up workers as individuals, making no claim on their wives and daughters, and honored the preannounced working hours that excluded evenings and Sundays.

Between land redistribution and changes in labor contracting, Villamaura's *braccianti* felt emboldened enough to adopt a nickname for the gentry. Respectfully calling them the *ceto civile* (civilized class) when we first met them in the 1960s, they now referred to their former landlords as the "so-called civili" (*cosi-detti civili*), or simply the "so-calleds" (*cosi-detti*). Reinforcing this shift in labels was the postwar migration of Sicilians that, from the early 1950s, took them to northern Italy, Germany, Switzerland, and the North Atlantic. In contrast to the earlier migration to America, men were accompanied for at least a part of their sojourn by their wives, who also worked abroad, and both were more likely than not to return, investing their earnings in Sicily. Overall, they encountered work situations more like the forestry project and the dam than like the earlier regime of large estates.

Also new in the lives of poor peasants was schooling, which became amendatory to age 14 following a national educational reform in 1962 (Barbagli, 1982, p. 271). Although the population of Villamaura declined from 8,054 to 7,229 between 1950 and 1970, the number of people with high school degrees or the equivalent increased from 125 to 345; the number with intermediate diplomas increased from 136 to 492. The proportion of girls to boys in school, formerly very low, was, by 1970, about equal. Intersecting this development was a transformation of production and consumption. Agricultural machinery, modestly expanding under Fascist policy, took off as the land-reform agency promoted cooperative and credit programs for the purchase of farm machines, reducing the demand for child labor in agriculture. Even shepherds, formerly recruited from among the youth of the *braccianti*, declined in number as imported, industrially produced feed and motorcycles restructured animal husbandry in a diminishing livestock sector. Overall, 64 percent of Villamaura's active population worked in agriculture in 1950, whereas only 44 percent did in 1970.

Machine-produced, presewn clothes began to enter local markets on a large scale in the 1950s, putting most of the remaining tailors and seamstresses out of work and forcing their emigration but also bringing "respectable" clothing within the reach of the peasant class. Electricity brought washing machines and other appliances into gentry households just as the land reform diminished their holdings and caused their erstwhile servants to reject "feudal relations." Perhaps the central symbol of the interconnected changes was the spread, after 1950, of "neo-technic" housing, much of it financed through emigration remittances and built with the labor of former peasants and returned migrants. For the class of landless laborers new housing had a special significance, because before the war they alone among social groups were likely to begin married life in a rented dwelling (Gabaccia, 1984, p. 24).

In Villamaura, as in the other towns of rural Sicily, houses are built on small plots in densely settled areas, although new neighborhoods now exist on the outskirts of town. Most of the peasant families in our sample could afford to either rennovate and expand an old dwelling or build or buy a new one only after years of working abroad and saving carefully. Yet all saw the house as a place where the wife, formerly compelled to disperse her energies, could retire to devote her labor and attentions to her own husband and children. In the recollection of both men and women, it was as if laborers' wives had organized a strike under the slogan *ognuno per i nostri mariti* ("every woman for her own husband"). *La casa è la prima cosa* ("the house is the first thing"), they insist. And "a clean house signifies a clean spirit, clean in all things."

Mass-produced imports helped to bring respectable housing, like respectable clothing, within the reach of the laboring class. Becoming ever more accessible locally were electric or gas-powered stoves, refrigerators, radios, and, since the late 1960s, televisions; reinforced concrete exteriors instead of the old blocks of limestone or stucco; and interiors finished with ceramic tiles – their colors, patterns, and the amount of coverage marking the owner's status. They especially wanted a floor plan based on an older gentry norm of civilized living, with separate spaces for separate functions. This meant, as a minimum, separate bedrooms for male and female children and for the married couple, a separate room for entertaining guests, and one or more rooms in which the family cooked, ate, and otherwise passed time. So important was the concept of separation that many houses include a corridor between rooms, even at the expense of living space.

The more or less new and neo-technic house, associated with the revolt against domestic service and the possibility for working-class respectability, plus the simultaneously rising cost of children (their birth, infancy, education, clothing, health care, and recreation became substantially more expensive), compelled family limitation in the landless laboring class. Indeed, Sicilian *braccianti* have a straightforward answer to the question of why they now practice contraception: it is the only way to have a decent life. Before their struggle and the land reform, no better life seemed possible. Until inexpensive, mass-produced clothes, floor tiles, and stoves appeared, these amenities of comfort and fashion seemed out of reach. In other words, a conjunction of machines and opportunities played for laborers the role that the two great depressions had played for the gentry and artisans. All were events that uprooted and overturned the earlier parameters of class relations and daily life, encouraging the rapid spread of new ideas about family, including the idea of limiting one's offspring through sexual sacrifice.

Earlier we compared the upper-class approach to coitus interruptus, in which the philandering husband made a martyr of his wife, with the artisans' companionate marriages and emphasis on cooperation between spouses. Among the *braccianti*, a third variation is detectable, also consistent with past gender relations. Unlike the artisans, people in this group resist the idea that they had a plan when they started – it was not a matter of deciding the right number of children in advance but of having them as circumstance permitted. Our sample of 30 *bracciante* couples who married in the 1950s and 1960s shows that 18 percent left a gap of five to 12 years between their first and second child. Artisan couples did the same in the depression years of the 1930s but not in the 1920s, when only 8 percent left such an interval. Moreover, 21 percent of the *bracciante* families who married in the 1950s, compared with 15 percent of the artisan couples who married in the 1920s, showed a gap of more than five years between their penultimate and last child (the maximum number of children being four). Although the *bracciante* figure declined to 15 percent in the 1960s, this was considerably higher than the 6 percent of artisan couples in the second decade of their transition.

Large gaps in birth spacing lengthened the number of years that a woman bore and raised children, making *bracciante* families appear less compact and generationally stratified than the "early-stopping" families of gentry and artisans (see M. Anderson, 1985). Moreover, although a long gap between the last and next-to-last child characterized a minority of families in this class, the last child is culturally marked. Parents refer to such last-born children as "accidents," even introducing them to outsiders as such. Explanations are consistent with older concepts of male sexual efficacy. Although one man attributed accidents to the effects of alcohol, others claimed they happen because, at a certain point, a man "wants to see if he can still do it." Women also hold men responsible, referring to them as *nervoso* (nervous). In the words of one woman, "The man is always nervous, so sometimes little drops spill out." Whereas men celebrate the accidents, to women they are a source of shame, above all in relation to their older children, whom they think should be innocent of conjugal intimacies.

Notwithstanding the somewhat greater distribution of "accidents" among *bracciante* families and the tendency for men to celebrate them as they once celebrated successive pregnancies, couples in this class convey a dynamic of cooperation and sacrifice that conforms in most other respects to the artisan model. Several women talked of withdrawal in terms that expressed gratitude to the husband who "had this much respect" or showed the same kind of "restraint" that keeps a man away from a woman after childbirth. One woman praised her husband for withdrawing each time "beautifully, precisely, exactly," another for having *tanto volontà* – so much will power. A frequent comment was that the husband was *cosciente* (had consciousness), not ignorant like some. Many husbands clearly intended that their wives be sexually gratified, but probably not all were. The woman whose husband's technique was beautiful and exact considered herself deprived but justified the sacrifice by noting that at age 54 she still looked like a maiden of 15, not all dried up (*sciupata*) as women were in the old days after a life of child-bearing.

Like artisan men, *bracciante* men took pride in their role in coitus inter-ruptus. Consistent with the "reverse gear" metaphor, they described the practice as their burden – as an indication of how scrupulous and determined they were in spite of the emotional burden: "At the most beautiful moment you have to pull out. The timing must be perfect because a second's delay means trouble." One man volunteered that the modern home with separate bedrooms made it easier to cultivate the art. In several conversations, men showed concern for the effects of withdrawal on women. Women's bodies, they thought, require a periodic release of pent-up libidinal energy (*dare sfogo*), otherwise they become ill. In the past the release came with repeated pregnancies as "blood flowed through its natural course," but the practice of coitus interruptus makes this problematic. Although some men spoke of their wives having taken the initiative to interrupt coitus, others claimed the ability to remain in control, even when their partner could not.

However they talked about coitus interruptus, both men and women touched on two themes: that of sacrificing pleasure – *fare sacrifici* – and that of social betterment or respectability. As with the other classes, betterment bred contempt for the sexuality of those whose multiple offspring proved them less controlled (see Wrigley, 1969, p. 199). A woman in our sample with six boys and girls reported that her neighbor, equally proletarian, had called her a rabbit to her face. Another couple with 12 children felt stigmatized as "mice." The latter family, one of only two in present-day Villamaura to have so many children, is indeed a target of local gossips (men as well as women), who chastise them for the *disgrazia* (disgrace) of not having thought before making such a *brutta figura* (bad impression). The prodigious parents, it is said, never look you in the eye and allow their children to skip school like gypsies. Needless to say, gypsies, rabbits, and mice are beyond the pale when it comes to local honor.

CONCLUSION

The approach to fertility decline that opposes "tradition" to "modernity" makes light of Western Europe's dependence on coitus interruptus for contraception. Assimilating this particular technique to the practice of birth control generally, then nesting both technique and practice in a cluster of values called "Western," allows us to think that the practice of withdrawal must everywhere signal individual, rational *self*-control. This essay has traced the adoption of coitus interruptus on the part of three classes in a rural Sicilian town – the gentry, artisan, and landless-peasant classes of Villamaura – using as a backdrop the boom and bust cycles of Sicily's political economy since 1860. Although couples in each class used withdrawal to control fertility, they did so in subtly different ways, consistent with past gender relations and habits of work and leisure. In no case did the dramatic fall in fertility presuppose the "Westernization" of all past values.

Among the classes considered, the landless laborers raise the most interesting challenge to the Westernization paradigm. This is because, on the eve of their transition to low fertility, their continued high birth rate coincided with characteristics that many demographers think constitute mental obstacles to birth control – in particular the patriarchal complex of honor and shame and the fatalism expressed in retrospective interviews regarding pregnancy and childbirth. Yet neither these nor any other cultural factor explains the high fertility of this particular class so compellingly as the wider context of their lives. This context included oppressive class relations that were not without demographic consequence, affecting as they did the ages at which the *braccianti* married, the birth intervals between their children, and their overall hopeless outlook. It is impressive that when, after World War II a land reform substantially improved their life chances, they quickly became adept at birth control.

If cultural patterns do not explain the timing of fertility decline in Villamaura's poorest class, which "lagged" behind the artisans by two decades and behind the gentry by five, neither are they irrelevant to the process of population change. In adopting coitus interruptus, *bracciante* couples did not eschew their patriarchal values of honor and shame but only adopted a technique that, as the other classes demonstrated, enhanced the possibility of fulfilling these values, in their case for the first time. For men there was a latent wish to escape from the trap of the beaten-down cuckold to a more honorable existence, and women (their mothers as well as their wives) appreciated the respect that they accrued in the process. This as much as "Western values" motivated the decline of fertility once the structure of opportunities changed.

In other words, certain of the (presumably) non-Western values that are often blamed for retarding transition to low fertility actually helped bring it about among the *braccianti*. This is not to say that Western hegemony is correspondingly absent. On the contrary, cultural phenomena from blue jeans to *Dallas*, from the practice of "dating" to "American" kitchens, are everywhere evident in Sicily, and one sees, as well, manifestations of "Western" ways of thinking about children, women's status, individual achievement, and autonomy from obligations to kin. Ironically, however, some Western-seeming patterns flow from the unintended consequences of the demographic transition itself, especially the experience of living in small families with children who are picky about meat and eggs, as compared with the "traditional" large family in which every child went off to work hungry. The notion that kin obligations are on the wane seems related to one elderly Sicilian man's image of modern youth as "having no other goal in life than to go to the pharmacy and buy beach clogs." Whatever their source, Western cultural elements interact with persistent Sicilian patterns and in ways that defy the expectations of dualistic, oppositional theories of population change.

NOTES

1 See also Giarrizzo (1976), p. 44; Giuffrida (1980), pp. 210–12.
2 See Mack Smith (1968), pp. 407–8; Brancato (1977), pp. 145–6; Corleo (1871); La Rosa (1977).
3 See also Giuffrida (1973), p. 45, and (1980), pp. 275ff.
4 See Lorenzoni (1910), pp. 128–45; Scrofani (1962), pp. 253–6; De Stefano and Oddo, 1963, p. 164.
5 See also Schneider and Schneider (1984).
6 See also Cornelisen (1977).

9

The History of Migration and Fertility Decline: The View from the Road

Leslie Page Moch

What is the relationship between the sweeps of migration that produced an urban world in late nineteenth-century Europe and the decline of fertility that occurred at the same time in history? What is the connection between the flood of men and women into the city and the decline of urban, then rural fertility? The history of migration in Europe offers insight into the fertility decline – but not the sort of insight that may have been expected a decade ago. The relationships between migration, urbanization, and the fertility decline are both more complex and more interesting than previously assumed.

The decline in marital fertility that swept Europe after 1870 occurred simultaneously with an impulse of urbanization – that is, an increase in the *proportion* of people living in cities. Much of this urbanization was caused precisely by the immigration of rurals into urban areas. Consequently, it is tempting to posit a causal link between urbanization and the decline of fertility. Although no particular city size seemed to set off fertility decline, fertility was higher in rural areas than in urban areas, and fertility declined in urban areas before it declined in rural areas (Sharlin, 1986, pp. 236–49).[1]

The dichotomous urban-rural perspective in which this finding is embedded is at odds with a somewhat puzzling, and very important, discovery about the European fertility decline – that differences among regions in fertility behavior were *greater* than those between urban and rural areas within the same region. Indeed, regional patterns of fertility and illegitimacy are most telling, and urban-rural differentials can be seen as "subsidiary differentials" within more significant regional patterns (Sharlin, 1986,

The author would like to thank the National Endowment for the Humanities for research support and members of the Conference on European Fertility Decline for comments on an earlier version of this essay.

p. 258).[2] How can we account for regionally defined behavior? Do shared language and the more general but less accountable term *culture* tell us all we need to know about what a region is? The history of European migration, embedded in a nuanced understanding of what distinguishes the regional community. This essay sketches out that history and relates it to the nineteenth-century fertility decline.

Initially, however, two assumptions about the history of migration must be left behind because they distort our understanding of fertility behavior (and much else) in European history. The first is that migration was new to Europeans in the industrial age; that during the nineteenth century Europeans picked up and left home as their ancestors had never done. As this essay demonstrates, Europeans have always moved. The assumption that mobility is a recent phenomenon is often manifested in the pernicious but persistent notion that to move toward urban areas is to become modern. Nothing could be farther from the truth, because migration is a much more enduring, widespread, and interesting phenomenon than a mere manifestation of "modernity" (B. Anderson, 1980). The second prevailing assumption about migration is that, historically, the act of migration was a permanent move, usually to the city – a one-way trip with an urban area as its destination; this impression does not reflect historical reality. Rather, much migration since the seventeenth century was a back-and-forth movement; some moves were rural-to-urban, others were not. This is especially important for understanding the fertility decline. Along with the tendency to think of migration as permanent, urban-bound moves comes the tendency to dichotomize rural and urban. This dichotomization reflects the assumption that urban and rural areas were populated by people distinct from each other, at least in occupation if not in temperament and worldview.

One fundamental fact marks most migration in European history: it was a social act (C. Tilly, 1978b, pp. 53–7). The decision to leave home was affected by village custom as well as by economic forces; some areas of Britain and the Continent developed migration traditions early on while others did not. Destination too was a collective choice as people together tried out work at particular destinations. For example, men from some villages of France's central highlands worked as masons in lowland cities every summer; men from nearby worked as shopkeepers in Spain for two years at a stretch; still others from a few kilometers away spent winters in the rural lowlands working as sawyers. Few people traveled alone, partly because to travel alone carried terrible risks. Thus migration was based and perpetuated by communities, through human networks (Baines, 1985, pp. 207–12; Poitrineau, 1962, pp. 5–14, 1983, pp. 149–81).

Although migration has long been part of Europeans' experiences, movers have been omitted from many fertility studies. The closest studies of fertility behavior before and during fertility decline are based on the reconstitution of village and city families and on German *Ortssipenbucher*; these unfortunately

necessitate the omission of those who are born, married, or deceased elsewhere (Knodel and Shorter, 1976, pp. 115–54). As a consequence, all but
the most sedentary are eliminated from study. Yet those who move are as
important as they are elusive, for a quarter to a third of many village populations moved and were thereby eliminated from reconstitution studies. The
problem remains of understanding the fertility behavior of whole populations from data concerning only those "who remain in place and [are] visible"
(C. Tilly, 1978c, p. 346).

We attempt to understand history in terms of sedentary populations at
our peril, for when only the sedentary are our subject the experiences of a
large proportion are lost. More important, we harbor the comforting but
erroneous illusion that we have studied the whole. Migration is unsettling.
After Laurence Wylie wrote about the French village of Peyrane in which he
had lived for two years, he discovered, to his dismay, that only about
one-tenth of the villagers had remained from 1946 to 1959 in the community
that he had described as a closed and tidy one. "At this point," he mused, "I
began to wonder what I mean when I refer to 'the people of Peyrane' " (1964,
pp. 351–2). He brought the *village* to his readers but not the *world of its
inhabitants*, who obviously saw beyond the commune that had been his focus.
To understand the world of historical actors we must look at their pere-
grinations. In this case it will help to make sense of the regional and quickly
diffused decline in fertility.

Yet it is difficult to write about human migration. Records of human
movement, particularly before the 1870s, are notoriously poor and scattered.
The parish registers for early modern Europe reveal nothing about movement from one place to another, except by noting the birthplace of a bride or
groom, for example; they give no indication of the fate of people who appear
at baptism or marriage but who then disappear from the record. The
censuses that came with the nineteenth century – even when they do list the
birthplace of each citizen – produce a still photograph that shows where
people are on a given day without giving any indication of the process or
timing of their movements (Jackson and Moch, 1989, pp. 27–8; Moch, 1986,
pp. 193–4). The best sources for studies of migration evolved, for the most
part, during the second half of the nineteenth century – the migration statistics gathered by the German government and the population registers
developed in Belgium, Italy, and Sweden. These sources must be used in
tandem with government inquiries, contemporary studies, care, and imagination. Together these sources allow the reconstruction of a rough history of
migration – a history that, by virtue of its ongoing and social nature, helps
interpret the fertility decline into the lived experience of historical actors.

MIGRATION IN THE SEVENTEENTH CENTURY

The seventeenth century was unmarked by the rural overpopulation that would push folk from the countryside or by widespread urban growth that would attract them in later centuries. Rural areas were relatively self-sufficient because the rural labor force had manufacturing and service functions, in addition to food and animal production. In fact, we infer from the autarchy of preindustrial Europe that country people lived out their lives in their natal village, "in earshot of the same parish bell" (Hufton, 1974, p. 72). Landholding patterns reinforce this impression, because the peasantry – that most sedentary of rural dwellers – was likely near its peak. In Western Europe a high proportion of rural dwellers had been released from the bonds of feudal manorialism. The peasantry would subsequently decline, yet in the seventeenth century the major depredations to the status of the free small-holder were yet to come.

Despite the autarchic nature of the rural world, moving around was an integral part of preindustrial life and rural folkways. Most crucial to the yearly round was the movements of harvest workers to cut grain; these were particularly massive to the breadbaskets near the great cities such as London and Paris. One vast system along the North Sea coast drew workers from Calais north to Bremen in western Germany into a Netherlands hungry for labor in its golden age (Lucassen, 1987, pp. 133–64). And just as Germans provided the muscle power to the Netherlands, so did the French to the kingdom of Spain. The Spanish invasion of the New World left a void of manpower exacerbated by the expulsion of the Moriscos. This void was partially filled by thousands of men from the central highlands of France – a massive migration of permanent and temporary workers that furnished the kingdom with manual labor. The most realistic estimate placed the number of French in Madrid at 40,000, and at 200,000 in all of Spain in 1655 (Poitrineau, 1985, p. 20). These are two of the seven systems of seasonal, long-distance migration that animated Western Europe, each composed of up to 20,000 men. Each one provided harvests for populous cities while feeding and maintaining hungry rustics. This kind of long-distance movement attracted workers to the Piedmont; southeastern England; central Italy; the coasts of Provence, Languedoc, and Catalonia; and the Netherlands and Spain (Lucassen, 1987, pp. 107–24).

It was common for preindustrial rural Europeans to move shorter distances than the crowds of harvest workers. Migration within one's region was part of marriage, family, and property systems in Western Europe. Throughout Europe the taboo on incest prevented men and women from marrying members of their own family. Couples often relocated at marriage, most commonly into a new household in the husband's parish. Much of this "marriage migration" was quite local, and female (Todd, 1985, pp. 19–21). Nonetheless, the fact that people moved at marriage, and that marriage was exogamous, signifies that if one spouse lived within earshot of the same village bell for a lifetime, that was unlikely to be true for the partner.

And the children of the peasant family were likely to leave home. As early as age ten, boys and girls began a series of one-year stints as what Americans would call "farm hands," the British "servants in husbandry," and the French "rural domestic service." Adolescents' annual moves account for the lion's share of the "striking...degree of individual mobility" that characterized peasant communities throughout seventeenth-century Europe (Macfarlane, 1984, p. 343). Between service and marriage, women were especially likely to leave their home village. And although adolescents generally served "their betters," many children of wealthy peasants too were sent out for training in another household. Young people in systems of strict primogeniture and in areas of de facto impartible inheritance (where only one child could marry and stay on the land) were particularly likely to leave home (Gaunt, 1977, pp. 183–210; Todd, 1975, pp. 729–30).

Families moved as well, as holdings were acquired or abandoned to align the household with new fortunes. Land was of central importance, but the particular landholding was less so. After searching through seventeenth-century English wills and legal cases, Alan Macfarlane concluded that precious little sentiment bound family to farm. For example, he found that fewer than half of the original 28 families of Lupton township in the north of England remained there in the two generations after 1642 (1984, p. 343).

If peasant families would move, the proletarian family was even more likely to do so. In early modern Sweden households were most likely to move in the manor-dominated parishes near Stockholm. Indeed, the primary demographic trait that distinguished manor-controlled cottager households from those in parishes where landowning peasants predominated were rates of mobility. "Real stability" in the sense of remaining in one's village of birth was not a general feature of Swedish society; it was, rather, characteristic only of males in areas where peasant ownership was common (Gaunt, 1977, p. 198). Sharecropping moved families in a similar fashion, because dissatisfaction with work and strained relations between estate manager and laborers put families in search of a new position (Todd, 1975, pp. 732–4).[3] To be sedentary was a privilege.

All those who left home did not stay in the country; indeed, the cities were a likely destination. This was especially the case for young women, who outnumbered men in towns, because there were so many menial urban tasks for which they could be hired. They chopped the vegetables, swept the floors, and sewed (Clark and Slack, 1976, p. 88; Souden, 1984a, pp. 159–61). Cityward movement was critical for both rural and urban areas. In fact, migration to the city in early modern Europe is distinguished by the fact that it was more crucial to populating the city than it would be in the centuries to come (de Vries, 1984, pp. 199–205). This is because preindustrial cities were deadly places. Only newcomers could replenish their populations, which would otherwise decrease. Moreover, the great port cities such as London and Amsterdam literally drained off thousands of young people each year who worked as sailors and indentured servants in the colonies, and who would die at sea or abroad.[4] Smaller towns were less deadly, but even they could not maintain their size without an influx of newcomers. In Frankfurt, for example, over half the burghers who received legal privileges in the seventeenth century were newcomers (Clark and Souden, 1982, p. 7; Soliday, 1974, p. 38; Zeller, 1983, p. 199).

Cityward migration was of particular importance to the rural population as well. This is because there were few "surplus" young people in the scarcely populated countryside; in conditions of high infant mortality, high child mortality, and late marriage, most couples would only replace themselves – if even that. In northern France, for example, only half the children born survived to age 20 (Goubert, 1960, pp. 41–5). Of those who survived, one in ten or 12 – from the Beauvais, which was without significant traditions of migration – left the home village. These departures had a greater impact on rural populations than they would have on a more populous countryside in later years.

The traditional countryside was bustling with movement – this was frequently local movement, but it nonetheless took people away from the parish where they were born. Even more important, the timing and the distance of their moves was related in a systematic way to the life cycle of rural folk and to their work and landowning status. To read the rurals of seventeenth-century Europe as a sedentary people is to misinterpret their experience seriously.

To be sure, in the relatively uncrowded countryside of the seventeenth century migration was due less to elements broadly affecting the social structure, such as rural overpopulation and the shift of capital and employment to urban areas, than it would be in subsequent years. Movement was more often due to factors that structured the individual life; these include the death of a father or sibling, birth order, and, of course, gender. If one desired, or was forced, to leave home, local traditions provided the means and the destination. For example, when Martin Guerre, a discontented young peasant from southern France, wanted out, he chose Spain – the same destination as thousands of young men from his region (Davis 1983, pp. 22–4).

What is the significance of the fact that so many people took to the road in preindustrial Europe? How can this help our understanding of the fertility decline that swept the Continent 200 years later? This widespread movement clears up several fundamental misunderstandings. First, people who have been labeled "premodern" folk were not unwilling to leave their birthplace. Indeed, in some areas, to leave home was part and parcel of a local tradition. And for women especially, leaving home usually came with marriage or, even earlier, with domestic service. Although our best records from the pre-industrial area are those of stayers, movers abounded as well. So powerful was the attraction of London that Peter Clark and Paul Slack estimate that a sixth of the entire English seventeenth-century population may have lived there at one time. Indeed, extraordinary records of a Shropshire village over 100 miles northwest of the capital show that one family in six had at least one member who had spent time in London (Clark and Slack, 1976, p. 87). Thus the scope of experience lived and reported was not altogether local; the world did indeed extend beyond the boundaries of the village and out from the city into its hinterland (which in the case of such cities as London and Amsterdam was vast). More broadly, regions were cemented by routine movements among villages, between countryside and city, uplands and plains. A shared population is the bedrock of regional cultures, and extensive migration created regional ties from common experience and location long before the industrial age and the era of most impressive urbanization.

Moreover, people's movement affected their fertility behavior. The childbearing patterns of women in the mountain villages of France, for example, from which men would depart annually for the lowlands or for Spain, echoed the rhythms of their husbands' seasons at home. Likewise, the long period in service for women delayed marriage while they earned a dowry in an urban household or on a farm – a delay that shortened their childbearing years in marriage. Just as migration and the creation of a regional culture date from the preindustrial era, so does the impact of geographical mobility on fertility.

MIGRATION IN THE EIGHTEENTH CENTURY

The patterns of migration that have been found for the seventeenth century were to be altered in the eighteenth, particularly after 1750, as the European countrysides filled with people. In the "long eighteenth century" that stretches from 1680 to 1820, the population of Western Europe grew by 62 percent, with most of the growth occurring after 1740. The growth was uneven: the German population expanded by 51 percent, the French population by 39 percent, the English population by an astounding 133 percent (Wrigley, 1983, p. 122).

The greatest increases in population are intimately tied with the proliferation of cottage industry.[5] In rural industrial areas such as Suffolk, Flanders, the Zurich highlands, and Normandy, spectacular increases in population accompanied the impulse of industrial wage-earning work for poor country folk. This expansion is attributed to the decline in marriage age that came with the proliferation of long-term, steady, rural employment for men, because earlier marriages allowed women about three additional years of childdearing. In other areas, the age of marriage did not fall, but other factors helped to increase numbers; for example, celibacy fell as employment created the means for more people to marry.[6]

In rural manufacturing areas, migration abetted population increase in two ways: a large proportion of the population could live in its natal village and therefore did not emigrate, and new folk arrived in the industrial village where they could earn a living. Indeed, comparative studies of cottage industry show that the freedom to migrate and settle in proto-industrial villages is at the heart of this form of work's success. Rural industrial village generally attracted and retained more people than villages with exclusively pastoral or agricultural economies (Souden, 1984b, p. 24; Berkner, 1973, pp. 288–91, 369–70; Kisch, 1981, pp. 179–82). For example, the Midlands village of Shepshed attracted singled people who married there during its industrial phase; the number of households in the Norman textile village of Auffay increased by 65 percent during its heyday; finally, the Belgian industrial villages near Verviers attracted newcomers during their initial expansion with annual net in-migration rates of 0.068 to 0.048 over a 30-year period (Gullickson, 1986, pp. 15–17; Gutmann, 1988, pp. 136–47; Levine, 1977, pp. 36–44).

What do these figures mean? Annual net migration rates are the proportion of the population that moves, net, in any given year; they signify that the balance of moves to and from the villages increased the village populations by 4.8 to 6.8 percent annually. In concrete terms they mean that, in a village of 1,000 people (about the size for Shepshed, Auffay, and each Belgian village), however many servants, young people, and families may have come and gone during the course of one year, 48 to 68 additional people would have remained at the year's end. Newcomers crowded into the manufacturing villages, attracted by year-round employment for several family members; in some areas lucrative seasonal harvest work sweetened the pot.

Not every region was so fortunate as northern France or the English Midlands. In fact, a very different migration scenario worked itself out in areas where cottage industry did not offer significant rural employment. In such regions the population increases of the eighteenth century resulted in the expansion of migration traditions. This was the case in France's central highlands, because population grew even in the sparsely populated uplands of central France. For nearly 50 years the number of people increased by a half percent annually, so that between 1740 and the end of the reign of Louis XV in 1774 the highlands came to support 30 percent more people. This increase in population brought many more mouths to feed than mountain families could support year-round. Emigration, for a season or for a few years, increased dramatically. The traditional avenues of seasonal movement for upland sawyers and peddlars, for example, were stretched to the limit. Because they could not export their products, mountain villages exported their people (Poitrineau, 1965, p. 120).

Mountains spilled over with people, cities grew, and the plains became full. Vagrants and beggars flooded the highways of France, Germany, and the Low Countries as the numbers of poor increased after 1750. Their children crowded orphanages and foundling homes; women and children begged on church steps and roadsides. Resources could not match the population in many areas, and so the line between migration and vagabondage was crossed by hundreds of thousands of Europeans (Hufton, 1974, pp. 107–27; Lis and Soly, 1979, pp. 116–29, 171–94; Schwartz, 1988).

The best way to understand rural production, on the one hand, and migration, on the other, is to focus on the people themselves – the poor of rural Europe who made their living by a variety of means, at home when they could and elsewhere when they could not, exploiting themselves and their kin, getting by on what Olwen Hufton calls an "economy of make-shifts" (1974, pp. 69–127). People used every expedient to survive until the next harvest, the next bout of taxation and manorial dues. In some areas those expedients were at hand in the form of cash-earning employment that could be done at home. Elsewhere one had to leave to subsist. What David Levine calls the cottage economy encompassed both strategies (1987, pp. 19–21). Generally speaking, the spread of cottage industry and population increase after 1750 divided Europe more sharply into people who were forced to leave home to subsist, on the one hand, and those who could stay at home in densely populated countrysides, on the other.

There were many variations between these two extreme situations, because the tasks of rural industries, like all others, were assigned either to women and children, or to men. Consequently, these could be left to one group while the others concentrated on agricultural work, and families could be deployed both at home and in labor elsewhere. For example, while the women and children of cottagers along the Ems River in western Germany worked linen, their men trekked to Holland for work. Indeed, Jan Lucassen's reconstruction of the migration system that supplied the North Sea coast includes a reconstruction of the cottage industries at home that complemented seasonal migrations (de Vries, 1984, p. 222; Lucassen, 1987, pp. 141–5; Schofield, 1970, pp. 265–6).

As the countryside filled to overflowing capacity in the eighteenth century, what role did cities play for this rural population that was turbulent in some areas and more settled in others? On the face of it, cities were less important to migrants, because urban areas were less deadly than in the previous century and the populous countryside could spare more young people than before. Yet cottage industry was a match between underemployed rurals on the one hand and urban capital on the other. The impulse of merchant capital underlay the putting out of raw materials and purchase of finished goods; without substantial investments, rural production would have remained small scale and local – or fragile, as it was in the central highlands of France (de Vries, 1984, pp. 206–7; Gullickson, 1986, pp. 16–18). Rural industry served to level rural-urban distinctions.

To understand movement to the urban node in an early industrial system, we must be especially attentive to the fact that the entire system was built on the complementarity of rural and urban areas and must look beyond city walls to adjacent settlements (i.e., the faubourgs in France) and the villages in the immediate vicinity (the *banlieux*). If we do not take account of outlying areas beyond the city proper, we are viewing urban populations in a vacuum (de Vries, 1984, pp. 101–2; Garden, 1982, pp. 267–75).

Jean-Pierre Bardet's study of Rouen, a hive of production and node in networks of international trade, highlights geographical patterns of urban population growth. The number of citizens housed within the walls of Rouen did not increase appreciably between the mid-seventeenth century and the outbreak of Revolution in 1789, but the population of the faubourgs and more distant *banlieux* increased. Of every 100 households added to greater Rouen between 1713 and 1772, 50 were added to the *banlieux*, where an estimated 2,000 new households appeared. The faubourgs grew at a similar rate, increasing their share of the total urban population by 50 percent (Bardet, 1983, p. 209; Mollat, 1979, pp. 209, 219, 221). Manufacturing transformed the *banlieux* and faubourgs. These were most desirable areas because people living in the *banlieux* were exempt from France's primary taxes, the *taille* and *droit de bourgage*; they also had easy access to markets for their goods and could bargain and sell on their own without a middle man. Like village folk, they could enrich their diet with the vegetables of their own gardens and take time for lucrative harvest work; like the inhabitants of *faubourgs*, they could sell the vegetables from their gardens at market as well (Bardet, 1983, p. 209).[7]

The modest growth of the early industrial city masks a vigorous population turnover. Bardet's close study of married males in the center city who had children shows that over one-fifth would move away from the city, even in the prosperous years between 1750 and 1789. In all, 21 percent of the couples in which the man was a native-born Rouennais and 37 percent of couples in which the man was born elsewhere would depart. This is particularly remarkable when we consider that these families with children were much more sedentary than young, single folk (Bardet, 1983, pp. 211, 216–17).[8]

Like most historical cities, Rouen stood at the confluence of migration streams that were primarily, but not exclusively, regional. This confluence of migration streams has been identified for Bordeaux by Jean-Pierre Poussou. A seaport and wine capital, eighteenth-century Bordeaux had a great period of prosperity and expansion that attracted migrants from greater southwestern France; the city grew from 45,000 to 111,000 between 1700 and 1800. As rural poverty deepened during the century of rising prices and population, migration to the city widened and intensified. The great majority of people who came to Bordeaux were from specific areas within southwestern France, primarily from the immediate hinterland – a dozen cantons within a radius of about 59.7 kilometers. These waves of immigrants from the immediate area, women in the majority, created a solid tie between city and hinterland. Others came from the region's river valleys; men came for seasonal work from the mountain sections of the greater Southwest. A smaller third contingent hailed from the other cities on France's Atlantic coast (Poussou, 1983, pp. 71–99, 104–14).

How does an understanding of human mobility in the eighteenth century elucidate the fertility decline that would follow? Cottage industry joined city and countryside, often in the financing, creation, finishing, and sale of a single product such as textiles. Consequently, the growth of cottage industry created a multiplicity of ties between countryside and town that were forged not simply by entrepreneurs but by common folk and workers as well. For example, the women of the Cauchois village of Auffay walked together weekly to market to sell their yarn; their market-town experiences were doubtless reinforced by the social act of group travel. If young people left that village, they were likely to set out for such a market town or for Rouen. Vintners' daughters from the Bordeaux region (like women from the outskirts of every large town and city) earned their dowry as urban servants. Every town had its demographic basin of nearby villages and small towns from which people came to the city, at least for a period of their lives; city walls were more often permeable membranes than barriers between unrelated lifeways and mutually hostile groups of strangers (Gullickson, 1986, p. 73; Fairchilds, 1984, pp. 61–2; Poussou, 1983, pp. 112–15; Moch, 1983, pp. 19–26, 33–9).

Whether people moved to a nearby town to take up industrial work or fled poor mountain regions, their migrations were a social matter, for destinations were shared. Men and women who left home entered a social experience that joined them with others via their destination and the region through which they traveled. Not everyone returned home; rather, migrants laced the landscape of Europe with webs linking homeplace with new settlement.

URBANIZATION, MIGRATION, AND FERTILITY DECLINE

After 1815 shifts in British and continental life struck at the ability of rural folk to make a living at home. None of these changes is exclusive to the nineteenth century and none affected Europeans evenly from region to region, yet they all dramatically diminished life chances in the countryside for a large proportion of rurals. The most fundamental of these was unprecedented population growth that proceeded on the eighteenth-century trajectory. Excluding the 52 million Europeans who departed the Continent in the nineteenth century, the population increased from 187 million to 468 million by 1913. Europe became far and away the most densely populated continent on earth. This growth was by no means even; in Great Britain, Denmark, and Finland the population more than tripled, but France grew by a mere 55 percent. The populations of Germany, Sweden, Austria-Hungary, Belgium, and Holland more than doubled while the Italian population doubled (Armengaud, 1976, pp. 28–30).[9]

In much of continental Europe rural areas held their maximum population around mid-century. They were then shaken by a variety of disasters: specific calamities, such as a plague on silkworms in the 1850s and an epidemic that decimated vineyards from the 1860s through the 1890s, befell regional cottage industries and agricultural systems. The implantation of the railroad dragged rural products into the world economy, where locally grown grain and locally produced rough wool, for example, could not compete. The collapse of prices for rural manufactured goods deindustrialized the country-side, dissolving the jobs that had enabled rural people to get by at home. In the words of Steve Hochstadt, "The protoindustrial balloon expanded and then burst in the nineteenth century, removing this crucial source of local income for the rural poor" (1985, p. 6). Indeed, the deindustrialization of the countryside is as much a key to migration in the nineteenth century as the growth of factory industry. Where rural industry collapsed, the people of whole regions groped to find other avenues of support. When prices for Belgian linen collapsed in the 1840s, hand-loom weavers entered the mills in northern France – some commuting from Belgium weekly – and harvested sugar beets in the summer. Between 1815 and 1914 (and earlier in Britain) countrysides that had been hives of industry became more exclusively agricultural or pastoral.

Rural crises varied in timing and intensity, but the net result was that, by the end of the century, fewer rural people could maintain themselves in village settings. Their movement to the cities contributed to the process of urbanization. In the long run, a metropolitan world was shaped by shifts in land ownership that completed proletarianization in the countryside, the movement of capital to urban areas, and the concomitant shifts in the labor force. But in the *short* run – from about 1850 to World War I – seasonal work and economic insecurity combined to inflate temporary movement. Close inspection of nineteenth-century migration records, in conjunction with local studies, suggests that migration reached an all-time high in this period but that a significant proportion of it was temporary.[10] The great volume of short-term moves responded to demands for temporary, rather than permanent, labor in both city and countryside.

The demand for seasonal agricultural work increased with the successes of large-scale capitalist crop agriculture. For example, expanding sugar beet production in northern France and Germany and the implantation of the wine industry in southern France called for more harvest and other short-term workers. Short-term agricultural labor worked to the detriment of rural domestics as year-round agricultural employment was on the wane. Ironically, greater opportunities for seasonal earning enabled some people to hang on in particularly underpaid sectors of cottage industry. For example, the hand-loom linen weavers near the French-Belgian border were reduced to buying their winter bread on credit by the 1890s; only summer work in the sugar beet harvest allowed families to bring in enough cash to subsist as weavers (Kussmaul, 1981, pp. 120–34).[11]

The construction of the railroad brought teams of temporary workers through countrysides in England, then France and Germany. Native-born workers were supplemented, and in some cases outnumbered by, foreign nationals – such as the Irish in England, the Polish in Prussia, and the Italians in Bavaria, France, and Switzerland. In addition, the railroad created new avenues for harvest work by enabling producers to capture distant markets for local goods. As Mediterranean France began to harvest spring fruit, vegetables, and flowers for shipment to northern cities, 15,000 Italians crossed the border annually to pick the crops (Chatelain, 1977, pp. 733–67; Hoerder, 1985a; Rosoli, 1985, pp. 95–116).

We associate harvest work with seasonal migration, but much urban work was seasonal as well, particularly during the great construction booms in urbanizing Europe. The summertime work of men in the building trades expanded the cities. Brickmakers, like those from Lippe in westernmost Germany who earlier had worked in the Netherlands, found plentiful, albeit backbreaking, work for a few months each year. Masons from Portugal who toiled in Spain, from the French highlands who helped to build Paris, and from Poland and Italy who worked in the Rhine-Ruhr zone all worked on a seasonal basis. Customarily, urban domestic servants, whose numbers peaked just before the outbreak of World War I, were hired for the winter between employers' summertime stays in the country. Although many urban domestics ultimately did not return to the countryside, most were newcomers to the city in their teens and twenties.[12]

Extractive and productive industries were also often seasonal employers. Mining – particularly in the beginning of shaft mining of coal – was an industry that initially could attract rural men only *outside* of the harvest season. Sugar-beet processing occupied only four to five months of the year and employed about 100,000 German workers in 1900. Textile mills were seasonal employers as well, laying off their workers in the dead season of summer. Dressmaking, which employed literal armies of female workers, rose and fell with the fashion season, pulling workers between 20-hour days during "high season" and complete lack of work during others. Many urban women who had no rural alternative were forced into prostitution by unemployment and underemployment (Hochstadt, 1985, p. 25; Stewart, 1987; Frey, 1978, pp. 816–19).

Between periods of employment many Europeans went home to villages, balancing between agricultural and urban work, between city and countryside, between proletarian and peasant. Michael Hanagan has sensitively reconstructed the movement of workers between their home villages over-looking the ironworks of the Stéphanois valley and the towns on the valley floor. James Jackson, Jr., has traced the well-beaten paths trod between the Rhineland industrial city of Duisburg and its rural hinterland; the city counted 720,000 arrivals and departures while it grew by 95,000 residents. The volume of moves is visible only in population registers and German migration statistics, which reveal intense, largely short-distance movement. Typical is the migration to and from Casalecchio, an outpost of Bologna. Almost a quarter of immigrants to this town between 1865 and 1915 emigrated within three years, and four-fifths of the townspeople departed for at least some period in their lifetime (Hanagan, 1986; J. Jackson, 1980, pp. 129, 155–60; Kertzer and Hogan, 1985; C. Tilly, 1984, pp. 44–7).

Insecurity accounts for much of this movement. Temporary migration of the late nineteenth century overruns the neat categories of traditional harvest migration, rural service, or temporary urban work. Young, single men and women were particularly vulnerable. Single men were the first fired with industrial layoffs, while young women were the hardest put to find perma-nent jobs that paid a living wage (Crew, 1979, pp. 63–4; Schomerus, 1981, pp. 178–9).

The insecurity of temporary work disrupted relations between men and women; it delayed marriage, rendered courtships unstable, and separated married couples. While peasants' sons went into the coal mines, their daughters worked as maids in other towns. While the spinners of the Caux worked in the riverside mills, male weavers from the same village entered Rouen factories. Such separations increased rural out-of-wedlock births and condemned many Europeans to celibacy. While women were at home, or in an exclusively female employment such as spinning mill or domestic service, men from their homeplace worked elsewhere. Mates of Italian and Polish women worked in another European country. In the case of the young women of Britain, Germany, Italy, and Portugal especially, "Their bonnies were over the ocean, their bonnies were over the sea."[13]

The departures of 52 million Europeans for the New World during the nineteenth century had much in common with the vast continental systems of temporary migration, because much of the trans-Atlantic migration was temporary as well. Indeed, particularly after the advent of the steamship in the 1860s, the migration that took Italians, Portuguese, Germans, and Britons to the Americas was often conceived of and executed as a short-term stay for cash-earning purposes. J. D. Gould reports that "an increasing frac-tion of those who migrated to the U.S.A. *never intended to remain perma-nently*" (1980, p. 51).[14] Between the turn of the century and World War I the repatriation ratio from the United States was 46.7 for the English, 47.1 for North Italians, 32.7 for Poles, 20.9 for German, and 16.3 for Irish immigrants, with patterns of return varying among migrant groups. More striking is the fact that the groups most likely to return home were the most *male* groups. In other words, it is men who traveled back and forth across the Atlantic while women either stayed at home or moved permanently to the New World. Among these were the Italian *golondrinas* (swallows) who harvested grain in Argentina from December to April, then returned home (Gould, 1980, pp. 52–60). Men's and women's lives were mismatched, and they were mismatched on a global scale.

For Europeans concerned about the homeland, the most visible form of migration was that to the city, which contributed to urbanization. Nineteenth-century Europeans witnessed an unprecedented growth of urban areas. Where there were only 23 cities of 100,000 or more in 1800, there were 135 a century later. By the 1890s small towns dotted the landscape and an unprecedented proportion of Europeans lived in cities of 20,000 or more. In England and Wales, more than half the population lived in such cities; more than a quarter of Belgians and Dutch did so. In Germany, France, and Denmark, more than one-fifth the population lived in cities of this size. Adna Weber echoed a generation of Europeans when he wrote in 1899 that "the most remarkable social phenomenon of the present century is the concentration of population in cities" (Weber, 1967, frontispiece, p. 1; Armengaud, 1976, pp. 32–3).[15] In every case the gain in proportion of people in cities and small towns came at the expense of those in the country-side, who came to figure less in each national population.[16] Although Britain was the most urbanized country in the world in 1900, unprecedented growth occurred in old commercial and administrative centers such as Paris, cities that added mechanized industry to their economic repertoire like Berlin, and new industrial towns like Roubaix in northern France – a manufacturing center of some 8,000 in 1815, a factory city of 125,000 in 1900. The greatest cities drew people from afar, but the majority of moves were regional. The most prodigious development of industrial centers occurred in the Ruhr zone, where villages and small towns like Essen, Düsseldorf, Dortmund, and Duisburg became cities of 200,000 to 350,000 by attracting Dutch and Poles, as well as Germans from both near and far.

The international migrations that expanded industrial cities, built Europe's railroads, and harvested its crops would come to an abrupt halt with the opening salvos of World War I. In 1914 migrants became foreigners trapped behind enemy lines; potential migrants stayed at home to fight or help in the war effort (see Bade, 1980, pp. 375–6). With the disasters of war, those who survived were needed for work at home. The movement of free labor across borders was nearly eliminated. In the 1920s and the Great Depression of the 1930s, internal migration and urbanization continued, but only France, with its population shortage, employed significant numbers of foreign nationals. The movement across national borders of forced laborers, concentration and extermination camp victims, refugees, and displaced persons between 1919 and 1950, however, was unprecedented (Kulischer, 1948). Not until the boom years of the 1960s and early 1970s would the movement of free labor across national borders resume and expand to workers from the Mediterranean basin and beyond.

CONCLUSION

How does this massive migration in an urbanizing age – much of it temporary and much of it regional – relate to the fertility decline that swept Europe at this time? It certainly had a disruptive effect on many a courtship, inflating the number of out-of-wedlock births and delaying or canceling marriage plans; temporary departures also affected the rhythm of childbirth for married couples.[17] However, an insight into the migration process is most valuable for the light it sheds on regional behaviors. Indeed, by 1900 regions had long been bound together by their people, who joined village with provincial capital and market town with webs of kin and friendship. With the heightened temporary movement of the nineteenth century, more people spent their adolescence and their twenties in *both* city and countryside; regions were internally bound more closely. If urban and rural people within regions exhibited similar fertility behaviors, it is partly because they were *the same people*, part of the same "regional network of economic opportunities and constraints, a system of shared knowledge and ramifying kinship networks" (Kertzer and Hogan, 1985, pp. 19–20). Couples married in the city might leave for the countryside, or marry in the countryside, then move back to the city where they had worked before marriage (Schiaffino, 1982, pp. 231–41). Their wedding witnesses were country cousins and urban friends alike. Given that kin and friends spanned rural and urban areas, cities and their hinterlands, we can expect that urban and rural people would exhibit similar fertility behaviors. Migration, neither a new phenomenon in the nineteenth century nor a single, one-way move, helped to create the regional cultures in which fertility behavior is embedded.

The history of migration challenges the perspectives of both the sentimentalist and the modernization theorist. On the one hand, it shows the necessity of revising our rather cozy vision of preindustrial life; it is simply not true that "everyone had his or her circle of affection," nor that "time was when the whole of life went forward in the family, in a circle of loved, familiar faces" (Laslett, 1983, pp. 5, 21). It may be more accurate to write that everyone *sought* a circle of affection. Those with land and fortunes could more easily remain with loved ones and could more easily find a place. For the landless, for young people, and for orphans, home was where work could be found. On the other hand, this was true in the seventeenth and eighteenth centuries as well as in the late nineteenth century. Mobility is neither unique to modern Europe nor did it ever necessarily indicate a forward-looking perspective. Rather, human mobility long has been part of family and landworking systems.

NOTES

1 The connection between migration and urban fertility is usually made in one of two ways that emphasize the composition of urban populations: (a) Migration increases the numbers of single persons in the city – and consequently lowers urban birth rates; and (b) Migration also lowers birth rates because newcomers to the city enter occupations that are themselves associated with low rates of nuptiality and birth. For example, Sharlin (1978) focused on the poverty of newcomers to the early modern city that kept them single. He hypothesized that they were a sort of demographic underclass that did not marry (and was relatively more susceptible to disease). They were therefore disproportionately responsible for the natural decrease that plagued early modern cities. Migrants have also been identified with the occupations of celibate people in an urban environment, such as soldiers and servants. When Knodel and Maynes (1976) found a large proportion of celibates in German cities, they looked to the newly arrived soldiers and serving girls for an explanation. It is certainly true that in cities of the past most newcomers were single. Moreover, studies of migrants in the nineteenth-century city during the fertility decline show that they not only dominated occupations for the celibate, such as domestic service, but were likely to be members of an occupational group that pioneered urban fertility declines: white-collar workers. See, for example, Dupeux (1973).

These observations identify occupational and demographic characteristics that distinguish the migrant population. They are ecological, insofar as they look at migrants in the structure of urban environments. Hence, although they are helpful and important to understanding the role of newcomers to urban demographic patterns, such observations do not contribute to our understanding of the historical process of fertility decline.

2 See also Knodel (1974), pp. 82–7, 89–106: Knodel (1977b); Livi-Bacci (1971), pp. 105–8, 112–14, 125–31; Livi-Bacci (1977), pp. 133–4, 61–9, 108–9: Lesthaeghe (1977), pp. 5–12; van de Walle (1974), chap. 7.

3 See the moving biography of sharecropper Etienne Bertin by Guillaumin (1983).

4 Clark and Slack (1976), pp. 87, 120; de Uries (1984), pp. 195, 210–12; Levine (1987), pp. 80–86; Wareing, (1975), pp. 356–78; Wrigley and Schofield (1981), tables 6.4 and 3.1; Wrigley (1967), pp. 44–70.

5 Levine (1977), pp. 58–87; Gullickson (1986), pp. 129–44; Braun (1978), pp. 289–334; Mendels (1972), 249–53; Terrier and Toutain (1979), pp. 19–26; Gutmann (1988), pp. 115–54. I avoid the term *proto-industry* in this essay because it is particularly inappropriate to a study of human mobility for two important reasons. First, "proto-industrialization" emphasizes the end of the process – that is, the replacement of rural manufacturing by machine industry. What was important for rural areas was the effect of rural industry as an alternative to migration, and the drastic consequences of rural deindustrialization for migration. Second, "proto-industrialization" is usually associated with rural work and thereby emphasizes rural processes and rural-urban differences rather than gives attention to the spread of capital and integration of the regional labor force.

6 Levine (1977), pp. 58–87; Mendels (1972); Terrier and Toutain, (1979); Braun (1978); Gullickson (1986), pp. 129–44; Gutmann (1988), pp. 115–54. See also Gutmann and Leboutte (1984), pp. 587–607; Houston and Snell (1984), pp. 479–84.

7 See also Guignet (1977), p. 214.

8 Studies of other cities (i.e., Caen, Geneva, Lyons, Marseilles) show a similar proportion of migrants among marriage partners. Terrisse has similar findings of population turnover for eighteenth-century Marseilles (1974, pp. 249–62).

9 Early French fertility decline is primarily responsible for relatively little population growth in that country (Wrigley, 1983).

10   Hochstadt (1981), pp. 445–68; Hochstadt (1987); Jackson (1980), chaps. 5 and 6; Hanagan (1986), pp. 77–107; Kertzer and Hogan (1985).

11   For an evocative biographical portrayal of the hand-loom weaving family, see Grafteaux (1985), pp. 16–31.

12   Bade (1980), pp. 366–70; Brettell (1986), chap. 2; Corbin (1975), pp. 177–225; Rosoli (1985); Lucassen (1987), pp. 78–81; Tilly and Scott (1978), pp. 107–8; A. Weber (1967), pp. 277–9.

13   Levine (1987), p. 185; Brettell (1986), chap. 5; Gullickson (1986), pp. 135–7, 178–94; Moch (1983), pp. 69–73, 142–8. For long-distance migration on the Continent, see Bade (1980) and Rosoli (1985).

14   For important work on the temporary migration systems between Europe and the New World, see Baines (1985), pp. 126–40; Brettell (1986), pp. 80–85; Hoerder (1985b), pp. 20–23. See also section 3, "Acculturation Twice: Return Migration," in Hoerder (1985a), pp. 353–434.

15   Migration was not exclusively responsible for the increase in the proportion of urban people. In fact, the relatively healthy city of the nineteenth century made natural increase a significant proportion of urban growth. Ironically, migration was less responsible for city growth than in had been in past centuries. See de Uries (1984), p. 233.

16   Rural populations were reduced in proportion of the total but not in numbers. Only in France, where natural increase was exceptionally low, did the growth of cities significantly detract from rural areas in absolute numbers. See White (1989), pp. 17–22.

17   For examples of the impact of migration on out-of-wedlock births and nuptiality, see Brettell (1986); for examples of the impact of temporary migration on the timing of births to married couples, see Corbin (1975), pp. 568–78.

10

Occupation and Social Class during Fertility Decline: Historical Perspectives

Michael R. Haines

INTRODUCTION

Studies of Europe's demographic transition, most recently by the European Fertility Project at Princeton University, have revealed that period fertility rates began to decline within a relatively brief period of time and within various levels of social and economic development[1] (Knodel and van de Walle, 1979; Watkins, 1986; Coale and Watkins, 1986). The notable exception was, of course, France, which had experienced fertility decline since the latter half of the eighteenth century. In conjunction with the European Fertility Project, Ansley Coale (1973) has delineated three preconditions for fertility decline. First, fertility must be within the calculus of conscious choice for individuals or couples. Second, reduced fertility must be socially and economically advantageous to the individuals making these decisions. And, third, effective techniques of fertility regulation must be available and not excessively costly.

A variety of explanations for the fertility transition have been proposed (see George Alter's essay in this volume). The modernization view essentially states that preconditions 1 and 3 had been generally fulfilled in Europe by the mid- to late nineteenth century and that the transition was precipitated by economic development and structural change. This explanation encounters

This essay is based on the paper "Social Class Differentials during Fertility Decline: England and Wales Revisited," originally prepared for presentation at the Conference on European Fertility Decline at the Ontario Institute for Studies in Education, Toronto, May 20–22, 1988. The paper was published in *Population Studies*, 43, no. 2 (July 1989), 305–23. This essay has benefited from comments made at the Conference on European Fertility Decline at Pembroke College, Cambridge, July 2–5, 1989.

the difficulty that, historically for Europe, declines in period fertility rates commenced within a short period of time (from about 1870 to 1910) in countries with vastly differing levels of socioeconomic development. For example, England (including Wales) was economically the most advanced nation in Europe by the late nineteenth century in terms of its urban population, the percentage of its labor force in agricultural or nonagricultural employment, or output per capita of key industrial commodities. Birth rates began to decline in England and Wales only after 1875. In contrast, Bulgaria was overwhelmingly rural and agrarian when it began its fertility transition merely 40 years later (ca. 1910–15).

Such facts would indicate that the second precondition might already have been met in some European nations by the late nineteenth or early twentieth century and that the first and third preconditions were, in fact, the binding constraints. Precondition 3, the availability and cost of fertility regulation, has often been assumed as not crucial, because traditional methods (including abortion) obviously sufficed in both the United States and France from the late eighteenth or early nineteenth century to enable some control of marital fertility. There is some debate, however, about the accessibility of this type of information in other nations to peasants and the working classes, in contrast to the middle and upper classes. The essay by Wally Seccombe in this volume supports this view for England in the late nineteenth and early twentieth centuries. Many working-class wives were motivated to restrict family size but had difficulty gaining access to safe and effective means of contraception.[1] There is also evidence from various areas in Europe about early declines among particular groups, including aristocrats, urban elites, and Jews, which indicates that preconditions 1 and 3 might have more relevance than has been thought (Livi-Bacci, 1986; Schneider and Schneider, 1984).

These facts lead to some reconsideration of fertility control seen as diffusion of an innovation versus adaptation to new material circumstances and also subject to an interaction of economic, cultural, and social circumstances and constraints (Carlsson, 1966; Schneider and Schneider, 1984). For instance, Ron Lesthaeghe has proposed the concept of "secularization" as an explanation for historical fertility decline (1977, 1983, 1989; Lesthaeghe and Wilson, 1986). This originated in the finding, for Belgium, that a good predictor of fertility levels and trends across Belgian arrondissements after 1800 was the degree of religious adherence as measured by the proportion of the area voting non-Catholic in 1919 and by the extent of Easter duty fulfillment. The strong differences in fertility levels and timing of decline across the language boundary of Belgium (separating Flemish- and French-speaking areas), despite similarities on other dimensions (e.g., literacy, urbanization, extent of nonagricultural employment), is also evidence in this direction. While not discounting the importance of material and economic incentives for smaller families, Lesthaeghe believes that the "historical transition in marital fertility and nuptiality" is a manifestation "of a long-term shift in the Western ideational system. The underlying dimension of this shift is the increasing centrality of individual goal attainment, that is, the individual's right and freedom of defining both goals and the means of achieving them" (1983, p. 429). Among the important historical factors are the emergence of capitalism and the rising role of the nuclear family in the West, reorienting behavior toward household well-being and away from community or kinship group welfare; an increasing emphasis on the welfare of children within households; and a more recent preoccupation with individual well-being, self-interest, and fulfillment.

The study of fertility decline by occupation or socioeconomic class can shed some light on these issues. Michael Teitelbaum has argued that fertility was probably ready to decline in England and Wales by the middle of the nineteenth century, based on such structural characteristics as the percent urban, literacy, and the extent of female employment outside the home, as well as contraceptive knowledge (1984, pp. 224–7). But prosperity and favorable economic conditions in the 1850s and 1860s delayed the fertility decline until the 1870s. Thereafter, the slower growth of incomes (after about 1873) and the growing scarcity and rising cost of domestic servants combined to precipitate the decline. The issue of servants was, of course, excessively an upper-class and upper-middle-class concern. Fertility decline was possibly accelerated by a growing public awareness of a greater variety of contraceptive practices consequent to the publicity surrounding the notorious 1877–9 trial of Charles Bradlaugh and Annie Besant for distributing Charles Knowlton's *Fruits of Philosophy*. This point is also made by James Banks (1954), who argues that a combination of rising expectations and slower income growth for the middle classes, along with the rising cost and increased scarcity of servants from the 1870s onward, led to reductions in family size. The distinction in timing of the English fertility decline does not go very far, however, to explain the much earlier declines in the more agricultural societies of France and the United States.

Jane and Peter Schneider have examined in detail the fertility declines of different social-class groups in rural Sicily in the late nineteenth and twentieth centuries. (Schneider and Schneider, 1984; see also their essay in this volume). They indeed found differential timing in the onset and pace of decline among the groups, and they also found class-specific differences in contraceptive practice. "Leading" the fertility decline was the group made up of gentry landowners, merchants, and professionals. Their fertility transition was followed by that of artisans and, finally, with a long delay, that of smallholders and landless laborers. But the timing of these changes in fertility behavior depended on a variety of factors – economic, social, and cultural – which cut across all of Coale's preconditions.

This essay presents evidence on the existence and relative size of fertility differentials during the demographic transition for several Western nations and seeks to explore the issue of "leading" groups in the fertility transition.

EVIDENCE FOR EUROPE AND THE UNITED STATES

The study of differential fertility by occupation and socioeconomic class is not novel. Much of the most instructive early work was done for England and Wales. T. H. C. Stevenson, the Registrar-General's superintendent of statistics who supervised the analysis of the 1911 Census of Marriage and Fertility of England and Wales (1923), prepared a paper in 1920 on class fertility differentials based on the retrospective reports on children ever born by married women (by marriage duration) in that census. Stevenson was instrumental in creating the system of social-class categories that is still used, albeit in considerably modified form.[2] One of his principal findings was that the "difference in fertility between the social classes is small for marriage contracted before 1861 and rapidly increases to a maximum for those of 1891–96" (1920, p. 431). In other words, class fertility differentials (based on categorization of husband's occupation) widened during the early stages of the fertility transition. Stevenson's results indicate that the middle and upper classes experienced earlier and more rapid fertility declines than manual workers, especially the semi-skilled and unskilled. The lowest fertility and the most rapid declines occurred among the professions, which Stevenson termed "the most purely middle class occupations" (p. 432). The trends held up (and indeed often were made more extreme) with stan-dardization for differences in age of marriage across social classes. Although the upper and middle classes also had lower child mortality, this only com-pensated in part for their lower fertility.

Some of this evidence is presented in table 10.1, where the parity data from the 1911 census are organized by marriage duration and several alter-native social-class groupings. This census is a rather remarkable social docu-ment. It was the first English census to ask questions (to married women) about children ever born (parity), children surviving, children dead, and the duration of marriage. To analyze this retrospective fertility information by social class, the Registrar-General used the occupation of the husband for all married women with husband present, of which there were 6,014,319 usable records in the census (out of a total of 6,630,284 married women counted in 1911). These women had more than 21 million births. The census published much detail, including extensive information on occupations of husbands and wives and geographic locations by marriage duration and age at marriage (England and Wales, 1923). A number of researchers have used these data for analysis of both fertility and child mortality.[3] Although there are problems with data of this sort, they can also be very revealing.[4]

Table 10.1 presents the results organized by the eight original social classes used by the Registrar-General for the 1911 census, as well as two other alternatives – the occupational groupings used in the 1950 U.S. Census and the five revised Registrar-General's social-class groups from the 1951

Table 10.1 England and Wales, 1911: average parity by social class and marriage duration (all ages of women)

	Years of marriage									60+ Before 1851	Relative decline
	0–4	5–9	10–14	15–19	20–24	25–9	30–39	40–49	50–59		
	1906–11	1901–6	1896–1901	1891–6	1886–91	1881–6	1871–81	1861–71	1851–61		1861–96
Social class: 1911 English census categories[a]											
I	0.6555	1.6247	2.2955	2.8670	3.3959	3.9522	4.7871	5.8942	6.3934	6.6458	1.056
II	0.7566	1.8647	2.6525	3.3168	3.8663	4.3975	5.2109	6.2914	7.1576	7.5933	0.897
III	0.8716	2.1459	3.2031	4.1371	4.9256	5.5702	6.2855	7.1216	7.5881	7.2000	0.721
IV	0.8988	2.1827	3.2178	4.1038	4.8925	5.5101	6.1755	6.9133	7.3143	7.9138	0.685
V	1.0249	2.4852	3.7269	4.7924	5.6035	6.1694	6.7372	7.3720	7.8358	7.9851	0.538
VI	0.7645	1.8199	2.6685	3.5808	4.3981	5.0931	5.8154	6.6973	7.2678	7.5000	0.870
VII	1.1251	2.7704	4.2316	5.5684	6.5781	7.2666	7.7921	8.2973	8.2819	9.2857	0.490
VIII	1.0140	2.4473	3.5599	4.6433	5.4520	6.1702	6.7037	7.2819	7.9372	8.1890	0.568
CV	0.168	0.167	0.186	0.198	0.194	0.179	0.142	0.098	0.072	0.093	
Index: social class I = 100											
I	100	100	100	100	100	100	100	100	100	100	100
II	115	115	116	116	114	111	109	107	112	114	85
III	133	132	140	144	145	141	131	121	119	108	68
IV	137	134	140	143	144	139	129	117	114	119	65
V	156	153	162	167	165	156	141	125	123	120	51
VI	117	112	118	125	130	129	121	114	114	113	82
VII	172	171	184	194	194	184	163	141	130	140	46
VIII	155	151	155	162	161	156	140	124	124	123	54
Social class: 1950 U.S. census categories[b]											
0	0.6374	1.5886	2.2192	2.7046	3.2022	3.7973	4.6586	5.9661	6.3971	5.7857	1.206
1	0.8440	2.1011	2.9764	3.7408	4.4206	5.0774	5.8882	6.8102	7.4913	8.4714	0.821

Table 10.1 (cont.)

	0-4	5-9	10-14	15-19	20-24	25-9	30-39	40-49	50-59	60+ Before	Relative decline
	1906-11	1901-6	1896-1901	1891-6	1886-91	1881-6	1871-81	1861-71	1851-61	1851	1861-96
2	0.7322	1.8143	2.6073	3.2900	3.8857	4.4751	5.4205	6.5574	7.1595	7.5200	0.993
3	0.6832	1.6836	2.3939	3.0527	3.6073	4.1583	4.9701	6.1364	7.0100	8.7143	1.010
4	0.7918	1.9148	2.7732	3.5151	4.1354	4.6724	5.4494	6.5809	7.0902	5.4545	0.872
5	0.8581	2.1071	3.0715	3.8936	4.5486	5.0771	5.7118	6.5167	7.2078	7.6046	0.674
6	0.9804	2.4028	3.6280	4.7173	5.6150	6.2425	6.8565	7.5566	7.8479	7.9524	0.602
7	0.8556	2.0164	2.8462	3.5865	4.2027	4.7564	5.5362	6.4805	6.9988	8.6667	0.807
8	1.0273	2.4988	3.7402	4.7990	5.5912	6.1359	6.6629	7.1976	7.5730	7.7101	0.500
9	0.5780	1.3164	1.6395	1.9416	2.4175	3.1471	4.4195	6.0311	7.0845	7.5570	2.106
10	1.0037	2.4376	3.5515	4.6367	5.4456	6.1646	6.7004	7.2793	7.9352	8.1890	0.570
CV	0.175	0.179	0.213	0.232	0.225	0.196	0.138	0.075	0.057	0.135	

Index: social class (o) = 100

	0-4	5-9	10-14	15-19	20-24	25-9	30-39	40-49	50-59	60+ Before	Relative decline
0	100	100	100	100	100	100	100	100	100	100	100
1	132	132	134	138	138	134	126	114	117	146	68
2	115	114	117	122	121	118	116	110	112	130	82
3	107	106	108	113	113	110	107	103	110	151	84
4	124	121	125	130	129	123	117	110	111	94	72
5	135	133	138	144	142	134	123	109	113	131	56
6	154	151	163	174	175	164	147	127	123	137	50
7	134	127	128	133	131	125	119	109	109	150	67
8	161	157	169	177	175	162	143	121	118	133	41
9	91	83	74	72	75	83	95	101	111	131	175
10	157	153	160	171	170	162	144	122	124	142	47

Social class: 1951 English census categories[c]

											CV
I	0.6313	1.5632	2.1700	2.6211	3.0874	3.6341	4.4673	5.6545	6.2675	6.9146	1.157
II	0.7484	1.5899	2.6680	3.3836	3.9881	4.5987	5.5448	6.6620	7.3546	7.7514	0.969
III	0.8755	2.1560	3.2173	4.1645	4.9712	5.6031	6.3054	7.1430	7.5981	7.1295	0.715
IV	0.9746	2.3556	3.4956	4.4861	5.2989	5.9113	6.5123	7.1795	7.6818	8.0000	0.600
V	1.0170	2.4752	3.7128	4.7906	5.5958	6.1519	6.7081	7.3141	7.7218	8.5714	0.527
CV	0.168	0.189	0.185	0.203	0.202	0.181	0.139	0.090	0.074	0.078	

Index: social class I = 100

I	100	100	100	100	100	100	100	100	100	100	100
II	119	102	123	129	129	127	124	118	117	112	84
III	139	138	148	159	161	154	141	126	121	103	62
IV	154	151	161	171	172	163	146	127	123	116	52
V	161	158	171	183	181	169	150	129	123	124	46
Total	0.8778	2.1543	3.1827	4.0712	4.8151	5.3866	6.0483	6.7864	7.2835	7.6065	0.667

a Registrar-General's original social-class grouping used for the 1911 census: (I) professional, clerical, higher white collar; (II) proprietors, mercantile, lower white collar; (III) skilled manual workers; (IV) semi-skilled manual workers; (V) unskilled manual workers; (VI) textile workers; (VII) miners and mine workers; (VIII) agricultural laborers

b Occupational classification used for the 1950 U.S. census: (o) professional and technical; (1) agricultural (except laborers); (2) managers, officials, proprietors; (3) clerical and kindred workers; (4) sales workers; (5) craftsmen, foremen, etc.; (6) operatives; (7) service workers; (8) laborers; (9) miscellaneous; (10) agricultural laborers

c Registrar-General's social-class grouping used for the 1951 census: (I) professional occupations; (II) intermediate occupations; (III) skilled occupations; (IV) partly skilled occupations; (V) unskilled occupations

CV = coefficient of variation (standard deviation divided by the mean)

Source: England and Wales, 1923, tables 30 and 35. All categories are based on reaggregations from the 190 nonoverlapping male occupational groups in the census. Hence parities for the 1911 social-class groupings will be slightly different from those in the census itself.

census. Briefly, the social-class categories for the 1911 census are (I) professional, clerical, and higher administrative; (II) proprietors, mercantile, commercial, farmers, and lower administrative; (III) skilled manual workers; (IV) semi-skilled manual workers; (V) unskilled workers; and the three special categories (excluded from the other categories) of (VI) textile workers, (VII) miners and mine workers, and (VIII) agricultural laborers. This scheme has been much criticized, and it was considerably modified for subsequent censuses. W. A. Armstrong has characterized it as "the wholesale assignment of occupations to social classes in a rough and ready way" (1972, p. 203), and both he and J. A. Banks have proposed use of the Registrar-General's 1951 census scheme (Armstrong, 1972, passim; Banks, 1978). Among other criticisms are the separate treatment of the last three occupation groups (textile workers, miners, and agricultural laborers) and various seemingly arbitrary classifications, such as placing business clerks in category I, above proprietors in category II. Simon Szreter (1984, esp. p. 540) has severely criticized the continued use of the Registrar-General's stratification categories based almost solely on occupation, particularly on the grounds that the scheme had been developed precisely to accentuate differences in fertility across groups. In addition, the true skill composition of such aggregations can be quite variable, complicating comparisons across countries. But because there is little consensus as to what should replace it, the original scheme, its 1951 replacement, and the more extensive and functional 1950 U.S. Census categories have been used in table 10.1 (and in tables 10.2 and 10.4). Nonetheless, it must be borne in mind that these are really occupational groupings without a solid underlying theoretical rationale for a characterization as social classes.

The 1911 census originally presented its results tabulated by the eight social-class categories. The recategorization of the data into the 1950 U.S. Census and 1951 Registrar-General's schema is possible because the published volume provided detailed listings of parity and child survivorship by marriage duration (and marriage age) for 206 husband's occupations or occupational groups.[5] When adjusted for duplication or overlap, this number is reduced to 190 groups. Although not all occupations and couples were thus covered, about 88 percent of the women used to tabulate the eight social classes in the original census are represented in table 10.1.[6] The detailed occupation listings from the 1950 U.S. Census and the work of J. A. Banks were used in mapping occupations into the new categories. In brief, the 1951 English social-class categories are (I) higher administrative and professional; (II) other administrative, professional, and managerial; proprietors; (III) clerks, shop assistants, personal service, foremen, skilled workers; (IV) semi-skilled workers; and (V) unskilled workers. The modified 1950 U.S. Census occupation categories are (0) professional and technical; (1) agricultural, excluding laborers; (2) managers, officials, proprietors; (3) clerical and kindred workers; (4) sales workers; (5) craftsmen, foremen, etc.; (6) operatives and kindred workers; (7) service workers; (8) laborers; (9) miscellaneous; and (10) agricultural laborers. In addition to average parities by marriage duration cohorts, all the groups are indexed to the highest social-class group (1 for the 1911 and 1951 English schema and 0 for the 1950 U.S. categories) within each marriage duration group (Graham, 1980; Banks, 1978).

Looking at women married in the 1850s and 1860s and comparing them to women married from 1871 to 1896, it is quite apparent that class fertility differentials had begun widening for the cohort marrying in the 1870s and that this widening peaked for the cohorts marrying between 1886 and 1896. It is difficult to make inferences for women marrying after 1896 because many were still bearing significant numbers of children. Furthermore, this phenomenon of widening class differentials is not obscured by the use of different social-class categories. Indeed, reorganizing the data into the more compact 1951 Registrar-General's social classes actually enhanced the phenomenon. Differentials across classes were actually wider, especially in the middle period when the relative gaps widened. This robustness of the results when alternative stratification schemes are used is very encouraging because it points to the strength of the underlying phenomena. Calculations of the relative decline in average completed parity between women married in the 1860s and those married from 1891 to 1896 reveal the largest declines among the highest socioeconomic groups (i.e., professionals, managers, clerical workers) and lowest among the least skilled manual workers, coal miners, and agricultural laborers. This phenomenon would produce, of course, widening differentials, because the groups with lowest fertility experienced the greatest relative declines. This may be seen in the second, fourth, and sixth panels of table 10.1, which index all average parities to those of Group I, or the professional and technical group (for the 1950 U.S. categories).

To help substantiate this impression, the data in table 10.1 and the underlying 190 disaggregated occupational categories were statistically analyzed. Most of the detailed results are reported elsewhere (Haines, 1989). In table 10.1 the coefficient of variation (the standard deviation divided by the mean, labeled CV) is given for each marriage-duration cohort for each of the three alternative social-class groupings. This statistical measure of dispersion showed that standardized variation across social classes or occupational groups increased from the oldest marriage cohorts and reached a peak among women married in 1891–6. For the most recent cohorts, variation was smaller but fairly stable. (Not too much should be inferred for the cohorts married less than 15 years, because many of these women were still having significant numbers of children.) The same set of calculations was performed for the 190 disaggregated occupational categories, and the same pattern emerged – greater variation in more recent marriage-duration cohorts.

An ordinary least squares regression analysis was performed on these data (Haines, 1989). The dependent variables were average parities for the 190 detailed husband's occupational groups for each marriage-duration category.

The independent variables were a series of categorical (dummy) variables for social classes to which each occupation was assigned. These regressions can clarify how well social class categories alone can "explain" (in a statistical sense) the variation in average parity across occupation groups. The summary measures were the R^2 value adjusted for degrees of freedom, which gives the proportion of variation in parity across occupation groups accounted for by the regressions, and the F-ratio, which gives a measure of goodness of fit. In general, simply knowing the social-class group of an occupation allowed one to account for half or more of variation in parity (within marriage duration cohorts), with the exception of the oldest cohorts – those married before 1871. Both the adjusted R^2 values and the F-ratios notably declined as one moves further back before the 1880s. This suggests (a) that social class was a good predictor of differential fertility, even for the most recent marriage cohorts with largely incomplete fertility, and (b) that this predictive power declined markedly for couples married before the 1870s, when period fertility rates began their decline. Overall, the statistical analysis substantially confirms the phenomenon of widening social-class and occupational fertility differentials during the decline. Again, the choice of these various stratification schema made little difference to the outcome.

The theme of social-class differentials during the English fertility decline was explored at greater length by J. W. Innes in 1938. He reviewed the evidence, both from vital statistics and retrospective reports from the 1911 census, and also added an analysis of London districts of varying socio-economic levels and composition. The conclusions were roughly the same as Stevenson's: an inverse correlation between fertility level and socioeconomic class or status and divergence of the differentials over the late nineteenth century. Subsequent work by Innes (1941), using vital statistics cross-classified by occupation of husband, seemed to show some convergence between 1921 and 1931, particularly for the large category of semi-skilled workers. He created a special subclass for clerical workers and noted that that group had had the greatest decline of all.

The issue of convergence of the differentials in the twentieth century was disputed by W. A. B. Hopkin and John Hajnal (1947), who argued that the statistical basis for this result was unclear. Although fertility *levels* for all socioeconomic groups had declined, vital statistics for 1939 and the use of alternative stratification schemes did not indicate much convergence. The 1939 data they used were of a rather different sort, however, being based on births by parity and not simply on overall period fertility rates.

More recent evidence has been provided by the 1946 family census, which was a 10 percent random sample of all married women in Great Britain taken when wartime ration books were exchanged. According to the retrospective reports of women in this census, it was clear that fertility had declined across all social classes and occupational groups, but the inverse association between social class and fertility remained. The gap between manual and nonmanual workers seemed to have remained constant with about 40 percent higher fertility among manual workers. Some anomalies did appear, however, with nonmanual salaried employees (largely clerks) having the lowest fertility and employers and self-employed nonmanual workers (excluding agriculture) having fertility above that for clerks and professionals (Glass and Grebenik, 1954, pt. 1, pp. 106–11). By the time of the 1961 census (which also asked for retrospective reports on children ever born), it was still true that intermediate and junior nonmanual workers had the lowest fertility and that self-employed professionals had higher birth rates. But now skilled manual workers had fertility very close to that of employers and managers. So, although the inverse gradient of fertility for unskilled, semi-skilled, and skilled manual workers still prevailed, the pattern had become less clear. Nonetheless, "despite these rather confusing differences, it looks as though... a broadly similar pattern of social class differentials to the traditional one is to be found in family-building amongst those married at 20–24 and still relatively young at the time of the 1961 Census" (Kelsall, 1967, p. 57). Thus the differentials that existed, and widened, in the late nineteenth century continued right up into the middle of the twentieth century, albeit at substantially lower levels of fertility.

Recent interest in the historical decline of fertility and mortality in England and Wales has produced a substantial amount of work. In particular, Robert Woods and his colleagues have been examining the changes in fertility, nuptiality, and mortality since the middle of the nineteenth century, using a variety of sources (Woods and Smith, 1983; Woods, 1985, 1987; Wood and Hinde, 1985). Woods's view is that, although differences in marital fertility clearly existed in the late nineteenth century across occupations and social class, there was little change in relative positions. Virtually all occupations experienced a decline in marital fertility together. An explicitly "diffusionist" view is rejected (Woods, 1987, pp. 287–90). An alternative perspective is provided in the work of J. A. Banks, who has maintained that there were "pioneer" groups in the upper and middle classes who, in general, preceded the working classes in the timing and extent of control of marital fertility in late Victorian England (1954; 1981, pp. 97–116). In one sense, this is a question of fact. The widening of differentials is at least consistent with a diffusionist hypothesis, although it is also consistent with other explanations. On the other hand, virtually simultaneous decline among all social classes and occupations would cast any diffusionist position into serious doubt. The results for England and Wales are, at least, consistent with the diffusionist hypothesis.

Similar results can be observed historically for some other nations. The pattern of widening differentials earlier in the process of fertility decline seems to have been true for Japan in the twentieth century (United Nations, 1973, p. 100) and for the United States in the late nineteenth century (Sallume and Notestein, 1932; Kiser, 1933; Grabill, Kiser, and Whelpton,

1958, pp. 180–82), although in both cases convergence seems to have followed. A number of censuses for various countries (including France, Norway, Sweden, Germany, Italy, Denmark, and Canada) report parity for women by occupation of husband (United Nations, 1953, pp. 87–8). Broadly similar results on differentials in levels of fertility may be observed, but the issue of changing differentials during the fertility transition has yet to be explored in most of these cases. (See tables 10.2–10.7 for evidence from several of these nations.)

Table 10.2 details average parities for different social-class groupings for women of different marriage durations for the United States in 1900. The parities were calculated from tabulations made from the public-use sample of the 1900 U.S. Census (Graham, 1980). This sample was taken from the original enumerators' schedules and consists 101,438 individuals. From the file of individuals, women were matched to their children and also to characteristics of their husbands and households. Of importance is that this census asked questions on children ever born, children surviving, and duration of current marriage.[7] These parity data were not published, but the existence of the public-use sample allows retabulation of the results in a way comparable to, and consistent with, those from the 1911 Census of Marriage and Fertility of England and Wales.

These retabulations are summarized in table 10.2. Only the 1911 English and the 1950 American social-class schema were used.[8] These tabulations are based on the records of 15,881 adult women who had borne 59,077 children. These were currently married women with husband present, for whom children ever born, children surviving, and marriage duration were known, for whom children surviving or own children present did not exceed children ever born, and for whom children ever born plus two were less than the number of years married. Some of these selection criteria were instituted to eliminate remarried women, because the census reported only duration of current marriage and, for remarried women, duration of current marriage is not a good proxy for exposure to risk of childbearing. The results for women married more than 50 years (i.e., married in 1850 and earlier) were based on very small cell sizes and were largely ignored. In additional, table 10.2 also presents results for the large subsamples of white and native white women.

It is to be noted that differentials in completed family size across occupational groups in the United States did exist well back into the nineteenth century. The differentials were not always of the same type, however, as found in England and Wales over roughly the same era. For the United States in 1900 there was, for example, not a smooth upward gradient in family size from category I to category V. This was particularly due to the high fertility of farmers (1950 U.S. occupational category 1), who had been placed in the 1911 English social-class category II. At this time farmers in the United States were more likely to have been family proprietors with modest-sized holdings, still becoming integrated into the market economy.

In contrast, England's farmers had a greater representation of larger, market-oriented renters and owners. Among the manual classes (III–V) in the United States, fertility gradients were not always clear or monotonic, although this was less likely to have been true among the most recent marriage cohorts. Relative declines (from the marriage cohorts of the 1850s to those of 1880–85) did, however, tend to reflect greater fertility reductions among the highest socioeconomic groups – professional and technical, clerical workers, and sales workers – but *not* among nonagricultural proprietors. The lowest rates of relative decline were found among farmers, craftsmen and foremen (skilled manual workers) and agricultural laborers. Calculation of coefficients of variation for the 1911 English social-class groupings in table 10.2 for various marriage duration cohorts did not reveal an increase followed by a decrease in variability as marriage duration rose. But there was such a curvilinear pattern for the 1950 U.S. occupational groups. This suggests that the latter may indeed have better reflected the occupational and class structure of the United States in the late nineteenth century. This curvilinear pattern was even more pronounced for white females. Thus there is evidence of widening occupational and class fertility differentials during later stages of the American fertility decline.

One of the problems with studying the American experience at this time is that the fertility decline had been under way since the late eighteenth or early nineteenth century. One might expect convergence rather than divergence of occupational and class differences in fertility after prolonged experience with family limitation. Further, there exists the issue of rather significant ethnic, racial, and regional differences in fertility levels and rates of decline. For example, blacks (except those in urban areas) had higher fertility than whites, while the family sizes of foreign-born white women exceeded that of native white women. The South had higher fertility and slower rates of decline than the Northeast or the Midwest (Tolnay, Graham, and Guest, 1982). In consequence, the results for native white women in table 10.2 are perhaps most meaningful.

One study that partially circumvents some of these problems is that of Sallume and Notestein (1932), which used a special sample of the manuscripts of the 1910 U.S. Census. The 1910 census also asked questions on children ever born, children surviving, and marriage duration. The sample consisted of more than 100,000 once-married women with husbands, present. Both husbands and wives were native white with native parents, and all lived outside the South. The nonagricultural occupations were sampled from 33 cities with populations between 100,000 and 500,000, while farm owners were sampled from the rural areas of 74 adjacent counties.

These tabulations, presented in table 10.3, are based on the experience of 24,526 women aged 45–69 in 1910 and use wife's age rather than marriage duration to identify cohorts. Although only four occupational categories were used by Sallume and Notestein (professional, business, skilled workers, and

Table 10.2 United States, 1900: average parity by social class and marriage duration (all ages of women)

	Years of marriage									Relative decline
	0–4	5–9	10–14	15–19	20–24	25–9	30–39	40–49	50+ Before 1850	1850–85
	1895–1900	1890–95	1885–90	1880–85	1875–80	1870–75	1860–70	1850–60	Before 1850	
Total Population										
Social class: 1911 English census categories[a]										
I	0.7222	1.7630	2.7508	3.2570	3.6512	4.2262	4.3519	5.7250	5.4286	0.431
II	0.9647	2.5964	3.8929	4.9889	5.8438	6.5185	6.5926	6.7719	6.6377	0.263
III	0.8601	2.0493	3.3363	4.2780	5.1617	5.7112	5.2069	5.4684	6.4444	0.218
IV	0.9109	2.3014	3.5779	4.5191	5.0299	5.3433	5.6232	6.3409	6.3333	0.287
V	0.9044	2.4881	3.7953	4.8500	5.3895	6.3197	6.4146	7.0833	7.3333	0.315
VI	0.8378	2.0930	4.5294	3.6667	6.5556	3.7500	5.2000	–	–	–
VII	0.9600	2.8148	4.3966	5.6486	6.5909	7.0714	9.2500	9.2000	–	0.386
VIII	0.8800	2.6142	3.7742	5.1356	6.0426	6.4000	5.8378	6.4545	9.0000	0.204
NC	0.8429	2.0615	3.2128	4.8649	4.9545	5.3158	4.6827	6.1111	6.5405	0.204
CV	0.083	0.141	0.141	0.162	0.163	0.192	0.228	0.419	0.607	
Index: social class I = 100										
I	100	100	100	100	100	100	100	100	100	100
II	134	147	142	153	160	154	151	118	122	61
III	119	116	121	131	141	135	120	96	119	50
IV	126	131	130	139	138	126	129	111	117	67
V	125	141	138	149	148	150	147	124	135	73
VI	116	119	165	113	180	89	119	–	–	90
VII	133	160	160	173	181	167	213	161	–	–
VIII	122	148	137	158	165	151	134	113	166	47
NC	117	117	117	149	136	126	108	107	120	47

Social class: 1950 U.S. census categories[b]

0	0.6789	1.7119	3.0366	2.7826	3.7000	2.9429	5.1509	5.2667	5.8000	0.472
1	1.0057	2.6645	4.0228	5.1532	6.0015	6.7152	6.8324	6.9150	6.7368	0.255
2	0.6772	1.9082	2.8223	3.6883	3.8649	4.9364	4.4959	5.1087	4.0000	0.278
3	0.7297	1.8810	2.4026	2.9455	3.5333	4.9524	3.4444	7.8182	—	0.623
4	0.7426	1.7010	2.7867	3.7778	3.6522	4.0625	4.3659	7.2667	3.0000	0.480
5	0.8692	2.0868	3.4733	4.3698	5.4286	5.5808	5.4842	5.6353	6.4706	0.225
6	0.9119	2.3504	3.7471	4.5825	5.5446	5.8816	5.7183	7.4737	6.0000	0.387
7	0.8061	1.9275	3.3281	3.9783	4.0000	5.1290	4.6207	5.0000	6.5000	0.204
8	0.9168	2.5390	3.8536	5.0246	5.4444	6.3235	6.3481	6.5476	7.0000	0.233
9	0.8421	2.1136	2.6905	3.6944	4.0313	4.3182	5.0000	6.8462	—	0.460
10	0.8607	2.5846	3.6630	5.1186	6.0426	6.2083	5.8378	6.4545	9.0000	0.207
99	0.8961	2.0541	3.1132	4.6170	4.7636	4.7222	4.5031	6.1161	6.4906	0.245
CV	0.122	0.156	0.158	0.192	0.208	0.205	0.177	0.148	0.558	

Index: social class (0) = 100

0	100	100	100	100	100	100	100	100	100	100
1	148	156	132	185	162	228	133	131	116	54
2	100	111	93	133	104	168	87	97	69	59
3	107	110	79	106	95	168	67	148	—	132
4	109	99	92	136	99	138	85	138	52	102
5	128	122	114	157	147	190	106	107	112	48
6	134	137	123	165	150	200	111	142	103	82
7	119	113	110	143	108	174	90	95	112	43
8	135	148	127	181	147	215	123	124	121	49
9	124	123	89	133	109	147	97	130	—	98
10	127	151	121	184	163	211	113	123	155	44
99	132	120	103	166	129	160	87	116	112	52
Total	0.8921	2.3346	3.6005	4.5937	5.3308	5.8947	5.8934	6.3842	6.4966	0.280

Table *10.2* (cont.)

	Years of marriage									
	0–4	5–9	10–14	15–19	20–24	25–9	30–39	40–49	50+ Before	Relative decline
	1895–1900	1890–95	1885–90	1880–85	1875–80	1870–75	1860–70	1850–60	1850	1850–85
White Population										
Social class: 1911 English census categories[a]										
I	0.7202	1.7737	2.7771	3.2305	3.6509	4.1506	4.3488	5.7975	5.4286	0.443
II	0.9630	2.4989	3.7581	4.8668	5.6278	6.2679	6.4153	6.6340	6.2500	0.266
III	0.8501	2.0491	3.3730	4.2630	5.1767	5.7135	5.1726	5.4545	6.4444	0.218
IV	0.8846	2.2862	3.4963	4.5136	4.8616	5.1250	5.5606	6.1429	6.3333	0.265
V	0.8924	2.4277	3.8475	4.8241	5.3176	6.1651	6.3446	7.4186	4.5000	0.350
VI	0.8611	2.0930	4.5294	3.3571	6.0000	3.7500	5.2000	—	—	—
VII	0.9796	2.8000	4.3396	5.6286	6.5909	7.0714	9.2500	9.2000	—	0.388
VIII	0.8797	2.4810	3.7742	4.4250	5.8611	5.8500	5.2308	5.2500	—	0.157
NC	0.8167	2.1864	3.0000	4.6452	4.7073	5.4118	4.6505	6.0531	6.3636	0.233
CV	0.084	0.131	0.138	0.169	0.153	0.189	0.236	0.431	0.791	
Index: social class I = 100										
I	100	100	100	100	100	100	100	100	100	100
II	134	141	135	151	154	151	148	114	115	60
III	118	116	121	132	142	138	119	94	119	49
IV	123	129	126	140	133	123	128	106	117	60
V	124	137	139	149	146	149	146	128	83	79
VI	120	118	163	104	164	90	120	—	—	—
VII	136	158	156	174	181	170	213	159	—	88
VIII	122	140	136	137	161	141	120	91	—	35
NC	113	123	108	144	129	130	107	104	117	53

Social class: 1950 U.S. census categories[b]

	(1)	(2)	(3)	(4)	(5)	(6)	(7)	(8)	(9)	(10)
0	0.6762	1.7456	3.0500	2.6769	3.7143	2.7059	5.1538	5.6429	5.8000	0.526
1	1.0039	2.5687	3.8903	5.0275	5.7667	6.4492	6.6547	6.7665	6.2708	0.257
2	0.6774	1.8923	2.8429	3.6776	3.9021	4.9259	4.4959	5.1087	4.0000	0.280
3	0.7182	1.8554	2.4026	2.9455	3.2759	4.9524	3.4444	7.8182	—	0.623
4	0.7500	1.7188	2.7867	3.7419	3.6522	4.0625	4.3659	7.2667	3.0000	0.485
5	0.8526	2.0656	3.4833	4.3648	5.4364	5.5474	5.4537	5.6353	6.4706	0.225
6	0.8834	2.3445	3.6816	4.5414	5.4019	5.7397	5.7183	7.1176	6.0000	0.362
7	0.7792	2.0175	3.6111	4.1190	3.9524	5.2759	4.6667	4.7500	6.5000	0.133
8	0.9275	2.4801	3.8608	5.0184	5.3495	6.0917	6.2733	6.8649	5.0000	0.269
9	0.8491	2.0000	2.6750	3.4706	3.9677	4.3182	4.5625	6.8462	—	0.493
10	0.8571	2.4390	3.6066	4.0000	5.8611	5.5000	5.2308	5.2500	—	0.162
99	0.8769	2.1818	2.9130	4.4146	4.5577	4.7400	4.4845	6.0728	6.3673	0.273
CV	0.123	0.138	0.153	0.185	0.204	0.198	0.172	0.156	0.666	

Index: social class (0) = 100

	(1)	(2)	(3)	(4)	(5)	(6)	(7)	(8)	(9)	(10)
0	100	100	100	100	100	100	100	100	100	100
1	148	147	128	188	155	238	129	120	108	49
2	100	108	93	137	105	182	87	91	69	53
3	106	106	79	110	88	183	67	139	—	119
4	111	98	91	140	98	150	85	129	52	92
5	126	118	114	163	146	205	106	100	112	43
6	131	134	121	170	145	212	111	126	103	69
7	115	116	118	154	106	195	91	84	112	25
8	137	142	127	187	144	225	122	122	86	51
9	126	115	88	130	107	160	89	121	—	94
10	127	140	118	164	158	203	101	93	—	31
99	130	125	96	165	123	175	87	108	110	52
Total	0.8824	2.2723	3.5378	4.4941	5.1713	5.7040	5.7523	6.3054	6.1923	0.287

Table 10.2 (cont.)

	Years of marriage								50+ Before	Relative decline
	0–4	5–9	10–14	15–19	20–24	25–9	30–39	40–49	1850	1850–85
	1895–1900	1890–95	1885–90	1880–85	1875–80	1870–75	1866–70	1850–60		
Native White Population										
Social class: 1911 English census categories[a]										
I	0.6994	1.7470	2.7420	2.9750	3.5480	3.8855	4.0407	4.9821	6.1000	0.403
II	0.9552	2.4620	3.6787	4.7421	5.4384	6.1886	6.2607	6.4433	5.9302	0.264
III	0.8243	1.9525	3.1515	4.0943	4.6776	5.4762	4.5887	4.9245	6.7273	0.169
IV	0.7939	2.1822	3.3424	4.2117	4.0286	5.1548	5.5250	5.1923	6.5000	0.189
V	0.8860	2.2933	3.6271	4.3162	4.9912	5.6471	5.8382	7.6364	4.5000	0.435
VI	0.7500	2.0000	2.7500	4.1667	8.0000	5.0000	4.3333	—	—	—
VII	0.9583	2.6207	4.2414	5.3913	6.5000	5.8889	8.0000	6.5000	—	0.171
VIII	0.8881	2.4348	3.7500	4.1818	6.1538	5.6111	5.5000	5.2000	—	0.196
NC	0.7442	2.0000	2.5667	4.5000	4.5484	4.9048	4.0597	5.3000	6.1364	0.151
CV	0.104	0.125	0.142	0.149	0.249	0.123	0.215	0.417	0.792	
Index: social class I = 100										
I	100	100	100	100	100	100	100	100	100	100
II	137	141	134	159	153	159	155	129	97	66
III	118	112	115	138	132	141	114	99	110	42
IV	114	125	122	142	114	133	137	104	107	47
V	127	131	132	145	141	145	144	153	74	108
VI	107	114	100	140	225	129	107	—	—	—
VII	137	150	155	181	183	152	198	130	—	42
VIII	127	139	137	141	173	144	136	104	—	49
NC	106	114	94	151	128	126	100	106	101	37
Social class: 1950 U.S. census categories[b]										
0	0.6632	1.7500	2.8657	2.6316	3.5128	2.6333	4.7143	5.0909	7.2500	0.483
1	0.9986	2.5201	3.8186	4.8783	5.5695	6.4017	6.5359	6.6048	6.1714	0.261
2	0.6489	1.8509	2.6879	3.5043	3.5948	4.6282	4.1250	4.9143	2.5000	0.287

									CV
4	0.7500	1.7722	2.6066	2.9512	3.6571	3.5238	3.9375	6.6667	3.0000	0.557
5	0.8277	2.0096	3.2872	4.1690	4.9149	5.2754	5.0224	5.0877	6.7273	0.181
6	0.8261	2.2367	3.3636	4.4793	4.9718	5.0976	5.3571	5.0000	–	0.186
7	0.7241	1.7143	3.2222	4.3571	3.8387	5.8500	4.5238	4.5714	7.0000	0.047
8	0.9069	2.2911	3.6806	4.4825	4.9597	5.8852	5.5325	6.7500	5.0000	0.336
9	0.6579	1.9688	2.6774	2.8261	2.9545	4.4667	4.5000	5.7143	–	0.505
10	0.8616	2.4110	3.6792	4.1515	6.1538	5.2222	5.5000	5.2000	–	0.202
99	0.6957	2.0179	2.5278	4.1111	4.4211	4.1176	3.8286	5.2813	6.0000	0.222
CV	0.138	0.137	0.146	0.214	0.233	0.214	0.191	0.132	0.864	

Index: social class (o) = 100

										CV
0	100	100	100	100	100	100	100	100	100	100
1	151	144	133	185	159	243	139	130	85	54
2	98	106	94	133	102	176	88	97	34	59
3	109	101	88	102	91	168	63	124	0	120
4	113	101	91	112	104	134	84	131	41	115
5	125	115	115	158	140	200	107	100	93	37
6	125	128	117	170	142	194	114	108	0	38
7	109	98	112	166	109	222	96	90	97	10
8	137	131	128	170	141	223	117	133	69	70
9	99	113	93	107	84	170	95	112	0	105
10	130	138	128	158	175	198	117	102	0	42
99	105	115	88	156	126	156	81	104	83	46
Total	0.8614	2.2055	3.3920	4.2905	5.5271	5.4778	5.8481	6.0778		0.266

a Registrar-General's original social-class grouping used for the 1911 census: (I) professional, clerical, higher white collar; (II) proprietors, mercantile, lower white collar; (III) skilled manual workers; (IV) semi-skilled manual workers; (V) unskilled manual workers; (VI) textile workers; (VII) miners and mine workers; (VIII) agricultural laborers

b Occupational classification used for the 1950 U.S. census: (o) professional and technical; (1) agricultural (except laborers); (2) managers, officials, proprietors; (3) clerical and kindred workers; (4) sales workers; (5) craftsmen, foremen, etc.; (6) operatives; (7) service workers; (8) laborers; (9) miscellaneous; (10) agricultural laborers

CV = coefficient of variation (standard deviation divided by the mean)

Source: Sample of census enumerators' manuscripts, U.S. census of 1900

Table 10.3   United States, 1910: average parity by occupation of husband and age of wife[a]

	Wife's age					
	45–9	50–54	55–9	60–64	65–9	Relative decline[b]
Children born						
Professional	2,695	2,173	1,526	1,044	751	
Business	5,755	5,071	3,477	2,442	1,293	
Skilled worker	4,318	3,898	2,946	1,652	808	
Farm owner	12,837	12,745	9,566	7,478	4,578	
TOTAL	25,605	23,887	17,515	12,616	7,430	
Women						
Professional	1,072	826	518	354	202	
Business	2,259	1,832	1,126	762	373	
Skilled worker	1,403	1,123	805	444	214	
Farm owner	3,202	3,045	2,227	1,709	1,030	
TOTAL	7,936	6,826	4,676	3,269	1,819	
Average parity						
Professional	2.5140	2.6308	2.9459	2.9492	3.7178	0.324
Business	2.5476	2.7680	3.0879	3.2047	3.4665	0.265
Skilled worker	3.0777	3.4711	3.6596	3.7207	3.7757	0.185
Farm owner	4.0091	4.1856	4.2955	4.3757	4.4447	0.098
TOTAL	3.2264	3.4994	3.7457	3.8593	4.0847	0.210
CV	0.199	0.190	0.152	0.153	0.094	
Index: professional = 100						
Professional	100	100	100	100	100	100
Business	101	105	105	109	93	82
Skilled worker	122	132	124	126	102	57
Farm owner	159	159	146	148	120	30

[a] The sample was of native white women of native white parents who had husband present. The husband was also native white of native parents. They were once married and lived outside the South. The nonagricultural workers came from 33 cities with populations between 100,000 and 500,000 in 1910. The farm owners came from the rural parts of 74 counties adjacent to these cities.

[b] The change in average parity from women aged 65–9 to women aged 45–9 relative to the parity of women aged 65–9

CV = coefficient of variation (standard deviation divided by the mean)

Source: Sallume and Notestein, 1932

farm owners), table 10.3 does indeed point to significant occupational fertility differentials and varying rates of decline. The gradients by occupational groups were in the expected direction, ranging from urban professional and business occupations with the lowest average parity to urban skilled manual workers and to rural farm owners with the largest family size. The relative declines (from the cohort of women born in 1841–5 to the cohort of women born in 1861–5) were largest for professional and business groups and smallest for farmers. Given the direction of the differentials, this would perforce lead to widening differentials. It is confirmed by the CV calculated for the average parities across occupational groups; these show increases from the oldest to the youngest age cohorts. These data, based on larger cell sizes and ethnically and geographically more homogeneous populations, provide much stronger evidence of widening class and occupational fertility differences during the American demographic transition.

The first French census to ask question on children ever born, children surviving, and marriage duration was taken in 1906 (France, 1912).[9] It provided tabulations of parity by broad marriage-duration categories for 126 separate occupational groups. The census itself allocated these occupations into three categories of employment status: owners, manager, employers, and proprietors (*patrons*); salaried employees (*employés*); and workers (*ouvriers*). The detailed occupational groups lend themselves, as in the English case, to recategorization into alternative stratification schema.

These results are found in table 10.4, where average parities by employment status, social class, occupational group, and marriage duration are tabulated. Unfortunately, this census only provided data by very broad marriage-duration intervals (0–4, 5–14, 15–24, and 25 years and over). Furthermore, France, as was the case for the United States, had already by 1906 been experiencing fertility decline for many decades. Hence fertility levels were relatively lower, and differentials absolutely smaller, than in other European nations. So, for example, comparing women with marriage durations 25 years and longer, average parity was 3.74 children per married woman in France in 1906, 5.98 in England and Wales in 1911, and 6.01 in the United States in 1900.

As is clear from table 10.4, there were, expectedly, marital fertility differentials across employment status, social class, and occupation groups by marriage-duration cohort. The category of owners, employers, managers, and proprietors (*patrons*) had consistently higher levels of completed marital fertility relative to salaried employees but not relative to manual workers. Salaried employees showed the highest rates of decline. A difficulty with the *patrons* category is that it comprised a mixture of owner-operator farmers, small-scale tradesmen and shopkeepers, and proprietors and managers of large establishments. Wealth and income likely varied enormously within this group.

When the detailed occupational groups are recategorized into the three different social-class and occupational-group schema, some of these anomalies disappear. For example, farmers (U.S. occupational category 1) exhibited *relatively* higher fertility levels and the lowest rate of decline.

Table 10.4   France, 1906: average parity by employment and social class of husband and marriage duration

| | Years of marriage | | | | | |
	0–4 1901–6	5–14 1891–1906	15–24 1881–91	25+ Before 1881	Total	Relative decline[a]
Employment status						
Owners, employers, managers	0.9369	2.3507	3.2702	3.6951	2.7420	0.115
Salaried employees	0.7294	1.7973	2.5553	3.1319	1.8378	0.184
Workers	0.9383	2.4100	3.6221	4.2213	2.5873	0.142
CV	0.113	0.126	0.141	0.121	0.165	
Index: owners, etc. = 100						
Owners, employers, managers	100	100	100	100	100	100
Salaried employees	78	76	78	85	67	160
Workers	100	103	111	114	94	123
Social classes						
Social class: 1911 English census categories[b]						
I	0.7924	1.9971	2.8792	3.5279	2.2728	0.184
II	0.9152	2.3137	3.2365	3.6747	2.6995	0.119
III	0.8826	2.2097	3.2248	3.8219	2.3466	0.156
IV	0.8912	2.2827	3.4267	4.1400	2.3624	0.172
V	0.9817	2.4570	3.6822	4.2987	2.6859	0.143
VI	1.0553	2.5879	4.0976	4.9576	2.9606	0.173
VII	1.2256	3.0388	4.8151	5.7224	3.1966	0.159
VIII	0.8996	2.4888	3.7522	4.2405	2.7323	0.115
CV	0.131	0.120	0.156	0.158	0.113	
Index: social class I = 100						
I	100	100	100	100	100	100
II	115	116	112	104	119	65

	Col 1	Col 2	Col 3	Col 4	Col 5	Col 6
III	111	111	112	108	103	85
IV	112	114	119	117	104	94
V	124	123	128	122	118	78
VI	133	130	142	141	130	94
VII	155	152	167	162	141	86
VIII	114	125	130	120	120	63

Social class: 1950 U.S. census categories[c]

	Col 1	Col 2	Col 3	Col 4	Col 5	Col 6
0	0.7319	1.8454	2.5674	3.0943	1.9772	0.170
1	0.9792	2.4893	3.4003	3.7062	2.9088	0.083
2	0.8709	2.1207	3.0032	3.6279	2.4392	0.172
3	0.7392	1.8145	2.6071	3.1963	1.8786	0.184
4	0.7282	1.7764	2.5443	3.1194	1.6628	0.184
5	0.8986	2.2527	3.2893	3.9117	2.3963	0.159
6	0.9978	2.4895	3.7973	4.4940	2.6219	0.155
7	0.7625	1.8713	2.7226	3.3048	2.0332	0.176
8	1.0349	2.5951	3.8778	4.4697	2.8678	0.132
9	0.7484	1.8440	2.6339	3.2503	1.4477	0.190
10	0.8996	2.4888	3.7522	4.2405	2.7323	0.115
CV	0.131	0.145	0.164	0.139	0.210	

Index: social class (0) = 100

	Col 1	Col 2	Col 3	Col 4	Col 5	Col 6
0	100	100	100	100	100	100
1	134	135	132	120	147	48
2	119	115	117	117	123	101
3	101	98	102	103	95	108
4	99	96	99	101	84	108
5	123	122	128	126	121	93
6	136	135	148	145	133	91
7	104	101	106	107	103	103
8	141	141	151	144	145	78
9	102	100	103	105	73	111
10	123	135	146	137	138	68

Table 10.4 (cont.)

		Years of marriage				
	0–4 1901–6	5–14 1891–1906	15–24 1881–91	25⁺ Before 1881	Total	Relative decline[a]
Social class: 1951 English census categories[d]						
I	0.7316	1.8201	2.5670	3.1279	1.9621	0.179
II	0.8504	2.0676	2.9060	3.5550	2.3271	0.183
III	0.8571	2.1482	3.1536	3.7805	2.2996	0.166
IV	0.9284	2.4385	3.6647	4.2314	2.6430	0.134
V	1.0491	2.6003	3.9259	4.5942	2.8563	0.145
CV	0.118	0.125	0.152	0.133	0.127	
Index: social class I = 100						
I	100	100	100	100	100	100
II	116	114	113	114	119	102
III	117	118	123	121	117	92
IV	127	134	143	135	135	75
V	143	143	153	147	146	81
France, 1906	0.9057	2.3010	3.2941	3.7396	2.7856	0.119

[a] From marriage duration over 25 years to marriage duration 15–24 years

[b] Registrar-General's original social-class grouping used for the 1911 census: (I) professional, clerical, higher white collar; (II) proprietors, mercantile, lower white collar; (III) skilled manual workers; (IV) semi-skilled manual workers; (V) unskilled manual workers; (VI) textile workers; (VII) miners and mine workers; (VIII) agricultural laborers

[c] Occupational classification used for the 1950 U.S. census: (O) professional and technical; (1) agricultural (except laborers); (2) managers, officials, proprietors; (3) clerical and kindred workers; (4) sales workers; (5) craftsmen, foremen, etc.; (6) operatives; (7) service workers; (8) laborers; (9) miscellaneous; (10) agricultural laborers

[d] Registrar-General's social-class grouping used for the 1951 census: (I) professional occupations; (II) intermediate occupations; (III) skilled occupations; (IV) partly skilled occupations; (V) unskilled occupations

CV = coefficient of variation (standard deviation divided by the mean)

Agricultural laborers (U.S. occupational category 10) also had higher levels and a low relative rate of fertility decline. The CV calculated for each marriage-duration group for the 1950 U.S. and 1951 English stratification schemes show that differentials widened between the marriage-duration cohort of 25 years and over the cohort of 15–24 years. This was also true for the CV computed for the 126 detailed occupation groups.[10] The 1951 English social-class categorization also demonstrated a more regular gradient, with fertility levels rising (within marriage-duration cohorts) from categories I through V and with categories I and II having had higher rates of relative decline in comparison to the manual classes (III–V). Fertility was generally lowest among professional and technical, clerical, sales, and service workers and highest among farmers, agricultural laborers, unskilled manual workers (laborers), operatives, and skilled manual workers (craftsmen, foremen). All this does not deviate from general expectations. For some specific occupations miners (1911 English social-class category VII) in France, as in England and Wales, had high fertility. French miners seem, however, to have experienced a more rapid fertility decline than their English counterparts in this era. In contrast to the English situation, however, French textile workers (1911 English category VI) had high fertility in relation to other occupational groups within France, although they also had relatively rapid decline.

A statistical analysis was performed on the 126 detailed occupational categories given in the 1906 French census similar in nature to that done for the disaggregated groups for England and Wales in 1911. For women married 15–24 and 25 or more years, about 30 to 45 percent of the variance in average parities across occupational groups could be explained by dummy variables for the social-class categories alone, when regressions were done using the unweighted observations. When the observations were weighted (by numbers of children ever born) to take into account the large differences in observations in these individual cells, the amount of the variance explained by these regressions using social-class categories rose to between 44 and 70 percent. In other words, simply knowing the social-class categories of the occupations can explain a great deal about fertility differentials. When the dependent variable was the relative decline in parity from marriage-duration cohort 25 years and over to marriage-duration cohort 15–24 years, these social-class and occupation categories could explain 77 to 92 percent of variation in a weighted regression.[11] Also of interest is the fact that the 1950 U.S. stratification scheme always explained more variation than the two English schema.

To summarize, despite the fact that France had, by 1906, long been undergoing a fertility transition, there is evidence of widening differentials by occupation and social class as the decline progressed. Completed French marital fertility was low by contemporary standards, probably the lowest in the world at that date. But the general pattern of differentials across socioeconomic strata was regular and in the expected direction, once the agricultural population had been properly taken into account. Statistical analysis supported the finding that knowledge of social class or occupational group alone can go a long way to explaining differential fertility and differential rates of fertility decline.

Another source capable of providing clues on this matter is Norway's 1930 census (Norway, 1935). Table 10.5 reproduces the tabulations of average parities for married women by husband's occupational group and rural-urban residence from the censuses of 1920 and 1930. These parities are for women who had been married 18 years or longer and had been married at ages 24 and 25. The basic comparison is the percent change between 1920 and 1930, recognizing that some of the same women who formed the basis for the 1920 calculations would also appear in the averages for 1930. With that in mind, the last three columns of table 10.5 are instructive. The percentage declines from 1920 to 1930 were higher in urban than in rural areas and were lower among fishermen, the agricultural population, sailors, and manual workers in general. Percent declines were greater among clerks, workers in public administration, and maritime officers. Note that the list of occupations in table 10.5 is ranked from highest to lowest by the level of achieved marital parity in 1920 for both rural and urban areas combined (column 2). In fact, there is a reasonable inverse correlation between the level of average parity in 1920 and the relative decline to 1930. This was true for the total and rural populations, but not for urban groups.[12]

The last pieces of evidence are taken from Germany, as reported by John Knodel in his monograph on the German fertility decline (1974). The first German census to ask a question on children ever born took place in 1933, but that census did not report results in a particularly usable form (Knodel, 1974, p. 120). The subsequent census of 1939 did provide useful detail, especially by tabulating the data by various marriage durations above 20 years.[13] This information is given in table 10.6, which lists average parities by marriage-duration groups for women married more than 20 years by size of place of residence, industry (agriculture versus nonagriculture), and occupation of husband (officials and salaried employees; self-employed and family workers, and workers). No greater detail on industry and occupational groups was published.[14]

As may be seen, there was usually a regular progression in average achieved marital parities from workers (highest) to officials and salaried employees (lowest), with self-employed and family workers in a middle position. One exception was for nonagricultural activities in the largest cities (over 100,000 in population), where white-collar employees (officials and salaried employees) and self-employed and family workers were close in level and showed reversals for women married 20–29 years. In general, however, it may be seen that certainly differentials by occupation existed and that these results accord with previous evidence. There was not, however, a

Table 10.5 Norway, 1920 and 1930: average parity by occupation of husband; marriages ≥ 18 years; wives married at ages 24–5

	1920			1930			% decline		
	Total	Rural	Urban	Total	Rural	Urban	Total	Rural	Urban
Fishermen	6.37	6.42	5.82	5.91	5.96	5.22	7.2	7.2	10.3
Agricultural laborers	6.41	6.41	6.63	5.94	5.94	5.11	7.3	7.3	22.9
Farmers	6.30	6.32	6.02	5.78	5.79	5.11	8.3	8.4	15.1
Factory workers	6.07	6.28	5.81	4.89	5.16	4.53	19.4	17.8	22.0
Construction, commerce, etc., workers	5.99	6.47	5.69	5.27	5.70	4.89	12.0	11.9	14.1
Artisans	5.91	6.07	5.77	5.01	5.36	4.62	15.2	11.7	19.9
Seamen	5.66	5.93	5.31	4.71	5.26	4.01	16.8	11.3	24.5
Professional, public administration workers	5.65	5.96	5.41	4.50	5.00	4.14	20.4	16.1	23.5
Subordinate officials, clerks	5.58	5.82	5.17	4.41	4.67	4.03	21.0	19.8	22.1
Proprietors: small industrial and commercial establishments	5.39	5.74	5.16	4.39	4.77	4.12	18.6	16.9	20.2
Maritime officers	5.16	5.22	5.10	4.13	4.26	4.02	20.0	18.4	21.2
Business and commercial clerks	4.94	5.14	4.81	3.89	4.19	3.63	21.3	18.5	24.5
Factory owners, wholesale merchants, etc.	4.82	5.15	4.61	4.12	4.41	3.91	14.5	14.4	15.2
Professional, public administration: self-employed and officials in superior services	3.80	4.12	3.65	3.27	3.35	3.23	13.9	18.7	11.5
Total	6.00	6.22	5.42	5.21	5.53	4.40	13.2	11.1	18.8

Source: Norway, 1935, table 6

Table 10.6 Germany, 1939: average parity in current marriages by industry and occupation of husband, residence, and marriage duration

Size of place	Industry	Occupation	Years of marriage				% decline	
			35+	30–34	25–9	20–24	From 35+	From 30–34
100,000+	A	Officials, salaried employees	3.18	2.57	2.13	1.85	41.8	28.0
		Self-employed, family workers	4.45	3.41	2.97	2.48	44.3	27.3
		Workers	4.66	3.76	3.12	2.66	42.9	29.3
		Total	4.47	3.48	2.96	2.49	44.3	28.4
	N	Officials, salaried employees	3.01	2.40	2.04	1.73	42.5	27.9
		Self-employed, family workers	3.30	2.40	1.98	1.61	51.2	32.9
		Workers	4.03	3.16	2.64	2.18	45.9	31.0
		Total	3.86	2.73	2.78	1.89	51.0	30.8
2,000–100,000	A	Officials, salaried employees	3.96	3.07	2.87	2.48	37.4	19.2
		Self-employed, family workers	5.44	4.51	3.97	3.37	38.1	25.3
		Workers	5.80	4.84	4.29	3.71	36.0	23.3
		Total	5.48	4.52	3.98	3.39	38.1	25.0
	N	Officials, salaried employees	3.73	3.07	2.62	2.23	40.2	27.4
		Self-employed, family workers	4.18	3.22	2.73	2.27	45.7	29.5
		Workers	4.88	4.05	3.49	2.91	40.4	28.1
		Total	4.70	3.57	3.05	2.56	45.5	28.3

<2,000	A	Officials, salaried employees	4.15	3.40	2.93	2.60	37.3	23.5
		Self-employed, family workers	5.42	4.64	4.10	3.52	35.1	24.1
		Workers	6.18	5.38	4.87	4.26	31.1	20.8
		Total	5.52	4.74	4.20	3.64	34.1	23.2
	N	Officials, salaried employees	4.32	3.63	3.17	2.67	38.2	26.4
		Self-employed, family workers	4.89	3.99	3.42	2.85	41.7	28.6
		Workers	5.38	4.62	4.04	3.51	34.8	24.0
		Total	5.16	4.13	3.65	3.16	38.8	23.5
All places	A	Officials, salaried employees	4.01	3.23	2.84	2.48	38.2	23.2
		Self-employed, family workers	5.40	4.59	4.06	3.48	35.6	24.2
		Workers	6.05	5.20	4.68	4.08	32.6	21.5
		Total	5.49	4.67	4.14	3.57	35.0	23.6
	N	Officials, salaried employees	3.44	2.80	2.39	2.03	41.0	27.5
		Self-employed, family workers	4.04	3.10	2.61	2.16	46.5	30.3
		Workers	4.67	3.82	3.27	2.76	40.9	27.7
		Total	4.52	3.35	2.84	2.40	46.9	28.4

A = agriculture

N = nonagricultural industry

Source: Knodel, 1974, tables 3.11 and 3.12, as reported from Germany, 1939

Table 10.7   Prussia, 1882–1924: male marital fertility rates by industry
and occupation[a]

Industry	Census date				% decline		
	1882	*1895*	*1907*	*1924*	From *1882*	From *1895*	From *1907*
Agriculture							
Farm owners, managers, clerks, officials			157	105			33.1
Workers			242	187			22.7
Total	204	203	190	134	34.3	34.0	29.5
Mining, manufacturing, construction							
Owners, white-collar employees			154	70			54.5
Workers			212	112			47.2
Total	224	215	197	99	55.8	54.0	49.7
Mining only (total)	239	276	278	156	34.7	43.5	43.9
Trade, transportation							
Owners, white-collar employees			133	67			49.6
Workers			197	98			50.3
Total	225	201	165	77	65.8	61.7	53.3
Civil service, military, professional							
Total	179	171	139	74	58.7	56.7	46.8

[a] The fertility rates are the number of legitimate births (including stillbirths) per 1,000 married men in each industry and occupation.

Source: Knodel, 1974, tables 3.9 and 3.10

strong pattern of differences in percentage declines (from marriage duration 35 years and over to marriage duration 20–24 years and from marriage duration 30–34 years to marriage duration 20–24 years) across occupation groups. Thus there is little here to support the case for a widening of socioeconomic differentials in Germany.

Additional information for Germany is given in table 10.7, where male marital fertility rates (legitimate births per 1,000 married men) are cross-tabulated by industry and occupation for the dates of the occupational censuses of 1882, 1895, 1907, and 1925 (Knodel, 1974, tables 3.9 and 3.10). The percentage declines in the last three columns of the table are from 1882, 1895, and 1907 to 1924. There were indeed differences in these current fertility rates across industries and occupation. Owners and white-collar employees had lower male marital fertility rates than nonagricultural workers, and, within agriculture, farm owners, managers, clerks, and officials had lower fertility than agricultural workers. Civil service, military, and professional occupations tended to have low fertility, although they were generally comparable to proprietors and white-collar employees in mining, manufacturing, construction, trade, and transportation. The low relative fertility of the agricultural sector overall was due to the preponderance of lower fertility proprietors (owner-operator farmers) within that sector.

Within table 10.7 there is a bit of support for the phenomenon of widening fertility differentials over time. Owners and white-collar employees in mining, manufacturing, and construction had larger percentage declines than workers over the period 1907–24. This was also true in agriculture. But it was not the case for trade and transport. And the group with one of the lowest fertility rates – civil service, military, and professional – did not show as great a percentage decline as did nonagricultural workers (except miners), who had much higher levels of fertility. It is notable, however, that agriculture exhibited the lowest percentage declines in fertility, a fact that has also appeared in the evidence from England and Wales, the United States, France, and Norway. This can be seen for Germany in both the 1939 census data and the male marital fertility rates for 1882–1924.

Overall, then, the German evidence does provide support for the existence of socioeconomic differentials but not much on divergence of the differentials during the fertility transition. It should be kept in mind, however, that the highly aggregated nature of the German occupational categories does not permit a very close examination of the phenomenon, as was the case for the other evidence presented here. In addition, infant and child mortality differentials across occupational groups may complicate the picture, because parents would take child survival into account in their childbearing decisions.

DISCUSSION AND CONCLUSIONS

The data in table 10.1 through 10.7 provide substantial confirmation for the view that social-class and occupational differentials did widen during the early stages of fertility decline in England and Wales, the United States, France, and Norway in the late nineteenth and early twentieth centuries. This result is relatively insensitive to the choice of alternative occupational groupings (of which three were used) to create social-class categories. When multiple-regression analysis of detailed occupational titles was used for England and Wales and for France, dummy variables for occupational group or social class were quite successful in explaining both fertility (parity) differentials within marriage-duration cohorts and also differential rates of decline across cohorts. For several of the cases studied, the CV across occupational groups or social classes also increased substantially more for more recent marriage cohorts. These findings all strongly support the view of increasing differentials during decline and are unlikely to be much changed by either standardization for differential age at marriage nor correction for any biases in retrospective parity reports. Evidence for England and Wales and for the United States does not indicate that differential child mortality by occupation group or social class even largely accounted for the difference in parity.

This returns us to the discussion of the origins of the fertility decline. It appears, for England and Wales, the United States, France, and Norway, at least, that fertility decline was "led" by the middle and upper classes. Social and economic elites apparently did act as leaders in modifying this most basic of activities – human reproduction. In contrast, the agrarian population was slower to change. It must be borne in mind that at least some fertility decline characterized almost all social classes from the earliest marriage-duration cohorts measurable from the retrospective census reports analyzed here. This is, in itself, not unusual, but it was the middle and upper classes that adjusted more rapidly.

The question then arises as to whether this was a new behavior, with innovation diffusing from the middle and upper classes, or whether it was an adjustment to changing socioeconomic circumstances. These results on occupational and class differentials during fertility decline are compatible with both views, and neither can be rejected. The ultimate explanation will undoubtedly include elements from both hypotheses. Prior to the fertility transition, control of overall reproduction was achieved through modifications of nuptiality, either through the age at marriage or the proportions of the population that never married. The basic change in behavior (i.e., control of fertility within marriage) occurred in France and the United States from the late eighteenth or early nineteenth century onwards but only from the late nineteenth century in many other Western societies (including those examined here – England and Wales, Norway, and Germany). If control of marital fertility quickly became the preferred behavior, it was because fertility control through nuptiality was either not sufficient or not desirable (or both). Control of fertility through nuptiality required considerable sacrifice in terms of deferred marriage and family formation by certain individuals, on whom it fell disproportionately. Control of fertility within marriage would require less sacrifice of that sort. It was, in some sense, more egalitarian – available to all if they wished to make the adjustments. Technology and wider diffusion of information about contraception made those adjustments less costly, but it remained for married couples to decide if it was in their interest to have smaller families.

Why then was control of marital fertility not adopted earlier in England and Wales? This is crucial, because it had been in France and the United

States, which were less advanced in terms of structural economic change. It is probably not coincidental that both France and the United States had experienced democratic political revolutions and were dominated by smaller-scale, owner-occupied agriculture. The timing of events in England and Wales seems unlikely to be related merely to changed economic circumstances. The slower economic growth of England and Wales after 1873 cannot fairly be described as a depression. Real measures of prosperity showed continued improvements (McCloskey, 1981). For example, real wages rose by about 34 percent (allowing for unemployment) between 1873 and 1896 (considered the period of the depression) (Mitchell and Deane, 1962, pp. 343–4). The shortage and rising cost of servants affected only a portion of the society. And fertility rates did decline after the 1860s for all groups, just more so among the upper and middle classes. Middle-class families had more economic security at an earlier date, but they also had more variable future prospects (Banks, 1954, 1981). If the wives of business clerks experienced one of the most rapid declines, it may well have been that they sought to emulate the more affluent among the middle class and could not, but they also had a more precarious socioeconomic status. Adjustment of marital fertility was a response to changing ideas and beliefs – that is, control of marital fertility was coming within the calculus of choice for much of the society. In addition, information regarding the technical means of achieving this end came much more in demand. But it was also more socially and economically advantageous to do so, lest couples would not have behaved in this way.

What seems apparent is that newer values, including an emphasis on individual choice and human capital and education, were being formed and diffused across various socioeconomic groups. As this process progressed, the lower middle and working classes ultimately began to reduce marital fertility with the lags observed. People needed a change in their basic outlook to consider substantial control of marital fertility as a possible and worthwhile strategy. The actual lags observed represented an interaction of the spread of these newer ideas, better and cheaper contraceptive knowledge and practice, and changing social and economic advantages (Caldwell, 1982; Schneider and Schneider, 1984). People change for "their own reasons," both material and cultural, which vary by group.

NOTES

1   For England and Wales, see also Teitelbaum (1984, chap. 8).
2   An extensive and critical account of the evolution of the Registrar-General's social stratification schema may be found in Szreter (1984). For other information and views, see Armstrong (1972), esp. pp. 203–5, and Banks (1978).
3   See, for example, Innes (1938); Woods (1985, 1987); Haines (1979), chap. 1; Banks (1981); Preston, Haines, and Pamuk (1981); Watterson (1986, 1988).

4   A number of the potential biases in the use of retrospective reports of parity are discussed in greater detail in Haines (1989). These would include the potential selectivity bias because, in order to report, both married women and their husbands must have survived up to the 1911 census. This is independent of any bias owing to differential under-enumeration. Also, different social groups had different ages at marriage. With such retrospective data, there may be problems of rounding and selective memory, especially for older women and those who had experienced one or more child deaths. Finally, the occupation of husband, the basis for social-class categorization, is not an immutable characteristic and can change with age. Nevertheless, census information on parity can be very useful if it can be shown that the biases are not too serious. This appears to be the case for the censuses used here.

5   England and Wales (1923). Table 30, for women below age 45 at the time of the census, and table 35, for women above age 45 at the time of the census, were combined.

6   The 190 nonoverlapping categories provided data on 5,297,161 women, or 88.1 percent of the 6,014,319 total women for whom information on occupation of husband was available.

7   The 1890 U.S. Census had also asked these same questions, but the original manuscripts were lost in a fire.

8   The reason is simply the great labor involved in recoding the numerous occupational titles. In principle, this could be done, but it would be unlikely to reveal anything unexpected.

9   Unusually the census asked the questions on children ever born, children surviving, and date of marriage of married male heads of household, but it appears to have been an effort at a complete count.

10 The CV calculated across the 126 occupational groups were duration 0–4 years, 0.128; duration 5–14 years, 0.138; duration 15–24 years, 0.163; and 25 years and over, 0.146.

11 The amount of variation explained in the unweighted regressions was much less, only about 3 to 12 percent depending on the categories used. This indicates a very important effect of certain very large categories such as farmers, clerks, agricultural laborers, and common laborers.

12 The zero-order correlations between fertility level in 1920 and the percent decline to 1930 across occupation groups in table 10.5 were total, −0.427; rural, −0.642; urban, 0.215. Spearman rank order correlations of the same variables were total, −0.543; rural, −0.728; urban, −0.068.

13 The 1939 census of Germany includes information on Austria and other territories acquired by Germany just before the outbreak of World War II.

14 Knodel did combine officials with salaried workers and the self-employed with family workers.

I I

Exploring a Case of Late French Fertility Decline: Two Contrasted Breton Examples

Martine Segalen

Two centuries ago, France invented voluntary limitation of births on a large scale: coitus interruptus was practiced not only by noble and bourgeois families but also by peasants. Consequently, from 1800 to 1914 French fertility was reduced by 40 percent. The discrepancy between French behavior and that of other European countries of particularly striking between 1800 and 1880, after which all European countries caught up with France on birth control. In 1835 the French birth rate was 19.5 percent; it was down to 12 percent in 1908, while in Great Britain at the same time it was still at 17.1 percent, and at 20 percent in Scandinavian countries. By another measure, the gross reproduction rate stood at 1.7 in France, 2.34 in England, and 2.15 in Sweden from 1850 to 1859.

This peculiarity, so full of consequences, did not pass unnoticed, and after 1870 *dénatalité* became a strong national, political, and ideological issue, especially in view of the revenge that was to be taken over Germany. How would France be able to win the inevitable war if it had so many empty cradles? Since the 1870s the French family situation has always had to be examined within the specific context of the early fall in fertility and the contemporaneous widespread criticism of the use of birth control to achieve small families, which has been a constant national concern for the past hundred years.

Stressing the French "invention" or "discovery" of birth limitation might sound provocative. Of course, *dénatalité* did not come all of a sudden and at once to all French men and women; it was a differentiated process that occurred amid various groups and with different timing.

The French fertility decline puzzles both demographers and social historians. Sociologists nowadays are at a loss when trying to explain the changes that occurred after 1964, when all European and North American countries, without exception, experienced a sharp fall in their fertility rates.

Despite sophisticated statistical analysis and sociological research, no single satisfactory cause can yet be set forth. When the birth rates for these Western countries started to fall, their divorce rates were still low, their economies flourishing, and their political prospects favorable. If we cannot explain recent changes, how can we account for past ones, for which full information is lacking?

Concerning the end of the eighteenth century, Jacques Dupâquier and Jean-Pierre Bardet set forth the hypothesis of a Parisian influence on peasant cultures, pointing to the fact that the rural areas where birth control was first acknowledged were close to Paris: the Vexin, and lower Normandy. They suggest that this was not caused by the Revolution, but that birth control and the Revolution were both products of cultural changes (Bardet and Dupâquier, 1986). Concerning the nineteenth century, purely demographic hypotheses have been suggested: assuming that the spread of contraception within marriage is accountable for the fall of fertility, Etienne van de Walle suggests that in some areas low birth rates were produced by late marriage and celibacy. In area where marriage occurred at a young age, birth control was adopted early. Accordingly, van de Walle contrasts the case of Brittany with that of the Garonne valley (1986). However, the Breton cases we shall examine are cases of high or very high birth rates produced by marriage patterns other than those described by van de Walle. His hypothesis, although mainly demographic, ties in cultural variables, implicitly linked to household and inheritance patterns.

Elucidating the causes of the fall of the birth rate is not only a contemporary concern. In the nineteenth century Frédéric Le Play attributed it to the Napoleonic Civil Code that ended primogeniture and mandated partible inheritance, which he believed forced peasants to divide their land, leading them to choose to give birth to a single heir (1855). A more systematic investigation of the correlation between inheritance patterns and fertility rates was conducted in 1901 by Alexandre de Brandt: its major finding was that a variety of inheritance patterns still prevailed throughout rural France at the turn of the century, despite a supposedly unified set of laws. It appeared that ancient customary laws were still much in use (de Brandt, 1901). H. J. Habakkuk (1955) and Lutz Berkner and Franklin Mendels (1976) again discussed these possible links: if there is any correlation between inheritance patterns and size of families, it is embedded in a complex set of ecological, economic, and cultural factors. The main difficulty lies with the variety of local patterns that endured throughout the nineteenth century. Van de Walle shows that, in 1901, residents of the three Breton *départements*, together with those of the Massif Central, the upper Alps, and the Savoy, did not practice birth control, whereas residents of the *départements* bordering the Seine valley or near the Gironde estuary did (van de Walle, 1986, p. 44).

Moreover, assessing the diversity of birth rates in France on a departmental basis is too crude. For instance, concerning the Southwest, which has known birth control since the end of the eighteenth century, Agnès Fine (1978) showed that family size was voluntarily limited in the plains of the Gers, in the Tarn and Garonne, and in the valley of the middle Garonne during the first half of the nineteenth century, whereas this limitation occurred only during the second half of the century in the Pyrenees.

The aim of this essay is thus twofold: to contrast two areas of Brittany where different inheritance and household patterns produced different levels in fertility, and to provide insights as to the causes and consequences of fertility decline in specific contexts of community organization. This will bring us to add the unexpected role of the Church in the process of family limitation to the already proposed causes.

THE RELEVANCE OF LOCAL STUDIES: THE BRETON CASE

Investigating the multiple aspects of fertility decline in Europe and particularly in France requires that we turn to local studies. However limited the conclusions we can draw from them, they can at least help us to formulate good questions so that we may understand how demographic, social, and historical changes are enmeshed in the process of birth limitation.

Exploring local cases serves many purposes. First, it highlights the particular mix of innovation and adjustment that went into this major demographic event. Second, it helps illuminate hypotheses on the important issue of timing in its spatial and temporal guises. It is important to emphasize that this study is set within the so-called modernization period after 1870, offering a local version of the general tune. Lastly, case studies should prevent us from imposing our rationality, our categories, and our logic on past cultures. The choices made about having children or limiting births cannot be considered from afar. The general result, observed on an aggregate statistical level, lumps together behaviors that are quite differentiated when observed at a local level. It is only by getting within the local groups' worldviews that changes in attitudes can be understood. "Starting to stop" must be studied in terms of local cultures, as they are embedded in close-knit communities. As Susan Watkins has rightly stated, cultural settings influenced the onset and the spread of fertility decline independently of socioeconomic conditions (1986).

This study of two Breton communities contributes to understanding the complex processes of family limitation. These cases are rather atypical of the general French pattern, because in them a very high fertility level endured until the beginning of the twentieth century. The two areas dealt with are located in Finistère, the westernmost *département* of Brittany (lower Brittany). It has been the most persistent Breton-speaking area (today Breton is still spoken there by people over 60). The *département* was densely populated during the nineteenth century, but in contrast to Côtes-du-Nord and Morbihan (the other two Breton *départements*), there was no out-migration until the 1920s. The two villages compared here are at opposite ends of Finistère and located in two different *pays*, regional divisions based on ethnic criteria. Saint-Jean-Trolimon in Pays Bigouden (south Finistère) is mainly an area of small farming where grain culture and cattle breeding were a common mixed occupation. The sea is dangerous and does not locally provide any resources, save for seaweed used as fertilizer. Fishing developed as a flourishing activity during the 1880s in the southernmost part of the area, providing new local job opportunities (Segalen, 1985).

The other commune studied is Sibiril in Pays Léonard (north Finistère), located west of the "golden belt" of Saint-Pol-de-Léon, which profits from a combination of fertile soils and the climate-moderating influence of the Gulf Stream. There polyculture slowly gave way during the second half of the century to intensive vegetable growing (artichokes, onions, cauliflowers). Sibiril (Pays Léonard) is slightly larger and more populated than Saint-Jean-Trolimon (Pays Bigouden), but both underwent a fairly similar population growth pattern, hovering around 1,000 inhabitants: a sharp increase from the beginning of the nineteenth century to the middle when it reached a kind of plateau; another increase starting at the beginning of the twentieth century; then a fall in the population, which began earlier in Saint-Jean-Trolimon and was much sharper than in Sibiril. This trend will be accounted for later on.

Both communities have been more similar than different, at least regarding ecological factors. Both were small communities by Breton standards (where communities are generally very large and encompass easily more than 2,000 inhabitants settled over a large territory). They both had a scattered habitat; the bourg was nothing more than a crossroad with a few shops around the church, and most economic transactions were conducted in the local regional capitals. People lived on farms clustered in hamlets of two to ten units. The community structure was thus strikingly different from that Jane and Peter Schneider describe for Sicily (see their essay in this volume). Although households were situated hierarchically according to the size of land they farmed, social classes were unheard of. Even the artisans, mainly tailors and seamstresses, belonged to the integrated local culture.

The scattered habitat shaped social relationships in a rather different manner from what was the case among clustered villages or small bourgs where the urban influence could develop. Our close-knit communities were rarely exposed to outside contacts until the second half of the nineteenth century, and national events came into the group chiefly through the mediation of the Church.

DIVERSITY OF CASES WITHIN FINISTÈRE

The Finistère birth rate was one of the highest of all French *départements.* The Finistère crude birth rate was 31.2 in 1851–5. In Saint-Jean-Trolimon (Pays Bigouden) it was 41.6 in 1853–62, and in Sibiril (Pays Léonard) 32.4 during this same period.* Thus in Pays Bigouden the birth rate was greater than the Finistère mean. This rate increased during the second half of the nineteenth century: in Saint-Jean-Trolimon it jumped to 48.1 between 1873 and 1882 and to 32.3 in Sibiril between 1863 and 1872.

We have developed a comparison between these two areas in order to contrast different responses set forth by local systems trying to cope with the problem of what we would describe as overpopulation (although this is probably an ethnocentric view of the question). We start by providing a few demographic figures, inasmuch as they can be tied to agricultural, inheritance, and residence patterns revealing different social systems. These figures show us that the fertility fall did not follow the same timing; because of the contrasting economic settings, further, the disruption that it caused on the household level did not result in the same social reorganization. The Breton examples thus exemplify Michael Hanagan's hypotheses (see his essay in this volume) on the variation of local ecological systems of production and reproduction.

Although the two rural communities display rather similar community and population patterns, there are striking demographic differences. As mentioned earlier, the birth rate was much higher in Saint-Jean-Trolimon than in Sibiril. The sharp decline in fertility took place in Saint-Jean-Trolimon after World War I: the crude birth rate decreased from 42.4 between 1903 and 1912 to 30.8 between 1913 and 1922. In Sibiril the decline occurred earlier, at the end of the nineteenth century. The crude birth rate fell from 31.6 in 1883–92 to 29.4 in 1903–12 and to 20.2 in 1913–22.

Another interesting demographic index is the nuptiality rate. Here again, as could be expected, the rate was much higher in Saint-Jean-Trolimon than in Sibiril, where it appears to be very low, and even to decline at the end of the century. Between 1861 and 1870, for instance, we have 21.4 marriages per 1,000 inhabitants in Saint-Jean-Trolimon, whereas it is only 15.2 in Sibiril. Armand du Châtellier, a nineteenth-century observer, noted this enduring difference, writing that in the Quimper arrondissement (where Saint-Jean-Trolimon is located) there was one marriage for 104 persons and in the Morlaix arrondissement (where Sibiril is located), only one for 126, the lowest rate in Finistère (du Châtellier, 1835–7, p. 23). A comparison of

---

* We are using crude birth rate (births per 1,000 inhabitants) because it is all that is available for these communes.

ages at marriage reveals it to be much lower in Saint-Jean-Trolimon (Pays Bigouden) than in Sibiril (Pays Léonard). Between 1861 and 1870 the mean age at first marriage for Saint-Jean-Trolimon was 25.7 for men and 22.3 for women. In Sibiril comparable figures were 27.2 and 24.9. The high fertility of Pays Bigouden is largely accounted for by the early age at marriage, which does not fit John Hajnal's European marriage pattern (1965). Pays Léonard, on the contrary, fits that pattern of late age at marriage; there it is associated with low birth and nuptiality rates. This is further supported by data about bachelors and spinsters. Absolutely nonexistent in Pays Bigouden, where it was a rule for all to marry, bachelors and spinsters were rather common in Pays Léonard. In Sibiril the census list of 1846 shows that among all men over 30 years of age, 11 percent were unmarried, and among women, 13 percent. This proportion remained remarkably stable throughout the century. In Sibiril marriage was the classical regulator of family size.

Thus if we examine statistical detail we discover striking local differences in population patterns. Statistics lumped together at the *département* level mask important cultural differences apparent at the *pays* level. These specific demographic patterns coexist with the inheritance patterns that again are superficially conceived to be "egalitarian" (Segalen, 1987).

EGALITARIAN: PARTIBLE OR IMPARTIBLE?

Discussions opposing partible to impartible systems have been numerous since 1976, and I shall not try to summarize the debates. Designating an area with a single label, however, is certainly too crude, and it indicates no more about the way a system works than does classifying ethnic groups as patrilineal or matrilineal.

Brittany has always been an enigma to observers. In the *Ancienne Coutume de Bretagne* (the traditional customal of Britanny) egalitarian inheritance was the rule, yet the eldest child was entitled to the choice of his share. Emmanuel Le Roy Ladurie, following Jean Yver's analysis, sees in the Breton areas an example of an egalitarian system associated with a type of "lineage" system, as opposed to the impartible system that prevailed in southern France, which is a system *à maison*, where the residence principle prevails over the kinship principle (Le Roy Ladurie, 1972). The Napoleonic Civil Code was supposedly based on the Breton egalitarian example. However, nineteenth-century observers, whether Breton landlords like Armand du Châtellier or German jurists like Alexandre de Brandt, observed a variety of local systems within Brittany that makes the area unclassifiable. Du Châtellier contrasted the "family customs" (*habitudes de famille*) of the Morlaix (Pays Léonard) and Quimper (Pays Bigouden) arrondissements:

Physical strength being the basic asset of farms, the idea that associating the family with the farm benefits the young farmer who comes of age must have presented itself naturally to the man who lives among the fields. This is why the usage of farms in *consorties* is so often encountered in the Morlaix arrondissement.... As most of the farms of the arrondissement and mainly in the cantons close to the coast are set up as associations between father and sons or sometimes two brothers or even two families that tie themselves together for that purpose, parents' retirement is not widespread....

[In the Quimper arrondissement], household heads have the habit of giving away their farms to their children. All the cantons of the Quimper arrondissements generally reject parcelling the land by giving the farm in its entirety to one of the children, generally the first married child, who will have to repay his co-heirs with cash. The Pont-l'Abbé canton is one of those where the practice is *least* often observed. (du Châtellier, 1835–7, pp. 18, 72)

Whereas du Châtellier was interested in the succession pattern between generations, Alexandre de Brandt stressed the diversity of partitioning patterns, in relation to the various types of economy:

While the type of activities linked to the vicinity of the sea and the vegetable output near the coast enable an egalitarian partition of rural land through inheritance, this is more difficult in the inland because farmsteads are isolated, land is less fertile and production less easy. These facts have resulted in farmsteads being passed along without division....[In the center of Finistère], the splitting of inherited goods is avoided by the continuation of the households between heirs. The privilege of the eldest is, where it stills prevails, so strongly rooted in people's minds that it is not considered as unfair, all the more so because many burdens are attached to it. Brothers and sisters remain on the farmstead in most cases until they find for themselves a chance to become a household head. (de Brandt, 1901, pp. 181, 186)

In the above descriptions we have opposed the Pays Bigouden to the Pays Léonard system, but these differences cannot be ascribed solely to *"habitudes familiales"* as du Châtellier qualifies them but to a number of social, economic, and ecological factors that combine to shape different coresidence, inheritance, and household patterns and eventually fertility rates.

DOMAINE CONGÉABLE AND HOUSEHOLD FORMATION:
THE PAYS BIGOUDEN CASE

In Pays Bigouden land was held under the archaic system of *domaine congéable*, which involved two owners: one of the land itself (a bourgeois or a noble in the nineteenth century) and the other of the *droits réparatoires, édifices et superfices*, house, outbuildings, and the surface of arable land (the farmer). The lease was unstable: the landlord could expel the farmer as if he were a tenant, provided he bought back from him "buildings, surfaces and compensatory rights," as the *notaires* (solicitors) expressed it. To take up a lease, one had to own these rights: thus if a son succeeded his father in a lease, he first had to buy back, with the landlord's permission, the compensatory rights from him. Some farmers had managed to accumulate, at the end of the eighteenth century, a number of those *droits réparatoires*, which they could sublet to other tenants. Upon their deaths, all children could thus inherit one or more of these property rights that were distributed equally among them. This egalitarian system impoverished the wealthiest families during the nineteenth century, but because the land remained within the hands of the families of the original bourgeois owners, the farms as working entities were not divided until much later, as we will see.

However, a difficult problem arose when a farmer owned only the *droits réparatoires* of the farm he was working, which was the most common case in the nineteenth century. In that situation, cash circulated between siblings, within a complicated system of shares, but only one child could succeed his father in the lease. Paradoxically, despite the fact that the number of farms was not expanding, marriages were not prevented, and households could find new niches, as E. Anthony Wrigley calls them (1985, p. 15) – that is, places in which to work and reproduce. It was held to be normal that everybody should marry, and Church influence was great in that local area. The Church criticized celibacy and encouraged young people to marry rather than take the risk of "living in sin." Indeed, there was no illegitimacy. The specific family cycle helped everybody marry and have children – and so increase pressure on the land. People married young, as we have seen, and coresided with their parents for a time until they found a farm for themselves. Each child coresided temporarily one after the other, until the last child generally succeeded the parents. A common household pattern included the household head and his wife, a couple of married children and their offspring temporarily coresiding, plus the younger unmarried children. But this composition was not fixed; the elder married children moved out of the house as they found farms for themselves, and they could be replaced by a younger child and spouse.

But where did people find new farms if the large ones were impartible? Demographic expansion took place through two different channels. The first was the farming of the very poor *palues*, sandy lands by the sea that had been used for communal grazing during the eighteenth century. Belonging to royal or noble estates, they were handed to the townships after the Revolution, and the townships in turn rented them to farmers. The second channel was the practice of oral sublet, which was very much in favor with the *pen-ty* (or end-house) sublet system.

Both practices created numerous very small farming units from which one could move to another location all over the southern Pays Bigouden. Population expansion was thus made possible through high mobility and by the acceptance of a specific category of landholding. We are accustomed to contrasting clear judicial categories of appropriation (ownership versus nonowner-ship); in this area of Brittany, however, history produced many categories between these two extremes. There was the landowner, the leaseholder himself, owner of the *droits réparatoires*, who could sublet to the *pen-ty* tenant with whom he was in the position of owner-farmer. Besides these informal arrangements, which enabled everyone to settle, the local economic context after 1880 facilitated the population increase without out-migration. The development of the fishing industry and its related canning and transportation activities called for manual labor. The poorer laborers went to Le Guilvinec or Penmarc'h on the southern coast of Pays Bigouden to engage in these new activities.

No matter how rigid the landowning system was, it did not impede the family reproduction system, quite in contrast to the case of Pays Léonard. The societal viewpoint was deeply egalitarian in that it provided each child part of a lease, a piece of rights, or a monetary compensation. The result, as we have seen, was low age at marriage and very high fertility rates. Mean number of children ever born to fertile women revolved around eight between 1830 and 1890.

THE SOCIÉTÉ DE MÉNAGE AND THE CELIBACY QUESTION: THE PAYS LÉONARD CASE

In Pays Léonard we find quite a different system, closer to ancien régime social organization. It is as though the Revolution did not take place there. Pays Léonard is dubbed *la terre des prêtres* ("the priests' land"), but it was also that of the *seigneurs* (local noble families), which owned important portions of land throughout the nineteenth century and still do today. But contrary to most of the landowners of Pays Bigouden, who lived in large cities such as Nantes, Rennes, or Paris, these *châtelains* remained on their land. Their local influence was all the more important, as was the influence of priests, who were numerous in the local capital of Saint-Pol-de-Léon, a city of churches and monasteries.

In the mid-nineteenth century three noble estate owners, de Cheffontaines, de Poulpiquet, and Le Stang du Rusquec, each owned more than 100 hectares (not counting their possessions in other communes in the area), which amounts to between 40 and 60 farms, out of a total of 220 farms in Sibiril. These farms were generally the largest in size (more than ten hectares); the rest of the land ownership was scattered among owners who had only 20 hectares each. Le Stang du Rusquec lived in his fifteenth-century castle of Kerouzéré and was the mayor or Sibiril.

The leases were not held under the complicated Pays Bigouden system of *domaine congéable*. They were regular *fermage* leases that were renewed every seven years at Michaelmas (September 29). The owners favored stability, and we have observed through the census lists a characteristic stability of family lines in total contrast with the mobility of Pays Bigouden domestic groups. The other side of the coin, however, was the total blockage of the economic and matrimonial system. The *pen-ty* sublet system was unknown here. As a rule, only two children among the siblings could marry – one who would be inheriting the lease and one who could find a farm through marriage. Moreover, marriage would take place at a much later age than in Pays Bigouden. The birth rate was thus lower because of powerful checks – late marriage and high rate of celibacy.

Genealogies confirmed by interviews show that the eldest son was preferred to succeed in the lease. Farmers' local habits were similar to (or were influenced by) the inheritance pattern of noble families. Farmers imitated the transmission pattern that gave the eldest male the title, and it is said that noble owners preferred not to see the name of the leaseholder change. It was acknowledged that one boy and one girl "go in-law" (*se marier belle-fille*); the other children knew that they would remain on the farmstead unmarried.

The double marriage of two sisters with two brothers or sister-brother/brother-sister marriage was preferred and quite apparent in our genealogical charts. It offered a twofold advantage: negotiation of dowries was easier (without having read Lévi-Strauss, Léonards dubbed this marriage *échange*); also, it was considered that in case of a *frérèche* household pattern, the two couples coresiding on the same farm would get along better than couples who were not close kin (this was believed especially true for wives who would have been strangers).

Young people wanted to marry, and every old spinster or bachelor nowadays can tell a story of a marriage that failed because the expected fiancé(e) had already found a boyfriend and a farm, or because the proposed dowry was too small. Parents made all the decisions, which were not even discussed with the children. This pattern of unquestioning obedience endured until 1960. At about age 27 or 28 the single youth would know that his or her time for marriage was over, the period for attending Sunday outings and dances past; his or her fate would be to work and remain on the farm.

Celibacy was not disparaged. It was believed that marriage brought distress and that bachelors were freer from family responsibilities. Sexuality was definitely foresworn by women (although there are traces of illegitimate births), whereas men could visit prostitutes – not in the local religious capital of Saint-Pol-de-Léon but in the larger city of Morlaix. One woman remembered her uncle saying that he was going "to grieve over his mother's tomb in Morlaix." Another old bachelor was reported to sleep in the stable so that he could return drunk at night or on Sundays without risking his brothers' and sisters' scolding. Generally they were considered to be happier and freer than their married siblings. Besides, in this area where the Church was also a solution for establishing children, and where the wealthier families could boast of having at least one priest or nun among the siblings, the celibate image was associated with education and civilization.

This one-successor system, together with a high rate of celibacy, reminds us very much of the impartible inheritance pattern described in 1855 by Frédéric Le Play for the Pyrenees and in 1962 by Pierre Bourdieu for the Béarn and in other areas of France or Germany later. But these similarities cannot be pushed further because the egalitarian Breton spirit still prevailed, and being a bachelor or a spinster did not entail any deprivation of one's rights. It is said that bachelor uncles and spinster aunts retained their authority over their nieces and nephews, threatening not to bequeath their possessions if they were not obeyed. They were not considered servants, as was the case in the Pyrenees, and they maintained their power and status (Comas d'Argemir, 1987). Aging at home meant being taken care of; many women remember that when they married they were expected to look after the old *tountouns*.

Upon the marriage of the chosen heir, the father/mother and the son/daughter-in-law would be associated in a *société de ménage*, which would give some advantages to the successor and yet protect the wealth of the unmarried children remaining on the farm. The wealth consisted only of movable goods, but given the fertility of the land, this wealth was often sizable.

The goods were said to be "green and dry" (*vert et sec*, or *glaz ha sec'h* in Breton) and consisted of furniture and all domestic items together with crops, farming implements, livestock, and grain stocks. On setting up the *société de ménage*, the old couple would give one-third of it to the married son and wife who were their associates, retaining a third for themselves and giving the last third to the other unmarried children together. This was a perfect example of *indivision*, undivided joint property. The money entering the household from the sale of vegetables or animals would also go into a common purse from which individuals would receive their share according to the percentage held in the *société de ménage*.

If children left the farm to marry and settled elsewhere they could sell their share of the *société de ménage* to the household head through a *cession de ménage* arranged with a *notaire*. So also could the parents upon retiring.

As unmarried children's shares in the *ménage* were well established, so were their rights in the leasehold. There unmarried siblings would also be designated as coresponsible, together with the brother, who was the main leaseholder. The owner would sign an undivided lease (*fermage indivis*) by which all adult children, married or not, would have their share, reserving the largest share for the married head of the household.

The common household pattern associating parents, the eldest son and his wife, their children, and unmarried brothers and sisters continued unchanged, save for births or deaths, for Pays Léonard domestic groups did not experience the constant change in household membership that the Pays Bigouden did. Task allocation was thus much more fixed.

We can contrast the two life cycles, that of Pays Bigouden and that of Pays Léonard. In the former, inheritance took place at the deaths of the parents, thus extending the cycles between new household formation. The cycles were shorter in Pays Léonard. Because parents settled the future of their farm and goods upon the marriage of the eldest child, the destiny of the younger children was more or less determined at that time. Interestingly enough, both Bigoudens and Léonards claimed that their typical cycle was "natural," that there was no other social choice; they therefore believed that it was best.

The Pays Bigouden partible system produced a high fertility level, whereas the Pays Léonard impartible system produced a lower rate. However, household size was rather large in both, averaging around six people. These figures clearly challenge any assertion that egalitarian systems are associated with nuclear households and show that there is no direct relationship between fertility rate and the size of households. What seem to us densely – or even overpopulated – households were obviously not considered so until the 1920s at least. The question is very relevant to the discussion of the causes of changes in attitudes about fertility control: When do people experience the feeling that they are too numerous?

When one examines the farming necessities in terms of labor power, it is quite clear that under both systems the farms were not overpopulated. From the economic point of view at least there was no rationality in curbing births, had this even been thinkable (God sent children and God took them back) or feasible. In a labor-intensive mode of production, children were not seen as a burden; rather, if they survived they were considered as both free hand labor and insurance against old age. In both the Bigouden and Léonard systems, it was the successor's duty to take care of the aging parents after they retired, providing them with food, fuel, clothing, and health care. This is why children were cherished and valued, and why there was no worse curse for a couple than sterility. Informal adoption prevailed freely within families, mainly through the systems of godparenthood.

During most of the nineteenth century, in both areas, there was no "internal" incentive in the partible Bigouden system to curb the number of births; cultural pressure based on the strong influence of the Church (and in Pays Léonard by the presence of noble families in their castles) reinforced the traditional large family pattern.

THE ECONOMIC, SOCIAL, AND CULTURAL SETTINGS OF THE DISCOVERY
OF BIRTH CONTROL IN PAYS BIGOUDEN AND PAYS LÉONARD

As our figures have shown, fertility started falling slowly at the end of the nineteenth century in Pays Léonard, and a sharp decline occurred in both areas after World War I. The emergence of entrepreneurial attitudes and the desire to curb the number of births came together, but one cannot assert that the economic changes induced this societal change. Both changes were part and parcel of the same trends.

The problem of population growth as it is related to birth control is not quite the same in the two systems, because the age at marriage in Saint-Jean-Trolimon (Pays Bigouden) was much lower than in Sibiril (Pays Léonard), where it already posed a check to family extension. It seems, however, that both areas at some point experienced the feeling of "fullness," which induced definite changing attitudes toward family size.

For the Bigouden area only, it is possible to trace the beginning of family limitation as observed through the lengthening of the intergenesic interval between the penultimate and last births. Among the many factors that can be set forth to explain this change are some purely demographic ones (i.e., the fall in infant mortality, which by prolonging the breast-feeding period would prevent a new pregnancy) and cultural ones (such as a change in agricultural techniques that would prevent women from working in the fields and reduce the number of miscarriages). The only sound hypothesis is linked to the age cohorts. Birth limitation first occurred among couples where the man was born after 1870 and drafted into the national army. In France it was after 1872 that all men were obliged to military service. The army was probably a place where men would learn about coitus interruptus techniques. This might support the hypothesis that husbands had to learn how to limit births before joining their wives in desiring and adopting fertility control.

In both the Bigouden and Léonard areas the impetus of fertility decline was bolstered by economic and cultural changes. After World War I both areas opened to the outside world through out-migration. From 1920 to 1960 the local culture worked steadily to integrate elements of modernity within the traditional framework.

The most striking economic change in Pays Bigouden took place near the coast where the fishing and canning industry expanded, offering jobs to the poorer farmers' sons and daughters, who experienced different working conditions (the fishing team for the men, the factory for the women). Moreover, when migrants returned from their first vacations (the most widespread social benefit of the Popular Front) after 1936 they brought back from the city cultural items from such realms as music (the accordion replaced the *biniou*) and fashion (men abandoned the traditional round hat for the worker's *casquette*). Between the world wars a number of stores and cafés opened – places where people talked and exchanged news and ideas. These were spread further through the development of the bicycle, which allowed social intercourse between people of the coast and people of the inland, mainly at dances and football matches.

World War II conveyed to many heads of farmstead households the feeling of their backwardness. Some of them, as prisoners of war, were sent to serve on farms in Germany where they discovered "modern" and "clean" farming. Mechanization had developed slowly after 1930 but spread fast after 1950 with the advent of sheaf-binding machines together with tractors, which made horses suddenly useless. At the very time farms were believed to be backward, a sense of a full outside world was felt. People remember that their main concern was that they "did not know where to go"; there was no more land for expansion and no more jobs on the seashore, where fishing was undergoing a severe cyclical crisis.

In the Pays Léonard modernity came from within, with the growing specialization in intensive vegetable production. Contrary to Pays Bigouden farmers, who were content until the 1960s with the occasional sale of a few calves, Léonard heads gradually increased their market orientation, thus developing entrepreneurial attitudes by taking account of the national and even international markets, competitive prices, and returns on investments. The Pays Léonard had always been more open to external influences, often mediated through the Church: there had been no local costumes; French was more often spoken among peasants; and local traditions of dances had long been overtaken by religious ceremonies. There economic modernity and birth control came together.

In the 1920s the effects of family limitation could be seen. Most families had five surviving children instead of the previous generation's eight. Attitudes within the population toward large families changed as these started to appear as the most marginal and poor. Mrs. R., an 80-year-old woman in Sibiril, explained that she had had six children within eight years of marriage and stopped only because of the death of her husband. Sleeping seven in the same room, she could not rebuff her husband, who was often drunk. She would not scream for fear of waking the children. She thus reluctantly endured successive pregnancies but would have much preferred to limit her offspring.

Birth-limitation methods adopted by the generation born after World War I were both feminine and masculine. Women interviewed nowadays about their mothers observe that the number of births in those times were in the neighborhood of four to six. Having an incentive to limit their offspring and enough authority within the household, women would send their husbands to sleep in the barn or in the room at the end of the corridor. Some women understand now why their fathers were said to be sick – an explanation for their sleeping alone. But men could also use coitus interruptus, called euphemistically "to have a good reverse gear" (*avoir une bonne marche arrière*) or "to know how to blow one's nose" (*savoir moucher son nez*).

THE AMBIGUOUS ROLE OF THE CHURCH

In the 1950s birth control came, paradoxically, through the influence of the Church, whose control was much tighter in Pays Léonard than in Pays

Bigouden, the Léonards being known for their deep faith and widespread religious practice.

Traditionally, the Catholic Church dictated the behavior of couples and taught them that the goal of marriage was procreation. Thus the first obviously successful attempts to limit the size of families ran contrary to Church rules. Any hint of family contraception was condemned by Catholic priests and could bring excommunication. Priests would visit families in which the last child was 24 months old; if no new pregnancy was announced, they would scold the head of the family for "not performing his duty," as has been reported as well among French Canadian priests. Many "missions" were carried on within parishes where priests would interfere boldly in these matters, going so far as to refuse absolution to couples who stopped at only two children. It was said that women would leave confession in tears during these "missions."

Notwithstanding Church condemnation, family limitation began gradually between the two world wars. After World War II the Catholic Church changed its position; it accepted the principle of family limitation in specific circumstances, but only particular methods were tolerated. Ironically, it may be that through the activities of Catholic local community associations, the Church itself became a propagandist for change.

The Jeunesses agricoles chrétiennes (JAC; Young Christian Agricultural Associations) and its female counterpart, the JACF, were created in 1929 but developed primarily after World War II. Their aim was to modernize the entire local society – agricultural techniques, residence, social relationships, and, more generally, worldviews. A true "modernization ideology" was spread within a Christian framework. Chief among the JAC's activities was to organize youth groups' leisuretime. At the parish or regional level youth gathered at regular meetings for festivals, discussion groups, and theater. The Christian movement thus both controlled young people and offered them a place to think for themselves. The organization of young women's associations was particularly new, giving them an outlet for discussion that could not be found within the family, where girls were brought up to obey and not to express their opinions. In the past feminine networks had been those of elder married women. The Church provided adolescent girls a place to exchange information. The JACF also organized visits to Paris for the annual Salon de l'Agriculture. These exhibits provided both symbolic and material signposts of the development of consumer society. Young farmers could see both the most modern agricultural machines and the newest domestic appliances. Modernization was available to the farm and to the home: one of the goals of change was to turn the household into a consumption unit.

Many brochures were circulated and discussed in the JAC youth groups which dealt with the nature of love. They promoted an image of free choice of the mate based on love. Psychological counseling was provided together with information on marriage. At the same time, young men were receiving information on the modernization of agriculture. The effort to modernize both agriculture and social relationships succeeded. The young men who organized the strong farmers' unions of the 1960s and turned the Pays Léonard into a rich belt of intensive market gardening were all trained within the JAC, as were local politicians.

The new attitudes of the Church in the 1950s must be considered within this context. While Pope Pius XI's 1930 encyclical Casti Connubii had forbidden the use of any contraceptive devices, Pope Pius XII tolerated the use of the Ogino and temperature (variations of rhythm) methods. Some widely circulated books such as *Foyers rayonnants* (*Radiant Hearths*) by Abbé Dantec (more than 200,000 copies sold) explained this position. Whereas Dantec's book recalled the traditional position of the Church regarding marriage – that is, procreation – a new emphasis was now set on the importance of "procreation education." This was the key concept: couples were to give birth to as many children as they could bring up decently; their fecundity should be "generous" but also "reasonable." There were three sets of legitimate reasons for limiting births. The first two were medical and economic reasons, including the scarcity of housing. This was a big issue after World War II, when the JAC campaigned for the modernization of agriculture, society, and family – and primarily for the independent housing of young couples. The third set of reasons concerned education. It was agreed that parents could hardly bring up more than five children properly. Couples were given the freedom to decide how many children they believed they were able to bring up as adults. Dantec wrote that "the duty of fertility varies with the various individual possibilities" (1964, p. 41).

The Church thus admitted the principle of family limitation (although the expression was never used as such), but it did not accept any means to reach that goal. Coitus interruptus was still forbidden, and the methods suggested were Ogino and temperature. Thus by enforcing the idea that sexual relationships could take place only during the supposedly infertile times of the feminine cycle, the Church remained faithful to its principles, because these methods are based on periodic continence.

The Church's new attitude toward fertility moved together with a new focus on the sanctity of marriage. As Antoine Prost wrote, "Sexuality gained a new dignity and beauty: it was no longer a shameful instinct that had to be controlled; it was a sign and the very language of love. Pleasure was not culpable among spouses as long as they loved each other and did not use contraceptive methods other than abstinence." Stressing now the importance of the conjugal bond, of conjugal love and happiness within the couple, the Church "advocated as always the large family, but as an extension of conjugal love. The notion of the large family thus changed in meaning: four or five children, not eight, ten or more. The ideal was no longer to reach the limit of natural fertility" (1988, p. 158).

This new doctrine was disseminated either locally (some priests asked the parishioners to "moderate their sexual drives" from the pulpit!) or during prenuptial classes attended by engaged couples to prepare them for their Christian life. These were very successful. Lectures on various spiritual, psychological, or religious themes were given on topics such as the nature of the marriage sacrament or the Christian meaning of conjugal relationships. A doctor in the local capital might give a lecture on the temperature method.

These JAC militants are nowadays 60 years old; a systematic survey of the number of their offspring would reveal the contradictions between the action of the Church and the matter of conscience it posed for many of them. For some the method offered by the Church achieved its goal: to conceive in full conscience, at the chosen time, the children they wanted. They are happy to remember that they had "a thoughtful and accepted" fertility, as opposed to former times when it was "instinctive and endured." Another couple admitted that they first made use of the temperature method, which gave them four children, and then turned to safer techniques, because the number of Ogino babies was well known. Another couple complained that this method was constraining and inefficient. After six children, Mr. C. said that he "did like the others," but not before making sure from his brother, a priest, that these methods did not put him into a position of sin.

In this very religious population, the Church's breach in its secular attitude toward fertility accompanied the desire of young people to limit the size of their offspring, and the JAC activities provided the ideological framework: modernizing agriculture and having smaller families went together. A large 1951 survey taken by JAC militants in all the communes of northern Finistère shows, from a host of data collected on a local basis, that the number of youth exceeded widely the number of empty niches (in terms of farming units). Stories were told of young couples who had had to wait for seven years before they could settle on a farm.

The desire to limit the size of the family had begun in the 1920s, but now in the 1950s it was openly expressed as a means to become modern – and survive. Thus the JAC and the Church initiated a movement that could not be resisted. In Brittany the first contraceptive revolution took place during the 1950s and 1960s. But after 1965 the new generation lost its interest in JAC activities and turned its attention to political action or regionalist movements. The short alliance between the Church and the faithful on the family-limitation issue was broken by the encyclical Humanae Vitae, promulgated by Paul VI during the very years when modern contraceptive methods could first be obtained from local doctors and pharmacists (Léridon, 1987). The local medical apostle of the temperature method was severely criticized in 1965 by fiancés who did not accept his description of what their sexual relationships should be and his stubborn rejection of new chemical contraceptive methods. A second contraceptive revolution began in Brittany after 1965 as couples regulated the number of their offspring within the intimacy of their sexuality and conscience.

In the Pays Léonard area it was in those years that the conditions mentioned by Ansley Coale to set a framework for a demographic change were met: fertility had become "within the calculus of a conscious choice," and "perceived social and economic circumstances" made reduced fertility seem advantageous to individual couples; and besides, "effective techniques of fertility reduction were available" (1973).

FERTILITY DECLINE AND ECONOMIC CONSEQUENCES

Fertility decline, combined with the specific inheritance patterns and agricultural systems, evolved into quite different social patterns in the two areas, as we can judge from the contemporary situation. In Pays Bigouden the outcome was the collapse of agriculture, whereas Pays Léonard reinforced its specialization in market gardening, always more labor intensive.

In Pays Bigouden mechanization, together with decline in fertility and out-migration, developed quickly. While farms were rapidly deserted by horses and men, machines spread even on the smallest ones. The family farm continued to be a production unit, but as of 1950 the paid help that had been so widespread and cheap disappeared along with the *pen-ty* system. Within 15 years hamlets were abandoned and farm units disappeared.

The problem here lies with the inheritance pattern. Farmers had managed to buy their farms after World War I, and as owners they carried on the accustomed partitioning practices. Three generations later, in the 1950s, at the very time that tractors were coming in, farm size had become so small that of the average family's five children none wanted to stay. In this period Bretons turned their backs on their culture and migrated to cities. The countryside was considered too backward; going to the city as a civil servant or a policeman was much preferred. The change in attitudes toward local culture, farming, and birth control were part and parcel of the same reversal of attitudes. The consequence was a steep fall in the number of farms and a total restructuring of the economy on a different basis. Fishing became the main economic resource of this area, while the modernization of agriculture that the farmers remaining on their lands belatedly undertook turned out to be a burden, because of financial changes and problems caused by the surplus within the European Economic Community. The agricultural future of this area, despite the land's fertility, is most uncertain. Saint-Jean-Trolimon had more than 150 farms throughout the nineteenth century and up to 1950; only three or four were left by 1990.

Contrary to Pays Bigouden, where the fertility decline occurred at a time when agricultural activity was stagnant, the fertility decline in Pays Léonard was accompanied by an extraordinarily rapid change in agricultural production. The 1960s saw the expansion of vegetable cultivation, together with the modernization of markets. Instead of being in the hands of merchants, as was the case in the past, the producers organized themselves to control the market and make their own prices. Saint-Pol-de-Léon became an extremely active local market town, and farmers enjoyed a boom. Some estates were sold by noble families to farmers, but an important part of the land was still held under the traditional lease system.

This new affluence can easily be perceived by visitors to the area. Everywhere new houses have been built to accommodate the young generation of farmers who decided to put an end to the practice of intergenerational coresidence. But the counterpart of this buoyant economy is much manual labor.

This labor-intensive activity developed at the very time birth-control methods began to be used and the size of households shrank dramatically. This led to a social reorganization of work. For the time being, help can be expected from four different sources:

1. Because the generation of people born between 1910 and 1930 is still rather numerous, it means that farmers can be helped by parents uncles, or aunts. It is rather strange to find old people working on their knees in the fields, but work here is a virtue, and they would be shocked not to be asked to help. This age group's contribution is bound, however, to disappear within a decade.

2. It is also striking to observe that, nowadays, farmers' wives are required to work in the fields, which was unheard of 50 years ago, when they were more often at home preparing meals. They do unskilled labor, working under their husbands' supervision, but some older women proudly boast of their competence in selecting and picking artichokes.

3. Because family labor is now insufficient and the number of farms has not declined as dramatically as is the case in Saint-Jean-Trolimon, farmers can call on neighborhood teams.

4. Labor teams are hired for summer work; they are composed either of students, young unemployed people, old people who are retired from agriculture or from the navy, or people from very small polyculture farms in the nearby area of Côtes-du-Nord.

The other important consequence in the fertility decline lies in the attitudes of farmers regarding the future: Will one of their children succeed them, and if so which one and when? Some pressure is put on the children, even as young as 11 or 12 years of age, to speak their minds. The situation is thus totally reversed from what prevailed only 50 years ago when there were too many children and not enough places to go. The assurance that a child will take over the farm keeps the parents working ceaselessly to modernize it and to cultivate new fields left by smaller farmers with no successors. Some couples even delay retirement until the time of their grandson's decision and keep on working the farm to hand it down to him.

Nowadays the birth of boys still matters more, even though this is not, strictly speaking, a patrilineal society. Boys have always been more valued than girls; with a large number of children, chances were high that at least one son would be born. If not, a son-in-law would be acquired through marriage. With only two or three children, the birth of a son is more haphazard. Besides, as is the case of many agricultural areas, girls stress that they prefer to receive a good education, find jobs, and marry outside agriculture while boys are expected to take over the farm.

When no children are available to inherit, farmers retire from the struggle; but they will fight to improve output and productivity as long as they see that their 12-year-old son enjoys riding the tractor more than playing football with his friends.

Lastly, and this is a consequence of the changes in the value of farms, inheritance appears more than ever as a critical passage, even though the number of children has been reduced. When a farm is inherited, it is a heavy burden for the successor to reimburse his brother's share, because of the increase in the value of land, equipment, and buildings. Paradoxically, it was much less difficult with many more brothers and sisters in the days of the systems of *société de ménage* and *cession de ménage*.

CONCLUSION

In both Pays Bigouden and Pays Léonard the fall in fertility meant a dramatic change in household size, with various consequences according to the type of economy. But it has also had the consequence, on the larger societal scale, of reducing the kin networks that are so typical of these Breton areas. Considered from the standpoint of a 25-year-old, there are still six or seven great-uncles in the 70-year-old generation, only four to five uncles in the 50-year-old generation, and in his or her own sibling group only two or three. Formerly, the wide kinship network could provide each individual with important help and social identification on a local basis. Nowadays the 45-year-old generation still enjoys these benefits. Many Breton migrants who left for Paris or Nantes plan to retire in their home villages; they have built a house to which they return regularly, and most social interaction takes place within the large kinship network. These networks facilitated out-migration to cities in the 1950s. But the young generation will experience a dramatic change as they cope with much smaller networks. If fertility continues to decline, the support offered by kinship networks may vanish. In the span of one generation these wide Breton kinship networks will shrink to the average size of French ones; many social relationships that were previously mediated through kinship will take place through social channels where class and formality replace long and deep acquaintance and informality.

At the end of the 1980s France had the highest fertility rate among European countries – over 1.8 – even though this figure is inadequate to ensure the renewal of generations. It is one of the countries in which political discussions on depopulation are more frequent and a major issue of public concern and debate. French governments, more than other European ones, have sought means to expand the number of three-child families. The effectiveness of such natalist policies is low because choosing the number of one's offspring is a basic freedom acquired by couples who are not ready to relinquish it, even for the sake of the nation's future. The "logic" of national economics is often contrary to the strategies pursued by families.

It would have been "logical" for Bigoudens and Léonards to limit the number of their offspring a century ago when farm were more difficult to find; it would be "logical" nowadays for Léonard farmers to have large families in order to supply labor and successors. Yet it is the reverse we observe. This is another regional paradox that is counter to the general French trends. After World War II welfare plans were favorable to families and accompanied the baby boom. These measures reached Brittany at the very time when family size was drastically curbed. There was a total contradiction between state policies and local cultural behaviors.

Once momentum was built into fertility decline, it achieved a causal significance of its own. There is no chance that couples and women will return to past behaviors, whatever the state's social or financial incentives. In Brittany as elsewhere in France, much attention nowadays is given to children; they have to be taken to specialized doctors, be taught tennis, dancing, pottery, or football. This is a total reversal of attitudes toward children that prevailed only 25 years ago. An old Breton woman who had borne six children asked a social anthropologist (a woman) about the number of her own children. To the reply that the anthropologist had only one daughter, the old woman exclaimed, "You are not very brave!" This reaction reveals the discrepancy between two worlds.

Our Breton examples show that decisions regarding the size of the family must be examined first from the point of view of the families themselves and that these decisions can never be dissociated from the social and economic contexts in which they are embedded. The complexity of fertility attitudes requires the simultaneous close scrutiny of both family and society.

IV

State and Politics

12

Constructing Families, Shaping Women's Lives: The Making of Italian Families between Market Economy and State Interventions

Chiara Saraceno

A TENTATIVE HISTORICAL AND THEORETICAL FRAMEWORK
FOR UNDERSTANDING THE DECLINE

The fertility decline in Central-North urban Italy occurred within a material and cultural context in which the entire normative and symbolic structure of the family, as well as many of its behavioral patterns, were changing. Since the last decades of the nineteenth century the Italian family, and foremost the urban one – its gender structure, generational relations, and responsibilities – has undergone a complex process of social construction, involving social and cultural agencies, labor-market forces, and the state. This was not a linear and totally intentional process. Multiple forces and processes constructed and shaped the family from within and without; outcomes not only differed for specific family members (men, women, children) and different social groups but also changed over time. What remained constant – and what may be unique to Italy during this period – was the explicit role state interventions played alongside economic and cultural changes. From this perspective, at least three different processes appear crucial in this reshaping of gender and generational relationships within the urban family:

1. State intervention in the area of reproduction, of gender and generational relations, through changes in the marriage law, laws affecting patterns of "growing up" (e.g., compulsory schooling, legal working age), and the development of redistributive measures (social policies). Through these different measures the state not only interfered with individual and

family behaviors, but it strongly contributed to shape social norms and attitudes, a function earlier achieved by local traditions and the Church.

2. Transformations in the labor market linked to the industrialization process and, later, to the development of a service economy. These processes, in fact, involved and promoted changes in family and individual strategies concerning women's and children's participation in the labor force, daughters' and sons' schooling, and so forth.

3. A diffuse cultural redefinition of family responsibilities toward children, therefore, a redefinition of the reciprocal statuses of children and parents, particularly mothers. Partly a consequence of the first two, this last process was also an autonomous one; it had started well before the period under consideration in selected groups of the urban intellectual aristocracy and bourgeoisie (Barbagli, 1988, chap. 8). One of the results of this process was the clear distinction between motherhood and fertility.

These three processes, in their content and in the outcome of their interaction on family-gender-generational relations and cultures, delineated two quite distinct phases: from the late 1870s to World War II and from the late 1940s to the early 1960s. During the first period state intervention was explicit and pervasive. Beginning with the Pisanelli code of 1861, which set the legal framework of unified Italy, adult married males were emancipated from the authority of their male elders, and their own authority over their wives was strengthened. The balance was therefore shifted from patriarchical power to the husband's power. Women were first and foremost defined as wives and mothers, and as such they were excluded from most political and civil rights.[1] This very focus on the importance and responsibility of motherhood, however, gave women motivations to reduce their fertility in the name of the needs of the children they already had and to resist Fascist pressure to bear more children. At the same time, the new role of the state (as employer and as service provider) opened up jobs to young, unmarried women of the middle classes.

During the second period legislation and direct state intervention in family relations played a less important role; instead, changes in consumption patterns, women's increased access to education, and the growth of the (private and public) service sector critically shaped family and individual behaviors and expectations. On the one hand, the "small family" – as an indicator of individual and social responsibility and as a means of achieving a decent standard of living – became a social and cultural norm. On the other hand, women were exposed to contradictory messages: while their full-time homemaking appeared crucial to their families' welfare, new educational and job opportunities opened up more diverse options.

DIFFERENTIAL TRENDS IN THE ITALIAN FERTILITY DECLINE, 1870–1950

In his 1977 study on Italian fertility, Massimo Livi-Bacci pointed out that for Italy as a whole the transition from high to low fertility occurred over a period of about 60 years, beginning at the end of the nineteenth century and ending in the 1950s (1977, chaps. 2 and 3). Succeeding cohorts of women consistently gave birth to fewer children – from about 5.5 children per (married) woman born before 1851 to the 2.3 children per woman born in 1921–5.[2] But, as Livi-Bacci further observed, this phenomenon had a different timing in the various Italian regions: in part of northern and central Italy fertility began to decline right after political unification in the 1860s; in the southern regions the existence of an intentional check on fertility became evident only in the 1930s and sometimes even later, during the 1950s.[3]

As a consequence, the fertility differential – particularly among married women – between the Center-North and the South increased in the period. Almost nonexistent at the beginning of this century, the fertility differential increased by more than 50 percent from the 1930s on. The fertility decline started specifically as an urban phenomenon in the Center-North, directly correlated with the population density: from 1871 to 1901 fertility decreased markedly in the large cities of the North and Center, widening the gap between town and country.[4] In Turin, Milan, Venice, Bologna, and Florence fertility for married women was about 34 percent lower than it was for the nearby rural population. At the same time, in these same towns, the fertility of the cohorts born in 1881–6 was almost one-third lower than that of the cohorts born before 1871 (while in Naples the cohort differential was 6 percent). This urban-rural gap further increased in the following two decades, to be reduced only in the period 1931–51, when fertility started to decline more rapidly in the rural population. In the southern regions, on the contrary, the rural-urban differential was not present: over the whole period fertility declined later, at about the same slow rate in large and small towns, as well as in cities and rural villages (Livi-Bacci, 1977, chap. 3).

Given these great differences in timing and trends, I focus only on the conditions in which fertility first started to decline in the urban Center-North.

THE DIFFUSION OF THE INTIMATE, ASYMMETRICAL FAMILY AS A SOCIAL
AND CULTURAL CONSTRUCT, 1870S TO WORLD WAR II

*The Construction of Dependent Family Members through Civil
and Social Legislation*

The newly unified Italian state focused many legislative measures on the regulation of family relations. This happened in two main directions: the revision and enforcement of the civil code (therefore of the new family law) in all previously politically separate regions and the development of a so-called social legislation aimed at regulating child and female labor.

The national civil code (Codice Pisanelli), approved in 1865 and largely inspired by Napoleon Bonaparte's Civil Code, delineated the family by sex and generation as a hierarchical structure. While adult men were freed from the authority of their elders, women were explicitly excluded from political rights and were expected to submit to marital authority in the name of family unity and of their duties as wives and mothers (Ungari, 1970; Galoppini, 1981).

The civil code, which remained almost unchanged up to 1940, regulated property relations within the family and concerned mostly the bourgeoisie and the artisan strata. Social legislation, starting in 1886, however, addressed the working-class family. Through a series of legislative revisions (culminating in the 1902 child and female labor law, which provoked strong disagreement not only among employers but also within the workers' movement and among feminists), child and female labor was regulated and "protected."[5] Women workers were officially declared minors, and lower pay for women and children, compared with what men earned, was legally established. At the same time, compulsory leave for pregnant women working in factories was introduced, together with a maternity benefit to be paid through the Casse di Maternita (state-managed maternity insurance agencies to which workers contributed).[6] This regulatory system permitted many exceptions, for both children and women, and most women and children (servants, clerks, at-home workers, workers in small artisan workshops, street vendors, shopkeepers, teachers, etc.) did not work in units covered by it and were therefore exploited. Nevertheless, these measures (accompanied also by laws concerning minimum compulsory schooling for children) and the debate they provoked had a great impact in defining the position of women and children not only within the labor force but within the working-class family as well: children were full dependents, but women were both dependents and those responsible for child care and housework. As they placed the marginalization of working women in a context of surplus labor (the ideal organization and division of gender and generational roles for the middle-class family), the laws also tended to extend that ideal to the working class.

Cultural Changes in the Family at the Turn of the Century

These state regulations of gender and generational relations within the family, and their focus on the importance of the family unit and of women's mother role, interacted with cultural changes and trends initiated well before, by the intellectual aristocracy that had supported the independence movement. These changes concerned mainly the new, affective dimension of the conjugal family and the promotion of the mother's role for women. This included an encouragement to breastfeed rather than enlist wet nurses, which in turn might have had the effect of reducing the fertility of women belonging to the upper classes (Barbagli, 1988, chap. 7).[7] During the first decades of the twentieth century these changes became apparent in the working class, whose members often translated them as a workingman's need for a wife who might keep his house and his children, instead of working long hours in a factory.[8]

Within this shifting cultural environment, where the changed family was to become also the privileged locus in which future citizens would be educated, the debate on women's right to education used the language of education for prospective mothers of future citizens and for prospective workers. An increasing number of women gained access to education based on their social role as mothers.[9]

The lower the social class involved in this educational program, the more the housekeeping/homemaking role of mothers was emphasized; being good mothers was equated with being first and foremost good and orderly homemakers. This was particularly evident in the housekeeping schools for women workers and for workers' wives organized within the *villagi operai* (workers' villages), established by paternalist employers in Vicenza, Sesto San Giovanni (near Milan), and other industrial districts. These schools were concerned almost exclusively with careful budgeting and good housekeeping. In them women's training consisted of nothing more than hygiene and regular habits. At the same time, women's role as teachers was extended to educating their husbands as well as their children through a "domestication" and "normalization" of their habits (such as drinking).

In the middle classes, in contrast, women's educational and managerial role as mothers and housekeepers was supported by domestic servants. Even a modest employee's family often had a live-in maid or at least a day servant to help with the heavy chores. Domestic labor was cheap, and servants' rights to space, adequate food, and even pay were fragile.

There was dual stress on children as objects of systematic education and on women as mothers and housekeepers. This constructed the family on the one hand as the responsible agency for good and healthy citizens and workers. On the other hand, it changed the place of children within the family and the life course of the individual adult, particularly the mother. Raising children increasingly required competence, energy, and time, as well as hard work.

Given this context, it is not surprising that the fertility decline in this period is closely associated with level of education. According to Luciano Ciucci and Anna De Sarno Prignano's analysis of retrospective data collected in Italy's 1961 census, the association between low fertility and high education was linear in the cohorts born before 1890; in the succeeding 1900–12 cohorts, however, and particularly in the large cities of the Center-North, the lowest fertility was that of women having a middle-school degree – a rising group in these areas (1974, esp. tables pp. 158–9). For these women, in contrast to better-educated upper-class women, housekeeping and child rais- ing involved a good deal of manual labor, notwithstanding the presence of servant help. And mothers were more liable to be the only persons respon- sible for their younger children's education. Therefore, even though mother- hood was increasingly distinguished from sheer fertility in both groups of educated women, for the less educated (and probably less prosperous) women motherhood and fertility might appear more contradictory: to be a good mother a woman had to bear few children. Cooperation to reduce fertility was probably a policy of middle-class couples, whose living stan- dards, aspirations, and strategies were constantly in tension between the style of living and consumption set by the upper classes, demands for respect- ability and distinctions imposed by a still highly class-conscious society, and the modest means white-collar salaries provided.[10]

Among women with little or no schooling, those belonging to the working class exhibited a declining fertility as well, although to a lesser degree than the middle and upper classes (Livi-Bacci, 1977, chaps. 3 and 6). Interviews indicate that in working-class families at the beginning of the century the new culture of the intimate family and motherhood, as well as of the rights of children, was not widespread. However, changes in legislation concerning child and female labor, and the access to some schooling for children, started to change the traditional framework of gender and generational relations within the working-class family as well: putting very young children to work became less usual and legitimate, and the woman's role as homemaker became crucial for family well-being and respectability in addition to her capacity to earn money if necessary. Unfortunately, there is no available data on fertility by the working status of women. Therefore we cannot say whether the clear, direct linkage between wage work and low fertility that appeared later was already in place during this period. Again, oral history and contemporary evidence about the working class suggest that women working in factories and small workshops were exposed not only to sexual abuse by men but also to sexual information from their women co-workers.[11] Moreover, women's organizations within the labor movement sometimes distributed leaflets giving information about contraception. In this way, women with little education who worked outside the home might be exposed to information that more advantaged women might receive in school or through intimate relations with their husbands.

Changes in Women's Labor-Market Participation

At the beginning of the century, in most large towns of the Center-North, women as well as children had a high labor-force participation rate. As manual workers they worked mostly in personal services, and in the garment-making, textile, paper, and tobacco industries. As professionals they were likely to be teachers, nurses, or midwives.[12] For newly migrated or longstanding urban working-class women, working for pay was part of the traditional family economy, but for many young middle-class women it was both a new necessity and a new option. Insofar as their families did not always have the necessary resources, young middle-class women might take a job to earn a dowry or to support themselves in the absence of marriage. At the same time, the newly unified state opened up jobs to women, particularly in elementary schools, which became compulsory and for which there were not enough trained men (women were already 70.5 percent of teachers in public schools in 1921); the paramedical professions; and the developing national bureaucratic offices.[13] Office work in the private sector also became available to women with some education.

The pattern of women's labor-force participation was somewhat different according to class and occupation. While middle-class women in service jobs (teachers, office workers) usually worked only before they married, and the same was true for servants (except for those who never married), manual workers in industries usually worked until the birth of their first child and sometimes even after; then they quit, although some returned to home work or day service. The consistent proportion of mothers working in factories was made possible by the introduction of measures such as the compulsory maternity leave and the Casse di maternita, as well as by the many initiatives in the area of child care (crêches, kindergartens, and so forth), which individual entrepreneurs or benevolent agencies began organizing at the turn of the century, and which continued into the Fascist regime, albeit within a different framework (Della Peruta, 1979).

During the period considered, there was no clear trend in women's labor-force participation. Scholars do not agree about the meaning of this. The total number of women employed in industries went through a series of declines and recoveries, but it was almost the same in 1936 as in 1911 (when the first decline appeared) (Ballestrero, 1979). The same period saw a significant increase in women's employment in commerce (reaching 28 percent of the total female labor force) and public and private administration (reaching 25 percent) (Pieroni Bortolotti, 1987). In the same period women's unemployment rates began to be higher than men's, and at the end of the 1930s adult women began to exit regularly from the official labor force (Sabbatucci Severini and Trento, 1975). By the mid 1930s an age-related pattern of women's labor-force participation became more firmly established; in all sectors women tended to remain officially in the labor force only when young and until they started their family, although a sizable minority remained longer. At the industrial census of 1936, the activity rates by age were 18.5 percent for girls 10–14, 49.8 percent for women 15–20, 47.2 percent for women 21–4, and 32.9 percent for women 25–44. The mean age at marriage was then 24.9 years.

These data suggest that an increasing number of young middle-class women were for the first time taking paid employment, which before had been only a lower-class phenomenon. At the same time, participation in the formal labor force became less likely for working-class married women.

Did the Fascist Regime Make a Difference?

It is well known that the Fascist regime developed a wide range of social policy addressing the family and particularly women's maternal role in an effort to reverse declining fertility where this process had started and was most visible: in the cities of the Center-North regions, among the new urban middle class and the industrial working class. These measures defined the normal place of adult women as wives and mothers in the home and encouraged both nuptiality and fertility.[14]

Various measures were taken to make the family into a quasi state institution – defining its organization and behavior in terms of the state's political and demographic aim. In turn, the state assumed some responsibility, not only for setting the rules but also for redistributing resources for reproduction.

The ideal family that it was hoped would result from this dual approach (regulation and redistribution) would be not only fertile but based on a distinct division of labor and responsibilities according to sex. Fatherhood and motherhood in particular were defined as different, albeit complementary, roles, with the father bearing the financial responsibility for the family and the mother abandoning any claim to financial autonomy. Marriage loans and tax rebates were given to men (and only men had to pay bachelors' taxes). Family allowances were instituted to supplement working fathers' wages. Even maternity benefits, which the regime at first gradually extended to cover more numerous groups of working mothers, were abolished in 1939. Substituted in their place were the fertility prizes given to fathers, thus clearly indicating that it was not a matter of compensating mothers for lost wages but of sustaining fathers in their role as breadwinners. Only unmarried mothers were entitled to receive directly the fertility prize. The state, however, encouraged them to find and persuade their child's father to marry them through the institution of a dowry.[15] Married women were discouraged from working; firing a woman because she married or after she had a child was not only legal but encouraged (and required in the public sector). Women also found it difficult to obtain higher education: they were charged double fees at the university. Moreover, many professions were barred to them, including some, like teaching in high schools, which previously had been open.[16]

Emerging patterns of fatherhood as well as motherhood within the most stable working class, with the best social security benefits, became the model for its more marginal, less protected sections, as well as the nucleus around which later policies developed.

Many working-class women continued to work – more or less intermittently – because of family needs. But the combined pressure of inadequate social security, low wages, the regime's hostility to married women's work, and its support of the wage gradually made the figure of the (officially) working mother an exception. High male and female unemployment rates following the 1930 economic crisis helped the regime to identify working married women as the cause of men's unemployment. Within the working class, and partly also within the struggling lower middle class, the regime's declaration that "women should go home and stay there" *(le donna a casa)* appeared to satisfy two of men's critical needs: a job and a domestic life. At the same time, it coincided with Catholic teaching. The regime's policy against married women's paid work apparently had its greatest impact on middle-class women, insofar as it disqualified married women from the new jobs and professions within state administration and bureaucracy. These measures, however, apparently did not keep young women from increasingly enrolling in institutes of higher education and applying for jobs in teaching and in the growing clerical and service sector. Even among women of this class who were friendly to Fascism, the regime's policy was debated and sometimes even criticized as a means for protecting men from women's competition.[17] Although they adhered to the sexual division of labor within the family and to the ideology of motherhood as a life job, these women also refused to bear more children. It is paradoxical that precisely that class which most strongly supported the regime – the urban middle class and the petty bourgeoisie – resisted its demographic message. Middle-class women were frequently the target of the regime's denunciations as too educated and too concerned with their own interests and with the welfare of their "small families" (see Meldini, 1975).

At the same time, the lack of social infrastructure and services in many working-class neighborhoods and the hard labor required to support a family in the city, together with the need to supplement meager male wages, made it increasingly likely that working-class married women would keep their traditional pattern of intermittent labor-force participation, responding to family needs.

The only policy specifically addressed to mothers and children – the institution in 1924 of the Opera Nazionale per la Maternità e Infanzia, the welfare agency for mothers and their infant children – contributed greatly to the definition to the duties of women as mothers. Its goal was to encourage numerous and healthy children for the nation and the "race"; its means were clinics and canteens for needy pregnant women and breastfeeding mothers and their children. Mothers were helped only if they agreed to breastfeed (exceptions were made only for medical reasons, and in this case mothers were provided with formula for their babies). Unwed mothers were also assisted, provided that they kept their baby and breastfed it.[18] Through its strong encouragement of breastfeeding, ONMI may have had the unintended consequence of reducing women's fertility.

ONMI also organized crêches for babies of working mothers, to help those who were obliged to work out of family need.

While defining women as mothers, these measures, and the cultural campaign that accompanied them, defined children as possessing needs and rights, for which both mothers and the state were responsible. This too might have had an unintended effect: insofar as it promoted children's needs, the program may have encouraged parents to have fewer of them.

The regime also increased penalties for induced abortion, defining it as an offense not only against morality but also against "the race" – that is, the nation's interest. The same applied to offering contraceptive information and devices. The impact of this strict legislation and the extent of its implementation is ambiguous, although it certainly made the medical and social circumstances under which women made their decisions concerning fertility more difficult.[19]

Other areas of children's experience and family status were affected by state policy in ways that further differentiated them not only by class but also along rural/urban and Center-North/South lines. In 1925 compulsory schooling was increased from 10 to 14 years of age, with different social classes assigned distinctive postelementary schools. Schools were scarce and unevenly distributed across the nation, however; most were concentrated in towns and in the Center-North. Lower-class children, therefore, were able to complete elementary school and to attend some kind of school up to age 14 only if they lived in cities and in the North. Lower-class children in rural areas either quit school altogether or repeated the last grade of elementary school until they reached the legal working age (Bertoni Jovine, 1963). Strategically, this meant that only in cities might a working-class family consider schooling for its children.

While dividing children by social class, the summer and health camps for children indicated the regime's interest in children's health and welfare. They became a resource for families of modest economic means. Although certainly aimed at indoctrination, the regime's measures concerning leisure (Opera Nazionale Dopolavoro, the free-time organization for workers; summer camps for families and so forth) generally constituted for the lower middle class and the stabler section of the working class the first opportunity to develop new consumption patterns, a dimension of domestic and private life beyond that linked to survival and reproduction. Most Italian families did not take a vacation (and this was true up to the 1970s). Many, however, started to do so during the 1930s, through the new regime's programs.

With Fascism, then, the state for the first time intervened systematically in the area of reproduction and domestic life, setting standards and allocating duties as well as certain rights. The motivations for these programs were both political (controlling the working class, attracting middle-class support) and demographic. Ironically, however, with the value they accorded to children's health and schooling, to families, and particularly to mothers' responsibilities and duties, these measures did not promote increased fertility but further motivated parents to devote themselves to their few children. From this perspective, the regime's failure in reversing declining fertility was directly proportional to its success in strengthening the already emerging twin agenda of childhood and motherhood.

THE GOLDEN AGE OF DOMESTIC LIFE: THE 1950S AND EARLY 1960S

The process initiated in the 1920s and 1930s was not culturally interrupted by the materially deprived experiences of war and reconstruction. Those experiences strengthened the appeal of domestic life as the "good life." This ideal was codified in the new Constitution, which declared that the Italian republic "acknowledges the rights of the family as a natural association based on marriage. Marriage is ruled by moral and juridical equality between spouses, within legal limitations established to grant family unity" (Article 29). All political groups adhered, although to different degrees, to this ideal of a family whose unity had to be based on only limited equality between the spouses and on a sexual division of labor (Gaiotti De Biase, 1979).[20]

Women, as wives and mothers, had improvised nutrition and developed survival strategies during the war. They now became concerned with the welfare and consumerism that timidly started in the late 1940s (when the first washing machines and refrigerators appeared on the market) but really developed in the late 1950s and early 1960s, beginning in the Center-North urban areas.

Reconstruction and Economic "Boom": An Uneven and Unequal Process

Parallel to the industrial reconstruction and economic recovery, the 1950s witnessed an unprecedented development in domestic technology and consumer goods; electricity, running water, washing machines, and refrigerators gradually penetrated the middle-class urban homes of the Center-North, changing the way domestic chores were performed. (They also introduced new needs and temporal planning for domestic appliances bought on the installment plan.) Given the still widespread poverty in Italy in the period, these phenomena deepened inequalities among regions and between social classes. A 1958 survey showed that 84 percent of Italian families did not have a refrigerator or a washing machine – goods that became an almost universal part of a household appliance package in Italy in the early 1970s (Luzzato Fegiz, 1956; D'Apice, 1981; Cacioppo, 1982).[21] Acquiring the domestic amenities available to the urban middle class became a cherished goal for many women. The concentration of industries in the North and the unequal economic development among Italy's various regions caused high rates of internal migrations, which continued into the 1960s. The social and cultural composition of cities like Turin and Milan changed greatly, which created social tensions among different groups, put pressure on urban services and schools, and increased costs for migrant groups. But it also sparked a mass resocialization process, both from rural to industrial work habits and from rural to urban family living and standards.[22] School attendance spread, and an educational level beyond elementary school gradually became a prerequisite for obtaining a minimally decent job even at the manual level. Children remained in school in higher numbers. This trend eventually lead in 1963 to unification of the different existing types of post elementary middle school. The school, therefore, became an important institution in relation not only to children but to family organization and values concerning children's education and behavior.

Along with the school, two other agencies became an increasingly important element in the shaping of domestic life and particularly women's roles. The first was the medical profession, through the extension of statutory health insurance. Doctors became the main interlocutors of mothers on the proper way of raising children – from feeding to deciding if and when to send them to a kindergarten. Urban women were almost all giving birth in the hospitals by the late 1940s. This experience exposed them to some kind of medical advice and screening, eventually integrated by ONMI services (which existed well into the 1960s) for those who had no access to a family pediatrician.

The second agency was the media. Radio listening and movie going were very popular in the 1930s: the regime had both used them skillfully and promoted their use (Mussolini's speeches were broadcast over loudspeakers in all Italian schools and in the central square of all cities and villages). In the late 1950s television appeared: many families, especially those with modest economic means, bought a TV before a more costly washing machine. And people who did not have a TV would go to cafés, parish houses, and relatives' and neighbors' houses to watch the most popular programs. Television not only constituted a kind of new domestic hearth, but it was a powerful means of mass socialization about consumer goods and behavior. Individuals and families learned through TV commercials about the new consumption patterns and life-styles to which they could aspire (Calabrese, 1975; Bimbi, 1985; Pitkin, 1985). Women began to hope for the nice house, the washing machine, the floor polisher, and the vacuum cleaner they saw on TV.

In the meantime, with or without these wonders, women worked diligently to construct a good domestic life for their families, struggling with limited budgets. It is now agreed that "occupation housewife" was the single female occupation that increased during the 1950s and 1960s, during which time a maximum number of adult women devoted themselves to full-time homemaking (Balbo, 1976; Zanuso, 1983). The standard of living that urban working- and middle-class families achieved in that period was due both to men's increasing real wages and to women's intensified domestic work (occasionally integrated with paid work in the informal or black economy). At the same time, in the more developed areas of Italy women's participation for at least part of their life in the regular labor market of industrial and particularly service work continued.[23]

While state intervention was crucial in helping economic development, social policies contributed very little to bettering family welfare. Social services were scarce and almost nonexistent for the elderly, infants, and handicapped persons. Child care and schools were organized in such a way (i.e., half-day attendance and no cafeterias) that a mother was needed at home to prepare the midday meal. Even workers often went home for the midday meal (many still do). Women's family work was therefore pivotal for their families' well-being. At the same time, the weakness of the public sphere in providing services and in setting standards and priorities strengthened the focus on families' private consumption, strategies, and interests (Balbo, 1976).

Conflicting Messages

The process by which "occupation housewife" emerged as the normal career of adult married women was neither linear nor unambiguous. The 1950s, which are often defined as a period of political and cultural conservatism, actually concealed tensions that eventually prepared the way for the social changes of the 1960s and 1970s (Gaiotti De Biase, 1957).

The mass of women, particularly urban women, were intensely socialized in this period to their "natural role" through messages addressed to them by women's magazines, family doctors, social workers, teachers, and media. In these messages the equation between motherhood and homemaking was obvious and direct. In those directed to more educated women, however, an effort had begun to distinguish and emphasize, in terms of values and gratification, the relational, affective dimension of motherhood rather than the housework one. This massive effort was variously supported by promises of "qualification" and "professionalization" of the homemaker role, through both the new domestic technology and access to bits and pieces of the "expert" culture. It resulted in an identification of women as pivotal not only in family care and children's education but in deciding what the family's economic strategies should be in a world where consumerism was becoming increasingly complex. Women became the "family consumers," as advertising agencies readily understood. Some scholars went so far as to interpret this in terms of women's emancipation (i.e., Ardigo, 1964), whereas the Church was at least ambivalent in its judgment of the impact of consumerism and economic improvements on family living (Ginsborg, 1989, pp. 327–8).

At the same time, old barriers to women's education were slowly being dismantled and formerly all-male professions were integrated by law: that is, while the adult world became, ideally and practically, increasingly divided along the family-home/work line, the world of schools became increasingly coeducational, exposing girls and boys to common experiences for longer periods. The same was true for youth associations. Even Catholic youth groups (the last to desegregate) located in schools or in the workplace in the late 1950s started to organize mixed-group membership. New curricula about growing up were developed for women, which pointed to new behaviors and future tensions in adult life.[24]

As the 1960s approached, full-time domestic help became increasingly less available to middle-class families for different reasons: a more sophisticated sense of privacy on the side of both potential servants and potential employees, and the job opportunities opening up in factories and offices for young women of rural, as well as urban, lower-class origin. The result was that for many young middle-class women, who often had a better schooling than their mothers and some work experience in the new professional jobs developing in the tertiary sector, starting a family in the late 1950s and 1960s meant entering full-time homemaking, which included total, or almost total, responsibility for housework. For working-class women, improvements in domestic technology might increase their status as housewives; for their middle-class counterparts, however, it was a dubious substitute for a maid.

The increasing stress on the conjugal, as well as on the mother's role, based on an ideology of domesticity as a protected shelter, also suggested different values and meanings. It led to expectations of reciprocity and equality within the couple, which were further reinforced, especially among the more educated, by shared experiences while growing up. But these expectations contrasted not only with existing family legislation and the rigid division of labor and power but also with the intense involvement of women in motherhood, as work and as a relationship. To have a couple relationship, to give attention to her husband's needs, a woman could not spend her life having and raising children. Catholic culture itself was developing ambivalence in this regard, indicated in the transition from the papal encyclical Casti Connubii of 1930, where the only aim of marriage and sexuality was procreation, to the encyclical Guadium et Specs of 1965, where sexuality was seen as a way of mutual happiness within the couple and the couple relationship was defined to be as important as procreation.[25] Motherhood was also partially changing its meaning and content in social imagery. Economic development, the modest expansion of social services, access to school, and to social security benefits by new social groups provoked public concern over increasing population, particularly in the overcrowded industrialized cities of the North. Increasingly, having "too many" children was equated with being a southerner – ignorant, socially irresponsible, and uncivilized. Of course, well-to-do large middle-class families of the North were excluded from this criticism. Nevertheless, large families became either an indicator of material "heroism" or an indicator of personal and social inadequacy. The problem was widely discussed in the media.

The mystique of motherhood increasingly diverged from the now-disputed value of high fertility, as indicated by the emerging concept/message of "responsible motherhood." In this period, however, information about contraception remained illegal. Women would speak of "Ogino-Knaus [rhythm] children," whisper to each other the name of the priest "who didn't ask," and were occasionally hospitalized for having had a *raschiamento*, the middle-class word for a "d and c" abortion.

Although the needs of working mothers and their children deviated from the ideal family model, they remained an issue that disturbed both Catholic consciences and the political Left. Legislation on maternity leave and benefits was slowly improved and extended to cover higher categories of women workers, and services for children of working mothers were extended, albeit inadequately, and within a social-assistance framework that labeled these children (and their mothers) as somehow deprived and marginalized. Nevertheless, the debate concerning these issues and the measures they provoked prepared the way for the more comprehensive measures of the 1970s, which acknowledged, and to some extent legitimized, the rights of working mothers and their children.

REDUCED FERTILITY: FROM DEPENDENT TO INDEPENDENT VARIABLE?

Increasing numbers of women living in the cities of the Center-North during the 1940s and 1950s lowered their fertility as compared to their mothers, as Italy's retrospective 1961 census data suggested the its 1971 census confirmed (Livi-Bacci and Santini, 1969; Ciucci and De Sarno Prignano, 1974). There was a small baby boom in the late 1950s and early 1960s, but it was mostly due to changed behavior in women under age 25. Women over 25, and especially those over 35, continued to reduce their fertility. Women who had already started childbearing were not affected, either because they had already postponed it during the difficult years of postwar reconstruction or because they were experiencing the difficulty of having both a satisfactory life-style and more than two or three children (Federici, 1984).

Moreover, although new job opportunities allowed many youths to escape family control and to marry young, the larger proportions of women staying in school longer raised the age of marriage above the average (which remained stable around 24) for these groups. Women exposed to increased education were also statistically associated with low fertility. In 1961 women who were completing their fertility and lived in the less-prolific northwestern regions had an average of 1.7 children if they had a middle-class degree, 2.2 if they had an elementary school degree, 2.6 if they had no school degree but were able to read, and 3.3 if they could not read. Similar differences can be found also in higher-fertility regions (Ciucci and De Sarno Prignano, 1974).[26] Fertility decline eventually resumed in all cohorts. Women who had started childbearing at an early age later reduced it sharply.

Research on differential fertility related to women's labor-force position started late in Italy – only in the late 1960s.[27] Married women with children who held regular jobs were a minority. But in this increasing minority there was a linear relationship between full-time wage work and low fertility. Part-time, irregular, and self-employed workers showed a similar but less marked relationship. Only agricultural work seemed not to have a similar impact. The cause-effect direction of this phenomenon is not clear, and probably there is no linear explanation. It is fairly clear that simultaneously holding a regular job and caring for a large family was almost impossible. On the other hand, women who had jobs, especially wage-earning ones, experimented with time and social organization, which can be understood not only as constraints but also as diversifications of their cultural and referential world.

Reduced fertility changed family relations, as well as family and women's life cycles, in homes with full-time mothers, although Italian women continued to experience more scattered pregnancy patterns than their European counterparts well into the 1970s (Federici, 1984, pp. 59–60). The time liberated from pregnancies and caring for very young children was filled with higher-quality housework and child care. Fewer children meant children in whom one might invest more. Increased schooling in all social classes, which started in the 1960s, cannot be read only as an adaptation to labor-market demands; it was also as a strategy of parents, particularly of working-class and often migrant parents, to spare their children the hardships they had suffered when young. This commitment to education meant longer childhood dependence. But fewer children also meant a shorter period of intensive childrearing and full-time homemaking and the reduction of time spent on small children's needs, although other family members continued to demand attention – meals had to be prepared according to different work and school schedules, beds had to be made, clothes had to be washed and ironed. The housework hidden in motherhood and wifehood became increasingly visible. This revelation prepared the way for later feminist analyses.

Increasing women's labor-force-participation rates in the mid 1960s and 1970s were due largely to the cohort of women who, having completed their childrearing years in their mid-forties, were now ready by busy themselves in some other way. They probably had not planned this outcome when they decided how many children they would have. It was rather a decision-in-progress, often motivated by a wish to increase family income or to obtain consumer goods (an apartment, a car, vacations) that were increasingly perceived as necessary for the good life.

Their daughters and other younger women observed the consequences of these women's demographic behavior: a different phasing of the life cycle and an expansion of the family's consumption. This message, together with the new personal independence achieved by many youths in the 1950s and early 1960s, was part of the symbolic world in which young women entering adulthood in the mid 1960s and 1970s faced their family, work, and fertility choices. Having few children was becoming a prerequisite for the life-course strategies of women and families.

NOTES

1 From this point of view, Fascism not only continued a conservative tradition, as De Grand (1977) suggests, but built on this tradition to make the family responsible to the state. On changes in family legislation after Italian unification, see Saraceno (1990).

2 Data are not totally comparable, because up to the 1886–91 birth cohort they refer to marital fertility, while for the succeeding cohorts they refer to total fertility (Livi-Bacci, 1977). I use the 1980 Italian edition (pp. 119–21). See also Livi-Bacci and Santini (1969), pp. 71–224, Ciucci and De Sarno Prignano (1974).

3 Italian political unification under the Savoy monarchy started in 1861. The formerly separated Italian regions were diverse not only in political system and legislation but also in level of economic development and labor-market structures. Family and gender cultures also differed (Barbagli, 1988). In some of the southern regions, such as Basilicata or Apulia, marital fertility declined in the 20 years preceding World War I. But the trend was reversed afterwards. According to Livi-Bacci, this phenomenon may not be explained by the diffusion of a contraceptive culture and practice but by the alteration of the population's sex ratio owing to emigration. Sicily is an exception within the southern regions with regard to the timing of the fertility decline: starting with quite high birth rates (41.4 in 1862–6, compared to a national 36.84 births per 1,000), it showed a continuous decline for over a century, more than halving its rate by 1960–62, although it still remained one of the highest in Italy. (See Jane and Peter Schneider's essay in this volume.)

4 At the same time, Center-North witnessed a much more intense urbanization following political unification. In 1861 towns with 100,000 or more inhabitants held 6.6 percent of the population in the North, 9.1 percent in the Center, and 7.6 percent in the South. A century later the figures were, respectively, 29, 39, and 22 percent. At the 1951 census 55 percent of the northern population was classified as "urban," 51 percent in the Center, and 34 percent in the South.

5 For a review of the debate, see Pieroni Bortolotti (1963), Ballestrero (1979), and Galoppini (1981).

6 On the history of the Casse di Maternita see Piva and Maddalena (1982). Paid maternity leaves at the beginning covered only the four weeks after delivery, and jobs were held for only three months after delivery.

7   On the new patterns of lower fertility in the aristocracy in the second half of the nine-
    teenth century, see Livi-Bacci (1977), chap. 1.
8   See, for instance, the examples quoted in Musso (1988).
9   Various political and intellectual groups were involved in the debate and with initiatives
    concerning women's education. Emerging feminist groups started to advocate a better
    education for girls as a road to economic autonomy and to full citizenship (Pieroni
    Bortolotti, 1963; Franchini 1986).
10 Some turn-of-the-century novels clearly depict the social impasse of this class. See for
    instance *Demetrio Pianelli*, by Emilio de Marchi. See also Scaraffia (1988) on the changing
    gender roles within the family. She uses a great deal of biographical material. To describe
    family cultural behavior, gender, and generational relationships in different social classes
    during the first three decades of the twentieth century (here and on the following pages),
    I also rely heavily on a study conducted by Barbagli of 801 women born in the Center-
    North between 1890 and 1901 and belonging to all social classes, who were inter-
    viewed between 1975 and 1979 (1988, chaps. 8 and 9). Women were interviewed about
    three periods of their life: age 10–12, early marriage, and ten years after marriage. Besides
    using Barbagli's own analysis, I also listened to many of the recorded interviews, which he
    graciously permitted. This and other oral-history material were analyzed in my study of
    working-class families and women's lives under Fascism (Saraceno 1979–80, 1981).
11 See, for instance, Merli (1972).
12 See, for instance, L. Tilly (1992) on Milan (esp. chap. 3). See also Pieroni Bortolotti
    (1963), Passerini (1984), and Guidetti Serra (1977). On Turin, see Maher (1983); on
    tailoresses, see Musso (1988).
13 Women teachers were also paid less than men.
14 For a review of the financial incentives available, see Livi-Bacci (1977), chap. 7.
15 This might even cause divisions among working-class women (Passerini, 1984).
16 Between 1931 and 1936 women declined from 70.5 percent of all teachers in public
    schools to 69 percent. But they increased their presence in private schools (from 65
    percent to 73 percent). See Pieroni Bortolotti (1987).
17 See evidence in De Grand (1976). Catholic young women's associations also developed in
    the 1920s and continued throughout the period, playing an ambivalent role in socializing
    women, insofar as they offered them experiences not solely focused on motherhood (Di
    Cori, 1979; Di Giorgio, 1979).
18 Most ONMI services were located in the cities, although there was an interesting exper-
    iment with "itinerant maternity services" in the rural areas, which taught women elemen-
    tal norms of hygiene and infant and child care. On ONMI see Fabbri (1934) and Corsi
    (1936). Jewish mothers' and children's (as well as fathers') rights were denied with the
    passing of racial legislation and internment in concentration camps.
19 See the study of the Turin Tribunal by Detragiache (1980). The family code approved by
    the regime in 1942 represents the culmination of this juridical construction. There the
    family is a hierarchical unit, with a male head and an economically and socially dependent
    wife and children. Wives' sexual offenses were punished more severely than men's
    (Cardia, 1975; Ungari, 1970). This code provided the juridical framework of family
    relationships for the succeeding 33 years: it was changed only in 1975.
20 On the opportunities (within a context of great risks and suffering) the war period offered
    women, see the testimonies gathered by Guidetti Serra (1977) and Mafai (1987). On the
    different political cultures in postwar Italy, see Ginsborg (1989), chaps. 5, 6, and 7. This
    work offers a good synthesis of recent Italian history.
21 I have written more extensively on these changes in Saraceno (1988).
22 Migrations sometimes caused the resettlement of entire kin networks, sometimes the
    dispersion of the nuclear family, as the father or even both parents moved to the North,
    leaving the children behind with their grandparents.

23 Società Umanitaria (1963), particularly the contribution by Federici, who maintains that since the mid 1950s women's labor-force participation increased in all sectors. It must be noted that during the 1950s there was an enormous diffusion of mostly irregular home work that, if taken into account, would greatly increase married women's labor-force participation rates. The scarcity and unreliability of data on this phenomenon are one of the causes of scholars' disagreements on the interpretation of women's labor-market participation in this period.

24 Piccone Stella (1981) developed this very suggestively.

25 On the evolution of and internal conflicts about the image of the woman within Italian Catholic culture, see Giuntella (1988).

26 See also the analysis developed by Bellettini (1972) on Bologna and Corsini (1967) on Florence with the same set of data.

27 See Bielli, Pinnelli, and Russo (1973); Bielli et al. (1975). See also Federici (1984), pp. 148–57.

13

Demographic Nationalism in Western Europe, 1870–1960

Susan Cotts Watkins

In this essay I show that between 1870 and 1960 national boundaries became more evident on the demographic map of Western Europe. In 1870 demographic behavior was largely local. By 1960 local diversity had diminished substantially, such that demographic behavior was much more uniform. Part of this greater uniformity was due to increased similarity among countries; even more important was an increased similarity among local areas within the same country. Country boundaries, in other words, increasingly distinguished distinct, national, demographic regimes. Although nationalism is usually discussed in political terms, it would appear to have had parallels in the most private of behaviors, births and marriages.

Those interested in demographic behavior in the last century have usually focused their attention on the demographic transition, the major declines in mortality and fertility. Here the question is different. The focus is not *levels* – not why fertility declined – but rather *variation*: With respect to their demographic behavior, how different were groups in 1870? How different were they in 1960? And what might account for the change?

Examining changes in demographic diversity leads directly to questions that have been at the heart of sociological inquiry at least since Emile Durkheim – questions that have to do with social integration (or its absence). Moreover, although the demographic data used here refer to aggregates rather than individuals, the demographic changes described appear to contradict the accounts of demographic behavior based on models of individual actors absorbed in cost-benefit calculations. Rather, as Granovetter (1985) has argued more generally for economic behavior, demographic behavior seems to be firmly embedded in social institutions; in particular, it seems to

Portions of this essay were previously published in "From Local Communities to National Communities," *Population and Development Review*, 16, no. 2 (1990), 241–72.

have responded to macro-level changes such as the integration of national markets and state formation (called by Charles Tilly the two great process of the modern era [1981, p. 44]) as well as to nation building. Here I present the evidence that led me to title this essay "Demographic Nationalism" and to conclude that demographic integration accompanied economic, political, and cultural integration – in short, that demographic integration reflects social integration.

I begin with the data and measures used and proceed to the description that is this essay's core. I try to account for the demographic changes that have been described by examining parallel changes in social institutions. Because the aggregate nature of the data casts an opaque veil over individuals as well as the smaller communities in which quotidien life went on, the correspondence between the activities of markets, states, and nations on the one hand and individuals in their bedrooms and courting parlors on the other is necessarily speculative. This correspondence does suggest, however, intriguing and unusual links between the structural transformations of the last century and demographic behavior.

DATA AND MEASURES

The social groups of interest here are defined spatially. The two levels of aggregation are the country and the province. The countries are the 15 countries of Western Europe. Eastern Europe is excluded because massive boundary changes over the century make precise comparison between 1870 and 1960 impossible. Provinces are *départements* in France, countries in England, cantons is Switzerland, and so on. Although demographic diversity would probably be even greater were smaller units (such as villages or parishes) included, these smaller units are more similar to each other when they are in the same province than when they are in different provinces (Watkins, 1990).

I use two measures of demographic behavior: marital fertility and nuptiality (marriage). Marriage and fertility are conceptually quite different, and the theories developed to explain them have been quite different: that the findings are similar increases the generality of the conclusions. The demographic measures are the indexes developed by Ansley Coale for the Princeton European Fertility Project and were calculated by collaborators on that project.[1] Marital fertility (I_g) is defined as $B_L/\Sigma m(i) F(i)$, where B_L is the number of legitimate births, $m(i)$ the number of currently married women in the population at age (i), and $F(i)$ the age-specific fertility rates of Hutterite women. The fertility of a group is thus standardized by the fertility of the Hutterites, an unusually prolific population. If a population had the same fertility as the Hutterites, it would have an I_g of 1; if all Hutterite women married young and remained married through their reproductive years, they would bear slightly more than 12 children. Nuptiality (I_m) is defined as $\Sigma m(i) \, F(i)/\Sigma w(i) \, F(i)$, where $w(i)$ is the total number of women in the population. I_m is thus a fertility-weighted measure of the proportion married. An I_m of 0.33 means that approximately a third of the women of reproductive age are married. Both indexes can in principle take on values between 0 and 1 (although I_g will be greater than 1 if fertility exceeds that of the Hutterites).

The indexes have three relevant drawbacks. First, they refer to groups defined spatially rather than by occupation, religion, and so forth. I show later, however, that there is reason to believe that the findings would be rather similar. Second, the indexes are rather large aggregates and thus may mask even more local diversity. Lastly, the indexes are summary measures; finer measures of nuptiality, for example, might show different patterns. The indexes are, however, the only demographic measures that can be calculated for all the provinces of Western Europe over this period. They are valuable because they permit a comparative analysis over a long period of time – usually from around 1870 to 1960.[2] I focus on two sets of comparisons. One is a comparison across countries: Which countries are more demographically diverse, and which less? The other is comparison over time: Is diversity greater or less in 1960 than it was in 1870?

I use two simple measures of diversity. The range (the difference between the maximum and minimum provincial values) gives a picture of the extent of diversity in 1870. For comparisons I rely on the midspread, the difference between the upper and lower quartiles of the provincial distribution (or interquartile range), which includes the central 50 percent of the values. I use the midspread rather than the range or the standard deviation as a measure of diversity because it is robust and because it can be relatively easily translated into numbers that have intuitive meaning (numbers of children or proportions married).

FINDINGS

Western Europe in 1870

The extent of pretransition local diversity within Western Europe is shown in Table 13.1. The maximum I_g, in the Flemish arrondissement of Dendermonde in Belgium, is higher than Hutterite standard; the minimum I_g, in the French *département* of the Lot-et-Garonne, is close to the average level for all of Western Europe in 1960. If marriage were early in these two provinces and out-of-wedlock births negligible, the range would be about eight children. The diversity of marriage patterns is also evident. In the southern province of Caceres in Spain, more than two-thirds of the women

Table 13.1   Indexes of marital fertility (I_g) and nuptiality (I_m) for all Western Europe provinces, 1870

	Median	Maximum	Minimum	Range	Midspread*
I_g	0.696	1.052	0.280	0.772	0.121
I_m ·	0.469	0.691	0.271	0.420	0.114

* The midspread is the distance between the upper quartile and the lower quartile.

of reproductive age were married, while in the Swedish *lan* of Stockholm and in Sutherland, in the Scottish Highlands, fewer than one-third were married.

Differences among local communities probably played a part in accounting for these local variations in demographic behavior. Historical demographers often have found that in the pretransition period differences in demographic behavior even among such communities as small villages or parishes were greater than differences by occupational group within these communities (Chaunu, 1973; Knodel, 1988). We can sketch several ways in which the local community might have influenced demographic behavior by examining plausible sources of variation among communities. Let us begin with marital fertility. Studies in both historical populations and in developing countries in which there is little use of contraception show that the duration and intensity of breastfeeding can explain much of the variation in marital fertility, with coital frequency, fetal mortality, and sterility playing lesser roles (Bongaarts and Menken, 1983; Casterline et al., 1984; C. Wilson, 1986). Whether or not women breastfeed seems likely to be associated more with the customs of the community than with individual characteristics. In some nineteenth-century German villages almost all of the women nursed their children for long periods, while in others few nursed for more than a brief time (Knodel and van de Walle, 1967; Knodel, 1988). In the areas of southern Bavaria where the practice of never breastfeeding was evident by the fifteenth century, exceptions to this practice "were subject to severe social sanctions, including ridicule from neighbors and threats from husbands" (Kintner, 1985, p. 168).

What was local about marriage? In Western Europe the age at which women married was largely a function of the age at which couples could afford to set up a new household (Dupâquier, 1972; Hajnal, 1965, 1982). The economic characteristics of the couple were important in the timing of marriage; thus local economic circumstances would have mattered, especially in agricultural communities where bad harvests would have delayed marriage for many. But there is also a role here for the local community. First, young people married those they had met, which means that the marriage market traced their movements. The parish registers consistently confirm the local

Table 13.2   Midspread and median of marital fertility (I_g) and nuptiality (I_m)
by country, 1870

	I_g		I_m	
	Midspread	*Median*	*Midspread*	*Median*
Northwest Europe				
Belgium	0.233	0.846	0.054	0.42
England and Wales	0.036	0.693	0.052	0.501
France	0.185	0.463	0.11	0.551
German	0.158	0.748	0.07	0.467
Ireland	0.031	0.718	0.069	0.386
Netherlands	0.111	0.83	0.051	0.448
Scotland	0.047	0.754	0.063	0.391
Switzerland	0.143	0.747	0.075	0.413
Scandinavia				
Denmark	0.064	0.653	0.043	0.464
Finland	0.153	0.692	0.063	0.504
Norway	0.047	0.767	0.024	0.41
Sweden	0.107	0.706	0.086	0.419
Mediterranean				
Italy	0.049	0.661	0.029	0.563
Portugal	0.065	0.711	0.089	0.471
Spain	0.076	0.667	0.1	0.618
Total	0.121	0.696	0.114	0.469

nature of marriage. In the *département* of Loir-et-Cher, for example, in only 13 percent of marriages between 1870 and 1877 did one of the spouses come from outside the *département* (Courgeau, 1970). In addition, what satisfied the prerequisites for a new household, and thus for marriage, seems more likely to have been defined by the group – community or class, neighbors or workmates – than by the individuals themselves.

Which countries were demographically most homogeneous, which most diverse? Table 13.2 shows the median and the midspread for each country. The rankings with respect to internal diversity on the two indexes are close, although not identical. In general the least diverse countries were those of the British Isles (England and Wales, Scotland and Ireland) and of Scandinavia.[3] The most diverse were usually Belgium, France, Germany, and Switzerland. Differences in marital fertility almost as extreme as those between any two Western European provinces can be found in a single country, Belgium, where (if marriage and out-of-wedlock birth were the same in these arrondissements) the results would be equivalent to a difference of nearly five children – surely a meaningful influence on the way life was lived in these provinces. The differences in Belgium were extreme, but they were approximated in France and in countries contiguous to France.

I am persuaded that the differences in the degree of demographic diversity are not accounted for by the quality of the data or by the varying number of the provinces.[4] Larger countries were generally more diverse than smaller, but size alone does not account for demographic diversity: England, for example, is more homogeneous than its size would predict, and France less. Nor do the differences in demographic diversity appear to owe to differences in the degree of economic development. For example, the Princeton European Fertility Project analyses showed only weak correlations at the provincial level between crude measures of economic circumstances (e.g., urbanization and the proportion in agriculture) and marital fertility at the onset of the fertility transition (Watkins, 1986).

Between 1870 and 1960 both declines in marital fertility and rises in nuptiality were widespread.[5] During a time of change we expect diversity to increase, as some provinces adopt the new behavior before others: thus it is possible that the diversity evident in 1870 was already a departure from a more uniform situation earlier. Only in France had a large number of provinces begun the fertility transition by 1870, and in France rises in nuptiality closely paralleled declines in fertility. Thus the high degree of demographic diversity in France may reflect its earlier fertility transition.[6] In the other countries, however, the midspread is not affected by early fertility decline.[7]

What to me is most striking is that the demographically most diverse countries are, by and large, those that were multilingual in the latter part of the nineteenth century.[8] Belgium was bilingual (Flemish and French); the provincial populations of Switzerland spoke French, German, Italian, or Romansch; in mid-nineteenth-century France, French was at best a second language for a substantial portion of the population, and some local dialects were unintelligible to those who spoke Parisian French (Levasseur, 1889; Weber, 1976). In contrast, English was the dominant language in all the English counties, Dutch in the Netherlands, and each of the Scandinavian countries was largely monolingual.[9] Italy is a puzzle: it is far more demographically homogeneous than the deep differences in dialect would suggest (Ascoli, 1910).

Language and demographic behavior would seem, a priori, to be related. Differences in language or dialect are typically taken by social scientists to be accompanied by other cultural differences (Geertz, 1971; Fishman, 1977; Parsons, 1975; A. D. Smith, 1986). Conventions about the proper age and circumstances for marriage, or the appropriate duration and intensity of breastfeeding, are more likely to be shared by those who talk to each other than by those who do not. If would be a mistake, however, to exaggerate the uniformity and isolation of local communities in nineteenth-century Western Europe. Class or occupation surely channeled conversations; religious networks were not necessarily congruent with political networks. There was considerable mobility and trade; religion and politics linked local communities to national and international networks (Gillis, 1974; Moch, this volume; Braudel, 1982; Macfarlane, 1977).

Nevertheless, the importance of the local community is seen in the measures of provincial demographic diversity. It was probably largely those who shared the same geographic space and the same language or dialect – those whose interactions were more frequent and regular because they were closer – who formed the reference group against which one's own behavior would be compared, thus providing models for behavior – models that rewarded the well-behaved and punished those who strayed.

Western Europe in 1960

By 1960 demographic diversity had diminished in Western Europe. There was less variation across all provinces, less variation among countries, and, particularly striking, less variation within countries.

Before examining the evidence to support this statement, a methodological digression is in order. Between 1870 and 1960 marital fertility decline was pronounced. We might expect that the measure of diversity (the midspread) would be related to this change in level and that we could thus account for at least some of the decline in the midspread simply by noting that fertility has fallen. In addition, we might expect that when the median is near either the upper or lower boundary (i.e., near either 1 or 0) variation might be reduced, because as the province values approach either a ceiling or a floor, they could be jammed together.

The relation between the median and the midspread is not, in these data, very close. Although, as we shall see, the midspread for marital fertility was smaller in 1961, when the median was low, than it was in 1871, when the median was high, during the early stages of the transition (while the median was falling) the midspread increased. In addition, and more significantly, we shall see that as the median level of marriage increased, the midspread decreased. Thus *both* the fall in marital fertility *and* the rise in marriage were accompanied, over the long run, by a decrease in variation. Nor do the index values closely approach either 0 or 1. However, a variety of measures intended to be less dependent on location were calculated, and all gave quite similar results. Here I present the logit transformation, which "stretches out the tails of the distribution" so that approaching the boundary is less of a constraint.

Table 13.3 shows the change when all provinces are considered together. Although the changes in level shown by the median were pervasive, they

Table 13.3   Median and measures of variation of marital fertility (I_g) and nuptiality (I_m) for all Western Europe provinces, 1870–1960

	I_g				I_m			
	1870	*1900*	*1930*	*1960*	*1870*	*1900*	*1930*	*1960*
Median	0.696	0.638	0.351	0.325	0.469	0.477	0.51	0.638
Range	0.772	0.738	0.643	0.494	0.42	0.411	0.402	0.399
Midspread	0.121	0.167	0.195	0.103	0.114	0.109	0.13	0.1
Midspread of the logit	0.574	0.721	0.846	0.462	0.46	0.438	0.525	0.43

were not synchronous; demographic changes were somewhat later in Italy, Portugal, and Spain than in the countries of Northwest Europe or Scandinavia. As a result the range, the midspread, and the midspread of the logit increased. They then diminished, and by 1960 there was less variation than there had been in 1870.

Diversity across all provinces could have decreased either because the countries became more similar to one another (a sort of demographic internationalism, or convergence) or because the provinces within a country came to be more alike. There are reasons to expect each. The convergence theories prominent in the 1950s and 1960s lead to the expectation that countries would converge demographically – that is, modern industrial societies would be more similar demographically than they had been in 1870.[10] The mobilization literature, in contrast, would lead us to expect greater demographic homogeneity within countries.

We can use analysis of variance first to examine the importance of country location over time and then to distinguish between the two possible sources of greater homogeneity. Two statistics are used to summarize this analysis: the R^2 and the F-value. The R^2 gives the proportion of the total variation in province values that is "explained" by differences among countries. If there is no difference in country means, then the R^2 will be 0 or close to it; if all province values cluster closely around their country mean and these country means do differ, however, then the R^2 will be close to 1. The F-value provides a measure of the extent to which country means vary over and above what would be expected if all actually had the same true mean but differed by chance or measurement error. An F-value close to 1 supports the hypothesis that the countries all have the same mean – that is, that country is unimportant as a determinant of province values. The higher the F-value the more important is country as an explanation for the differences in province values. In addition, a high F-value shows that the R^2 (the proportion of total variation that is explained by country differences) is significantly different from 0.

Table 13.4   Analysis of variance of marital fertility (I_g) and nuptiality (I_m), by country, separately for 1870, 1900, 1930, and 1960*

	1870	*1900*	*1930*	*1960*
Marital fertility (I_g)				
R^2	0.57	0.57	0.64	0.68
F-value[†]	41.79	43	55.81	68.21
Sum of squares				
Between country	4.25	5.37	5.52	3.09
Within country	3.26	3.99	3.16	1.45
Total	7.51	9.36	8.68	4.54
Degrees of freedom				
Between country	13	13	13	13
Within country	416	416	416	416
Total	429	429	429	429
Nuptiality (I_m)				
R^2	0.59	0.67	0.76	0.75
F-value[†]	45.68	64.68	98.74	94.81
Sum of squares				
Between country	1.95	2.37	2.76	1.67
Within country	1.36	1.17	0.89	0.56
Total	3.31	3.54	3.65	2.23
Degrees of freedom				
Between country	13	13	13	13
Within country	416	416	416	416
Total	429	429	429	429

* This table uses all provinces with data available at the date. This analysis omits Germany.

[†] F-values are significant at the 0.0001 level or better.

The analysis of variance in table 13.4 shows that the R^2 increased over time. We can interpret this to mean that in 1870 country boundaries already tended to enclose national demographic regimes but that these boundaries became increasingly important over the century. The F-values also increase, showing that the R^2s are statistically significant. The between-country and within-country sums of squares show the two components of these changes: the former tells us what happened to differences among countries, and the latter tells us what happened to differences within countries. Both for martial fertility and for nuptiality the between-country sum of squares increased as the countries diverged and then diminished, such that countries were closer to each other in 1960 than they had been in 1870. The decline in the within-country sum of squares was even greater: from 3.26 to 1.45 for I_g, and from 1.36 to 0.56 for I_m.[11]

To summarize, when 1960 and 1870 are compared, between-country variation did diminish, but within-country variation decreased even more. Country location was statistically more important in accounting for demographic behavior in 1960 than it had been in 1870, largely because the provinces within a country had become increasingly similar. It is this finding that gives statistical meaning to the term *demographic nationalism*.

Analysis of variance is a statement about aggregates, about all provinces and all boundaries, rather than about any particular provinces on any particular boundary. We would like to know, for example, what happened in the Basque region: Did the border that separated the French Basque provinces from the Spanish Basque provinces become more evident as well? An analysis of provinces in different countries that shared the same border showed that in general the borders became statistically more evident (Watkins, 1991).

Now let us look more closely at variation within each country. The comparison between 1870 and 1960 can be summarized by a simple ratio of the midspread in 1960 to the midspread in 1870. If the ratio is greater than 1, variation was greater at the later date than at the earlier; if the ratio is less than 1, variation has diminished. Figure 13.1 shows these ratios graphically and separately for Northwest Europe, Scandinavia, and the Mediterranean (the medians and midspreads are given in Watkins, 1991).

In most countries variation was less in 1960 than in 1870. This generalization holds least for the three Mediterranean countries, where the transition was later than in the rest of Western Europe, and somewhat better for the Scandinavian countries. Of the Mediterranean countries, Italy – where variation was surprisingly little in 1870 – is again quite unusual. The midspread is five times larger for marital fertility (I_g), more than three times larger for nuptiality (I_m). In Scandinavia it is Norway that is the most unusual, with greater diversity both in marital fertility and in marriage in 1960 than earlier. It is likely that the greater diversity of the Mediterranean countries in 1960 than in 1870 owed largely to the later fertility decline there; examinations of diversity in Portugal in 1970 and in Italy in the 1980s showed that fertility subsequently declined (Watkins, 1990).

Variation diminished in almost all of the eight countries of Northwest Europe, often by 25 to 50 percent. The exceptions are Ireland – including the counties of Eire and Northern Ireland – where variation in marital fertility was slightly greater in 1960, and Belgium, where variation in marriage was slightly greater in 1960.

Up to now attention has been focused on demographic differentials among groups defined by geographical location. A set of comparative fertility surveys done in Western Europe in the mid 1970s permits us to examine fertility differentials among groups defined by religion, education, occupation,

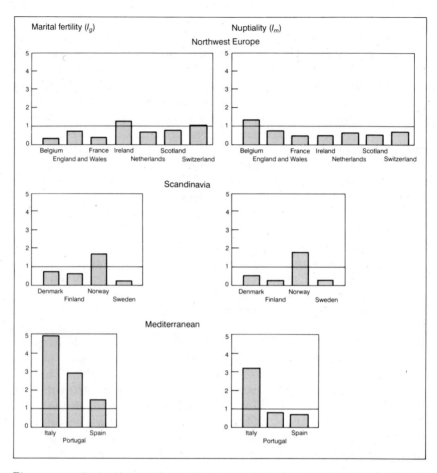

Figure 13.1   Ratio of the midspread in the provincial indexes of marital fertility (I_g) and the index of nuptiality (I_m) for 1960 to the corresponding measure in 1870

income, and urban-rural residence, although equivalent information is not available for the nineteenth century.[12] Table 13.5 shows how many children, on average, had been born to women in various social groups.[13]

"Large" and "small" are obviously matters of degree. When differences are seen relative to the mean, they appear large because the mean is so low. In terms of the childbearing experience of couples in different socioeconomic categories, however, table 13.5 shows that in the 1970s the differences are rarely more than half a child. This is a large percentage difference but a small absolute difference. Even when smaller and potentially more extreme categories are chosen, the differentials are still rather modest.[14]

Table 13.5   Average number of live births per married woman (standardized by marriage duration) by socioeconomic characteristics and country, ca. 1975

	Current residence		Religion		Wife's education		Husband's occupation		Husband's income	
	R	U	C	N	E1	PS	A	NWOA	VL	VH
Northwest Europe										
Belgium (Flemish)	1.9	1.8	1.8	1.5	1.8	1.9	2.2	1.8	1.7	2
France	2.2	1.9	2	2	2.5	1.7	2	1.8	2.2	1.8
Great Britain	–	–	2.1	1.7	2.2	1.7	2	1.7	–	–
Scandinavia										
Denmark	2.2	1.9	–	–	2.2	1.9	–	–	2.2	1.1
Finland	2.1	1.7	–	–	2	1.6	2.1	1.8	1.6	1.8
Norway	2.2	1.9	–	–	2.4	1.9	2.3	1.9	1.9	2
Mediterranean										
Italy	2	1.9	2	1.5	2.5	1.5	2.3	1.9	–	–
Spain	2.5	2.4	2.4	2.5	2.6	2.4	2.6	2.4	–	–

R = rural
U = urban
C = Catholic
N = none
E1 = both those who have not completed elementary school and those who have completed only elementary school (= only those who have not completed elementary school in France, Italy, and Spain)
PS = some postsecondary education
A = agricultural workers
NWOA = nonmanual workers outside of agriculture
VL = very low (bottom income-distribution quintile)
VH = very high (top income-distribution quintile)
Source: Jones, 1982, tables 2 and 4

The strongest support for viewing the reduction in demographic diversity within countries as a consequence of increased social integration within national boundaries comes from an examination of parallel changes in linguistic diversity. Personal networks depend on a shared language, and those who do not speak the same language are less likely to be influenced by patterns and norms emanating from outside the local community. Although Switzerland shows that a common language is not a sine qua non for a sense of identification with compatriots, it is reasonable to expect that social integration is more easily achieved when the population does speak the same language.

The reduction in demographic differentials among inhabitants of provinces is usually matched by a reduction in linguistic diversity. In most

Western European countries with only one official language, mother-tongue diversity declined, and by 1960 there were few who were not able to speak and read that language (Lieberson, Dalto, and Marsden, 1981; Stephens, 1976; Trudgill, 1983). Because both the demographic and the linguistic data are aggregated, it is not possible to show that demographic differences are associated with linguistic differences at the level of the individual. But there is reason to believe that at the level of the province the relationship holds. In France, where both linguistic and demographic diversity diminished considerably between 1870 and 1960, the *départements* that remained demographically distinctive in 1960 were usually those that had been linguistically distinctive a century earlier (Watkins, 1990). Brittany – the *départements* of which retained high fertility and low nuptiality until the very end of the nineteenth century – appears to have persisted longest in maintaining its own language. But by 1927 only the aged were monolingual in Breton, while the children were monolingual in French (Dauzat, 1927).

What had happened? Pierre-Jakez Helias, in his autobiography, *The Horse of Pride: Life in a Breton Village* (1978), suggests an answer. Returning from his first weeks at school in French, just after World War I, he complained to his parents,

"But you, my own parents, never speak French. Nobody in town or in the country speaks French, except for poor Madam Poirier."

"We don't need to," said my parents, "but *you* will need to.... *You* will need to speak French all the time."

"But what happened?"

"It's the world that has changed, from one generation to another." (1978, p. 145)

Helias's grandfather put it more pithily: "With French, you can go everywhere. With only Breton, you're tied to a short rope, like a cow to a post. You have to graze around your tether, and the meadow grass is never plentiful" (p. 135).

DISCUSSION

What might account for the increased importance of national boundaries for demographic behavior? I think it is possible to distinguish three processes that would produce greater demographic uniformity: market integration, state formation, and nation building. All three processes are like "distant thunder" – they are public and institutional, apparently far removed from birth and marriage. We cannot interrogate individuals – and, indeed, even if we could, it is unlikely that they could be articulate about the influence of these processes on their private lives. Nor can we enter each of the provinces one by one. But an examination of the parallels between these processes and demographic behavior suggests links between them.

It is hardly necessary to argue that modern demographic behavior is responsive to economic circumstances. A vast literature attempts to account for the decline in fertility by calling on economic development or industrialization and to account for cross-sectional demographic differentials by stressing differences in income, occupation, and so forth. Although the results of the empirical analyses conducted in this framework have not been impressive, the framework itself is so familiar that it cannot be easily disregarded. More important for increasing demographic homogeneity, however, would seem to be not the changes in income levels but the changes in regional economic inequality and the integration of national markets. Both are part of the stylized facts of economic history. A comprehensive analysis shows that regional economic inequality typically increases during the first stages of industrialization and then diminishes.[15]

There are two market levels for us to consider: the between–country market (Western Europe) and the within–country market. Although the economic exchange across both provincial and country boundaries in the nineteenth century was considerable, it is unarguable that there was far more of both kinds of exchange in 1960 than in 1870. The increase in within-country exchange, however, seems to have been greater than the increase in between-country exchange. Particularly after 1870 economic integration in Western Europe was overbalanced by state-driven moves toward national economic autarchy. In the late nineteenth century and on into the twentieth, national economies were defined by tariff walls, the removal of internal customs barriers, and other policies and programs, such as the payment of national subsidies (Pollard, 1981). Both world wars vastly enhanced the nation-states' power over their economies. There would almost certainly have been more national market integration without war, but there was almost certainly more yet as a result of the mobilization of the civilian economy in wartime.

How might the decline in regional economic inequality and the increase in national market integration affect demographic behavior? To the degree that economic circumstances affect demographic behavior, we would expect the decline in regional economic inequality to be evident in reduced demographic inequality. It marriages and children can indeed be considered as consumer durables, it would not be surprising that provincial populations bought similar family packages. National labor-market integration increased internal migration, and thus the possibility of direct interaction among those from different provinces within the same country. France provides a good example. By 1910 railroads had reached that country's most distant and inaccessible towns (Pinchemel, 1969, p. 222), and presumably as a consequence long-distance migration increased much more than did short-distance migration. An analysis of migration in France found that the probability of short-distance migration (from one *département* to an adjacent one) increased about 1.5 times between 1891 and 1956, but that long-distance migration (from one *département* to another at least 600 kilometers away) increased fivefold (Courgeau, 1970, p. 85).

The development of improved transport made a greater difference for the migration of women than of men; women rarely accompanied male migrants in the first half of the century but increasingly moved as workers (many as domestic servants) or as wives (Chatelain, 1977). Leslie Page Moch writes that the marriage records for three French villages "provide an extraordinary picture of the broadening of geographic horizons for women in the last half of the nineteenth century. Marriage records attest to women's legendary eagerness to leave the mountains and rural life succinctly expressed in the proverb from Western Languedoc: Goats ascend, girls descend. The women of the *belle époque* simply went further than their mothers" (1983, p. 68).

Once the women came down from the mountainside, they were more likely to marry someone from a different province than would have been the case earlier. In the *département* of Loir-et-Cher, for example, 12.8 percent of the marriages between 1870 and 1877 involved one spouse from Loir-et-Cher and the other from another *département*; in 1946–54, 28.2 percent fell in this category (Sutter, 1958; Sutter and Tabah, 1955). Marrying away did not necessarily rupture the relations between the individual and his or her family. The temporary migrants of the late 18th and 19th century forged links between their new residence and their old, much as migrants did in the 20th century. Writing about contemporary France, Laurence Wylie noted that virtually everyone in the village of Chanzeaux has relatives, close friends, neighbors, and landlords who are emigrants, and it is through them that the village gains "intimate and personal contact with the 'New France,' which in many other respects has bypassed the small villages" (1966, p. 183).

Lastly, and more speculatively, the distribution of goods across all of the national territory would have meant that people in one part of the country could eat the same foods, wear the same clothes, and buy the same cars as those in another. This means that when one encountered someone from another. This means that when one encountered someone from another province within the same country he or she would appear, at least outwardly, to be more like oneself than would have been the case in the nineteenth century. The more general point is that market integration would have contributed to a sense of participation in a national community.

The state's role went beyond that of sculpting national economies. Although governments rarely implemented policies intended to directly affect either fertility or marriage (Fascist Italy and Nazi Germany are obvious exceptions), in all countries the state increasingly substituted for the family as a source of social security. The welfare community became increasingly national, with marked differences among countries. The last quarter of the nineteenth century and the first quarter of the twentieth saw the "collectivization of providence": social welfare became collective, compulsory, and nationwide (de Swaan, 1988). In France, for example, public assistance had been funded almost entirely at the local level, but during the Third Republic (1870–1940) these responsibilities were increasingly interpreted as national obligations. France has also had distinctive pronatalist policies (Weiss, 1983). Expanded welfare schemes during the Great Depression must have further increased people's perceptions that not only their prosperity but their survival was directly linked to national policies, thus enhancing the consciousness of interdependence within the national community and enlarging the distance to communities on the other side of the border (Pollard, 1981, p. 74).

State functions expanded enormously, increasing what Fernand Braudel called its "'diabolical' power of penetration" (1984, p. 51). Compulsory military service gave to all a direct interest in state affairs, and the expansion of tax liability directly linked all groups above the indigent to the state (Anderson and Anderson, 1967, p. 24). One measure of the state's expansion is the growth in state budgets as a percentage of gross national product. The general trend was upward, with the sharpest sustained increases in central government expenditure from late 1890s to 1930 (Grew, 1984). Another measure of the state's expansion is an enlarged bureaucracy. Compared to the middle of the nineteenth century, the number of points at which individuals came in contact with state bureaucrats increased enormously. Bureacrats and budgets do much to make the state more visible in daily life, thus surely enhancing the sense of belonging to a national community in addition to – or even instead of – a local community.

While state formation began well before the nineteenth century, nation building was largely concentrated in the period after 1800, and mass identification with a nation almost certainly grew after 1870 (C. Tilly, 1975; Hobsbawm, 1987, p. 146). Nation building includes the insistence by the state that everyone be able to communicate in the official language (or languages) and the invention of national traditions such as coronation rituals and anthems (Hobsbawm, 1983; Agulhon, 1981). In time of war, the group that was living and dying together was seen to be the nation, thus heightening intergroup solidarity (Simmel, 1955). In time of peace, the enemies of the nation were international (e.g., the Catholic Church and international socialism) and regional (e.g., users of dialect and regional patriots) (Hobsbawm, 1987; Grew, 1984).

More important, I think, in nation building was education. It is not only the higher levels of education that are demographically relevant but also that students attended either state schools or schools subject to a considerable degree of state regulation. Schools taught national history and deliberately sought to inculcate civic loyalty (Katznelson and Weir, 1985). Ernest Gellner has argued that in the modern, industrial nation-state this must be so:

The *nation* is now supremely important, thanks both to the erosion of sub-groupings and the vastly increased importance of a shared, literary-dependent culture. The state, inevitably, is charged with the maintenance and supervision of an enormous social infrastructure (the cost of which characteristically comes close to one half of the total income of the society). The educational system becomes a very crucial part of it, and the maintenance of the cultural/linguistic medium now becomes the central role of education. The citizens can only breathe conceptually and operate within that medium, which is co-extensive with the territory of the state and its educational and cultural apparatus, and which needs to be protected, sustained and cherished. (1983, pp. 63–4)

The exceptions to the general pattern of increasing demographic homogeneity suggest the importance of nation-building in accounting for diminished demographic diversity within countries. Belgium, Ireland, and to some degree Norway are countries for which there is reason to believe that a sense of national community was less than in the other countries of northwest Europe and Scandinavia. In both Ireland and Belgium political divisions seem to be paralleled by demographic divisions. In Switzerland, where religious and linguistic differences are contained by a common political culture, demographic diversity diminished.

National economic integration, state expansion, and nation building are obviously not entirely separable. The growth of capitalism was managed by the state, which saw the encouragement of industrialization as its responsibility, and an autonomous market was one of the goals of nationalist leaders (Grew, 1984; A. D. Smith, 1981; Haines, this volume). The adoption of national welfare policies and programs indicates an expansion of the morally relevant community from kin and neighbors to the nation-state. This expansion of the morally relevant boundaries is a prerequisite for the functioning of a national market economy (Kohli, 1986).

Nor should the list of processes that may reasonably be associated with the growth of a national community be confined to the economy, the state, or the nation. In 1898 Gabriel Tarde emphasized the role of the press in penetrating provincial boundaries. The effective influence of newspapers, however, stops at the frontiers of the language in which they are written:

It is surprising to see that as nations intermingle and imitate one another, assimilate, and morally unite, the demarcation of nationalities becomes deeper, and their oppositions appear more irreconcilable. At first glance one cannot understand this contrast of the nationalistic 19th century with the cosmopolitanism of the previous century. But this result, however, paradoxical, is actually very logical. While between neighboring or distant peoples the exchange of merchandise, ideas, all kinds of items multiplied, the exchange of ideas, in particular, between people speaking the same language progressed even more rapidly, thanks to newspapers. Therefore, even though the *absolute* difference between nations diminished, their relative and conscious differences grew. (1969 [1898], p. 306)

A similar argument was made by Benedict Anderson, who emphasized the interactions of capitalism, printing, and the growth of standard vernacular languages in the formation of what he calls "imagined communities" (1983). One of Anderson's central images is that of a newspaper – this one-day best-seller, out of date tomorrow, read in privacy: "Yet each communicant is well aware that the ceremony he performs is being replicated simultaneously by thousands (or millions) of others of whose existence he is confident, yet of whose identity he has not the slightest notion....What more vivid figure for the secular, historically-clocked, imagined community can be envisioned?" (1983, p. 39). Imagined communities are not necessarily harmonious, but when there was conflict rather than consensus, these conflicts increasingly were fought out at the national rather than the local level. Expanded suffrage increasingly focused political discussions at the national rather than the local level. As politics nationalized, power centralized and communications among dissident groups improved, the protest of local groups (such as guilds) being replaced by the protest of trade unions and political parties (C. Tilly, 1981, p. 106).

We think of the decision to marry or to conceive a child as intensely private acts, much like the decision to take one's own life. Certainly the rhetoric that surrounds them is the language of individualism, a manifestation of what Emile Durkheim called the "cult of the individual." Market integration, state formation, and nation building would seem to go on at a public level far removed from birth and marriage, and the connections between the public and the private remain speculative. These three processes would have made the circumstances that influence demographic behavior more similar. If prices and incomes are important determinants of demographic behavior, then the greater homogeneity in prices and income that can be expected to follow from the integration of national markets and the development of state welfare programs would result in greater demographic homogeneity.

Market integration, state expansion, and nation building presumably also knit together local personal networks into larger national networks. If couples also take into account what other couples are doing – if, for example, they observe the demographic behavior of their friends, neighbors, and acquaintances – then the integration of diverse local communities into a national community would expand the geographical extent of these social networks. The increased importance of national boundaries in 1960 suggests that the relevant community for demographic behavior had become the national one.

Will national boundaries be less significant for demographic behavior in the future? There are two reasons to expect that this might be the case. The first derives from the resurgence of ethnic movements of the 1970s and 1980s, which usually focus on communities smaller than the nation-state; the second derives from economic and political integration over a larger area than the nation, specifically the European Community, as well as from the crossing of national boundaries by the media.

William McNeill (1986) has argued that the period between the French Revolution and World War I was unusual in the degree of national ethnic homogeneity that was aimed for and achieved. Earlier empires were likely to be multi-ethnic, and modern societies, he says, may be multi-ethnic as well. The prosperity of the 1950s and 1960s drew migrants to Western Europe from farther and farther away, and the idea that these immigrants can be assimilated has faded. Others have proposed that ethnic identification becomes increasingly attractive in a sterile modern world, that ethnic identification becomes important because it is a basis of claims on state resources, or that in an age of global realignments nation-states mean less (Bell, 1975; Hannan, 1979; Nagel and Olzak, 1982; Beer, 1980).

It seems highly unlikely, however, that vigorous ethnic movements would attempt a pronatalist policy, which would appear to be even more difficult than a language policy (which most movements have eschewed), or that such movements would have the unintended consequences of raising fertility levels. Since the late nineteenth century fertility rates have almost without exception become lower. Even deliberate and expensive pronatalist policies have not had the desired effect of simply halting or reversing fertility decline. Low fertility appears to be irresistible in modern societies, and I see little reason to expect that the leaders of the Basque, Breton, or Scottish nationalist movements would attempt to reverse this trend, or that they would be successful at it if they did.

What about convergence within Western Europe, which would also reduce the salience of national boundaries? Marx and Engels (1967 [1848]) predicted that some national differences would diminish with the advance of capitalism. Differences between countries were less in 1960 than they had been in 1870, but only slightly. What about the future? Economic boundaries are, I think, less likely to coincide with national boundaries. Levels of economic integration are higher now than they were when the European Coal and Steel Community was formed in 1950 and are likely to be higher yet after 1992, when all trade restrictions between European Community countries are removed. While political integration has lagged behind economic integration, analyses of a series of surveys in EC countries reveal increasing support for supranational organizations over national ones (Inglehart, 1977). And, significantly, Lesthaeghe and Meekers (1986) have found some evidence for a connection between support for internationalization and demographic behavior. But despite neoligisms such as "Euro-dollar," "Euro-TV," and "Euro-babble," I detect little of the passion for European integration that one can find for nation building in many of the histories of particular countries. And linguistic differences among the European countries are likely to remain, despite organizations that attempt to standardize languages across countries. It seems likely, however, that linguistic differences will become less salient, at least for some. Ernest Gellner notes that among such groups as the upper professions, there is little need to adjust when visiting each others' lands: "They already 'speak each other's language,' even if they do not speak each other's language" (1983, p. 188).

Based on the analysis of demographic nationalism in Western Europe between 1870 and 1960, I predict that national boundaries will be less deeply etched on the demographic map of Western Europe. But just as those *départements* in which many spoke languages other than French in the nineteenth century were the demographically distinctive ones in 1960, I would expect that national demographic differences will persist as shadings of tone, if not of color, on the demographic map of Western Europe.

NOTES

1   These collaborators were E. Harm (Finland); J. Knodel (Germany); R. Lesthaeghe (Belgium); M. Livi-Bacci (Italy, Portugal, Spain); P. Mathiessen (Denmark); C. Mosk (Sweden); M. Teitelbaum (England, Ireland, Scotland); E. van de Walle (France, Norway, the Netherlands); F. van de Walle (Switzerland). Roy Treadway prepared a computer tape containing these indexes; it is available from the Office of Population Research, Princeton University. They have also been published as Appendix A of Coale and Treadway (1986). Where more than one series was published for a country, series 0 was used except in the case of Italy, where series 1 (corrected for male out-migration) was used, and Spain, where series 1 (smaller provinces) was used.

2   The indexes are based on the information most widely available: vital registration of births by legitimacy status and census distributions of women by marital status (single, married, widowed, and divorced). They are described more fully in Coale and Treadway (1986). The Princeton European Fertility Project gave considerable attention to correcting these indexes. There is a full discussion of the sources of the data and the corrections made to them in Appendix C of Coale and Treadway (1986). In most countries the data required to calculate the indexes are available at the level of the province starting around 1870. The analysis ends in 1960 because subsequently some of the countries did not publish all the requisite data. Because of boundary changes, the number of provinces varies slightly over time. Unless otherwise noted, only those provinces for which data are available in 1870, 1900, 1930, and 1960 were included in this analysis. In a few countries the indexes cannot be calculated until 1880 or 1890. Germany is included in the comparisons across countries in 1870, and in the analyses of all provinces at all dates; it is excluded from comparisons by country between 1870 and 1960 because boundary changes affected the number of provinces at these dates substantially.

3   England and Wales are treated together, as are Eire and the six counties of Northern Ireland.

4   Watkins (1991). Cormack O'Grada (1988) has argued that the European Fertility Project underestimated marital fertility in Ireland. Comparing his estimates for 1881 with those based on the project's, the range and midspread would be larger than those shown here. The midspread is still, however, one of the smallest in Western Europe.

5   For a summary of the findings of the Princeton European Fertility Project, see Coale and Watkins (1986).

6   There is reason to believe, however, that France was demographically diverse before the fertility transition began. David Weir has calculated I_g for a sample of 40 villages for the period 1740–90; The midspread for his sample, 0.157, is virtually identical to the 0.159 midspread of French *départements* in 1831 (Weir, personal communication). Similarly, I have found that variation in nuptiality (as measured by the proportion remaining

unmarried at age 50) was about the same for cohorts born in 1756 (before the beginning of the transition) as for cohorts born 1796–1801 (after the beginning of the transition). Because the marriage patterns of the earlier cohort were probably unaffected by the fertility transition, this suggests that departmental differences in nuptiality were long-standing (Watkins, 1980).

7   An analysis that compares diversity among countries at the first date for which data are available (as early as 1831 in France) shows only slightly less diversity than in 1870.

8   By multilingual I mean that there was more than one national language or that some people were monolingual in a language other than the national language (or languages). I stretch the term *language* to include dialects that were incomprehensible to outsiders. For a comprehensive compilation of language data around the turn of the century, see Tesnière (1928).

9   In Wales in 1871 about a quarter of the population was monolingual in Welsh (Verdery, 1976), but excluding Wales from the analysis changes the measures only negligibly.

10   The theorists of convergence (e.g., Moore, 1965, 1979; Levy, 1966; for a review, see Weinberg, 1976) do not discuss demographic behavior directly, except to predict that fertility will be low in modern societies. But because many of the aspects of modern industrial societies that they expect to converge are those which are often considered to influence demographic behavior, predictions about demographic convergence among countries follow easily.

11   Excluding the Mediterranean countries from the analysis changes the numerical results somewhat, but not the overall findings.

12   The aristocracies, and presumably the more broadly defined upper classes as well, were among the forerunners of the fertility transition (Livi Bacci, 1986) and in many countries may have begun the transition before the first date that the indexes can be calculated. Because at that first date class variation is likely to have been large, a comparison of variation then with variation in the modern period would surely show a decline in variation. The same is true for rural/urban comparisons, because urban marital fertility decline generally preceded rural declines (Sharlin, 1986). See also Haines (this volume).

13   The measure of fertility is based on women of all ages, controlling for differences in marital duration (Jones, 1982).

14   For example, in France the difference between those who express strong and weak religious feeling is 0.48 (about half a child), between those living in a village and those in a city is 0.42, by family income is 1.02, and by women's employment (currently working vs. worked only before marriage or never) is 0.70 (Jones, 1982).

15   Most of the series of economic indicators on which Williamson based this conclusion are not long enough to adequately represent regional economic inequalities before industrialization, but in France, where an agricultural wage series begins in 1862, regional variation was less in 1953 than in 1862 (Williamson, 1965, pp. 29–30). In England regional wage differentials declined after the 1860s (Hunt, 1973; O'Grada, 1981; O'Brien and Engerman, 1981).

14

War, Family, and Fertility
in Twentieth-Century Europe

J. M. Winter

The separation of political history from demographic history – each in majestic isolation on its own peak – impoverishes them both. One illustration of the need to bring them together is the case of the demographic history of the two world wars. Military conflict in this century has twice transformed the political, social, and economic context in which demographic change has taken place. Indeed, there are few better examples of the ways in which cultural norms and material forces are in constant tension than in wartime.[1]

Most historians would not quarrel with this statement, but few have integrated it into their analyses of population history or political history. Responsibility for this omission rests on both sides. The close alignment of demographic history with economic history has led in some quarters to a kind of economic determinism, which declares that the broad broom of industrialization inexorably sweeps away high fertility rates. The upheaval of war simply doesn't enter into the equation.

Political historians too must accept some of the blame for the narrowness with which these issues have been studied in the past. The recognition that the experience of total war has marked European history in profound ways – evident to anyone who explores the formative years of European politicians from Kurt Waldheim up – is bound to remain mere rhetoric until scholars fully explore the realm of civil society, and especially the sphere of personal life and family formation. Then and only then can political and demographic history merge into something resembling the history of human communities.

This preliminary sketch suggests one – and certainly not the only – place to start. It is in the exploration of the impact of war on women's lives, on the burdens they bore, and on the functions they fulfilled or were supposed to fulfill, both at home and in their communities.

In this essay I argue that the experience of war first expanded and then severely contracted responsibilities and opportunities open to women in twentieth-century Europe. The call to arms of millions of men and the mobilization of female labor in wartime twice coincided with a reinvigorated pronatalist campaign, sponsored by both state agencies and interest groups. The immediate effects of these developments are clear. First, there was a profound distortion of the population's sex ratio and age distribution, leading to adjustments in both the short and long term, in family life, and in some patterns of demographic behavior. Second, there was a change in the gender and skill composition of the labor force, which (to a degree) challenged some prewar conventions and assumptions about the gender division of labor. Third, there was an upsurge of both the rhetoric and the political will behind what was called the politics of the family. This phrase was shorthand for a political movement, both lay and secular, both in and out of governments, composed of those who advocated measures to increase the birth rate and to shore up the family as the center of social life. The politics of the family gathered supporters from all parts of the ideological spectrum. In the period of both world wars, and in many countries, such groups formed a consensus behind measures to encourage childrearing and to protect the health of mothers and children.

My argument is that total war first undermined prewar forms of family life and gender roles and then substantially strengthened the politics of domesticity. Wartime mobilization by necessity multiplied the social roles and economic opportunities of women; postwar demobilization drastically reduced them.

The demographic consequences of this twofold process of advance and retreat for women were different in the two postwar periods. In the aftermath of World War I, economic disorder and decline further pushed back the threshold of female independence outside the home, and in some cases inside the home too. Women left the heavy manufacturing sector in which they had worked during the conflict. But it was difficult to go back to the prewar world, because the highly unstable conditions of the immediate postwar period undermined many of the traditional trades in which women had worked, primarily (but not only) in textiles. Mass unemployment in the interwar years for both men and women was bound to negate much of the force of the pronatalist campaign to increase the birth rate. After a brief postwar recovery, fertility rates continued on a downward path.

After 1940 in some countries and after 1945 virtually everywhere, the decline in the birth rate was reversed. The mix of cultural and economic pressures leading to this dramatic reversal of demographic trends was striking. A second burst of support for the politics of the family coincided with a very different postwar settlement, in which full employment (understood as full *male* employment) was a conscious aim of most governments. Their stated intention was not to repeat the mistakes of 1918, and in this they largely succeeded. This time the restoration of the family took place against the backdrop of economic conditions as favorable as any that had existed for 40 years. The cultural campaign of the 1940s to strengthen the family and to restore women to their "rightful" place firmly within the home coincided with one of the most remarkable periods of European economic growth. This was the backdrop to the European phase of the post–1945 baby boom, which extended in several waves until the mid 1960s.

These considerations may also help put in perspective the end of the baby boom in the 1960s. By then, both the cultural and economic supports for above-replacement fertility were significantly weakened. The politics of the family looked more and more like a fading anachronism of another age. The beginnings of a new women's movement coincided, first, with the appearance and dissemination of effective contraceptive devices and, second, with a set of changes in the legal status of women affecting both their reproductive and working lives. In addition, the momentum of the postwar economic boom was checked, and a new and more austere phase of European economic life began. Inflation, economic instability, and mass unemployment returned, not in the same form as in the 1920s and 1930s but with the same demographic effect, namely in (in association with social pressures) leading to a decline in the total fertility rate to below replacement levels throughout Europe (Teitelbaum and Winter, 1985).

This interpretation is of course deliberately general and stylized. The history of family forms and fertility in each European country varied considerably and defies any general explanation. In addition, there is a danger of conflating the history of the baby boom in the United States, Canada, Australia, and New Zealand, with the lesser but still substantial European baby boom. Different processes may very well have yielded similar demographic outcomes. All I claim here is that there is merit in locating some of the special features of the one period in European history over the past century in which the decline of fertility was temporarily arrested. The postwar generation of young adults came of age after the most destructive armed conflict the world has ever known. They came to childbearing years at a time when the cult of the family was an established cultural and political force. They proceeded to raise European fertility levels to heights no one could have foreseen before 1939. But at least in this domain, they did not leave a lasting legacy to their children, born in a world fortunately undisfigured by the abominations of total war. In the mid 1960s they resumed the century-long decline in fertility, which persists to this day.

At this state of our knowledge of recent history, such an interpretation must remain in the realm of the suggestive and the speculative. But it is hoped that it will draw much needed attention to some of the ways the second Thirty Years War has had a bearing on the history of women, the family, and fertility in twentieth-century Europe.

THE MOBILIZATION OF MANPOWER, MILITARY LOSSES,
AND THE SEX RATIO OF EUROPEAN POPULATIONS

First let us consider the extent to which the two world wars disturbed the sex ratio of European populations. The mobilization of military manpower in both conflicts was a stunning achievement. In many continental states, pre-1914 conscription had created structures for the swift processing of millions of men at a time of national emergency. But no one could have been certain that the machine would operate smoothly in 1914, in part because of what Carl von Clausewitz called "friction," or the tendency of things to come unstuck in wartime, and in part because of the threat of a strike against war by the parties of the Socialist International. In the event, socialists chose nation over class and joined their compatriots in a flood of recruits in August 1914. These men were joined by millions of volunteers from Britain and from the overseas dominions of the major imperial powers. By 1918 a staggering total of 70 million men were under arms. This constituted nearly 30 percent of all men aged 15–49 in the major combatant countries.

Of those who served in the Great War, approximately 9.5 million were killed or died in active service. Casualty rates varied substantially among countries. The most severely hit populations were in Eastern and southern Europe, where the war crisis had arisen. Of 750,000 men mobilized in Serbia, approximately 280,000 – 37 percent of those mobilized and 23 percent of the nation's male population aged 15–49 in 1914 – were killed. The Romanian figures were similarly appalling: 250,000 men killed – 25 percent of men mobilized and 13 percent of the nation's male population of military age.

Among other major powers, Britain and France lost respectively one in eight and one in six of the men who served in their forces. On the other side, casualties were similarly astronomical. One in eight of the Austro-Hungarian army's 9 million-plus men was killed; one in six of the German army's 13 million-plus men was killed. In all countries, about 70 percent of the men killed were under age 30 (Winter, 1986, chap. 3).

This brief sketch of some military statistics should suggest the extent to which war transformed the sex ratio and age distribution of the home front of the major combatants. This was apparent from the very first days of the conflict. In many rural areas, the old, the infirm, children, and women tried resolutely to gather the first harvest of the war in August 1914. This they succeeded in doing, but only slowly did they learn that they had to face alone the second, the third, the fourth, and the fifth harvest of an extended war (J.-J. Becker, 1986, pt. 1). At times prisoners of war (POWs) or bored troops billeted in an area helped with farm work, but the bulk of the burden rested on the young, the old, and women. Some men returned, but their wounds precluded their resuming their prewar place in village or family life. And each month brought news of additional losses, which are memorialized in lists inscribed in stone in many parts of rural Europe (Prost, 1986).

In all areas the family form of male wage earner as the head of household and wife as housekeeper and subordinate partner was challenged or undermined. This family form had probably been realized only in middle-class communities. In some working-class areas, this form was an ideal; in others, especially in rural areas, it was unachievable and possibly undesired. Despite these variations, the subordinate and economically dependent position of women within families was the rule in 1914.

The war presented in a variety of ways a real or imagined threat both to the cohesion of family life and to patterns of authority and independence within families. In many parts of Eastern Europe, in Italy, and in Belgium and northern France, refugees – frequently women, children, and the elderly – streamed away from combat zones. All too often they lost their homes and lost touch with their families. In addition, leave arrangements for mobilized men were highly irregular. Separations owing to migration of women workers to war industries were also common. Those families who remained intact were the lucky ones.

Millions of women were paid a separation allowance in all major combatant countries, partly to provide for dependents whose well-being was threatened by mobilization, and partly to keep intact the households whose male heads were temporarily removed for active military service (Pedersen, 1990). The maintenance of some semblance of domestic stability required considerable ingenuity, frequently backed by the support of kin, neighbors, and friends. The results varied considerably depending on a host of circumstances and luck as much as on national developments. In some areas the economic condition of families did not suffer substantially during the war. This was true in Britain and France but not in most parts of Belgium, Germany, Austria-Hungary, Italy, or on the Eastern Front. The war increasingly meant deprivation, hunger, and disease (Winter, 1988). In oral testimonies women who lived through these years on the Continent have spoken of dreariness, anxiety, and exhaustion; of having to cope alone with children and aged dependents; of having to make ends meet on severely restricted rations, obtained after hours on endless queues or on the black market; and of having to face each day with the gnawing possibility that a cable or a knock on the door would bring the official form of gratitude for the "ultimate sacrifice." Women faced multiple burdens in wartime: the "normal" household tasks were only a small part of a day's work, coming before or after paid labor and the daily search for provisions (Sieder, 1988).

Additional problems arose out of the fact that in central and Eastern Europe the fighting did not end in 1918. Civil war and revolution merged in a period of uncertainty and confusion – the human texture of which can be conveyed perhaps only in art or literature. Boris Pasternak's *Doctor Zhivago* and Alfred Doblin's *November 1918* are two very different visions of the cold, bleak postwar period in which families all too frequently disintegrated or disappeared. Furthermore, the lithographs of Kathe Kollwitz speak for the mute grief of millions of mothers bereaved in a war of unparalleled carnage.

If memory, imaginative literature, and art are the only means adequately to convey the upheaval of family life during World War I, the same is even more apparent with respect to World War II. But here the key difference is that by 1939 the distinction between military and civilian targets in warfare had been completely obliterated. Weakening the enemy included strategic bombing to destroy its cities, and hence the families therein, as with the German blitz of London and the Allies' fire bombing of Dresden. The Nazis' Final Solution applied this annihilation strategy to whole peoples. Of course the Turks had already laid the groundwork for this kind of war crime in their policy of extermination of the Armenian population in World War I, but before Hitler's war, this was the exception and not the rule.

In the case of the 1939–45 conflict, again we must distinguish between quiet areas, where the war left intact much of village life but removed the bulk of the adult male population, as in France between 1940 and 1943 and in parts of Germany until 1945, and areas that were scenes of aerial bombardment or direct assault, such as Rotterdam, Dresden, Warsaw, and most of European Russia. Here everyone was a potential victim, and given the catalog of atrocities inflicted on civilians, both inside and outside the concentration camps, family life was fall too frequently reduced to a struggle against arrest or starvation and to a search – frequently futile – to retain the barest minimum of human dignity.

Again, the scale of the direct military effort of the major European combatants was monumental. Approximately 20 percent of the male labor force of the major combatant nations was mobilized (Milward, 1977, p. 216). This may have constituted a slightly lower proportion in the armed forces than in the 1914–18 war. One reason is that World War II was much more highly mechanized than the earlier war, requiring greater attention to maintaining a balance between the manpower needs of the military and of industry. In addition, the Nazis learned from the mistakes of the German war effort in the 1914–18 war, when the needs of the civilian population were ignored by a cartel of army and industry. The Nazis consequently paid careful attention to the condition of the Aryan population at home (Borchardt, 1984).

Casualty statistics are rarely reliable, and with respect to World War II, the totals are so vast that even if a true record could be constructed, it would probably defy the imagination. All we can do is present the outlines of the catastrophe. Of perhaps 110 million men in uniform, perhaps 22 million were killed, either in combat or in the archipelago of POW camps strung out across the world (Urlanis, 1971, p. 293).

Estimates of civilian deaths can only remain notional. No one can say with any precision how many Japanese civilians died as a result of Allied bombing: it all depends on how you measure radiation-related disease and mortality. No one knows how many Russians perished in the siege of Leningrad: perhaps one million, perhaps more. One Soviet demographer claims that 10 million Soviet civilians died during the war, equalling the total of 10 million men in uniform who perished. To these 20 million Soviets must be added 30 million people of other nationalities whose deaths were war related, producing a global total of 50 million victims of the 1939–45 war. Of these, perhaps 12 million perished in concentration camps or were otherwise exterminated; 1.5 million died in aerial bombardment; and 14.5 million perished as a result of blockade, starvation, and war-related disease (Urlanis, 1971, p. 294).

The effect of these staggering losses on the sex ratio of European populations was phenomenal. In the Soviet Union in 1959, there were 20 million more women than men at ages 20–80. At ages 35–50, the female-to-male sex ratio was seven to four. At ages 55–59, when men would have been old enough to face both world wars, the ratio was two to one (Urlanis, 1971, p. 286; Milward, 1977, p. 212). There were only 605 Russian males aged 36–40 for every 1,000 females in 1959. The sex ratio among the population of Asian Soviet republics was similarly distorted, leading to ethnic intermarriage and "Russification" in the postwar years. Given the staggering nature of Soviet war losses, the effect of casualties on demographic patterns was bound to be greater than elsewhere in Europe (Anderson and Silver, 1988, pp. 212, 234). It will take another 50 years for this imbalance in the sex ratio to pass through the age structure of the Soviet population.

In central Europe the absence of males was equally severe in the immediate postwar period. One survey disclosed that approximately one-third of all German families in 1950 – years after refugees and POWs had returned – were headed by a woman (Moeller, 1988). Under conditions of scarcity and uncertainty, it was a very untraditional family structure that had to pick up the pieces in the aftermath of Hitler's war.

WAR AND WOMEN'S WORK

So far we have briefly sketched the outline of the disturbance to the sex ratio of European populations attributable to the two world wars. But these conflicts also brought about a change in gender roles at work, by feminizing the labor force and by undermining restrictions on women's access to skilled work. We should not exaggerate either of these two developments. Between 30 and 40 percent of the female population of Britain, France, and Germany worked in extradomestic labor prior to World War I. While there was a shift upwards in the number of working women and in the proportion of the female population in the labor force, the primary effect of war was to redistribute female labor and to convert part-time and occasional workers into full-time workers.

Some data on the German labor force are instructive in this context. In 1913 the general category of "females and youths under 16" (a revealing reflection of official thinking) constituted 13 percent of the labor force in heavy industry. By 1918 the figure is 34 percent, representing an increase of approximately one million women workers. By 1920 17 percent of this sector was female – more than before the war, but substantially less than during the conflict. In the more traditionally feminized textile trades, the figure is 58 percent of the labor force in 1913 and 76 percent of a substantially reduced labor force in 1918 (B. Moore, 1978, table 10).[2]

In Britain there was a similarly impressive shift of women from one branch of industry to another, but an even more spectacular growth in women's employment in commerce, finance, and banking. Approximately 500,000 women were drafted into this sector, and, unlike women working in heavy industry, they stayed there after the war (Kirkaldy, 1921, table 8).

The redistribution of the female labor force in France was similarly striking. After the war women stayed in the white-collar labor force, but their numbers dwindled in other traditional sectors of female labor-force participation, such as textiles. As Jean-Louis Robert has noted, the war's effects were twofold. In the short term, the war marked the zenith of the upward secular trend of women's participation in the labor force and in the proportion of the labor force that was female. But it was also the point of departure for a 50-year decline in the role played by women in the French labor force (Robert, 1988).

The trends set by World War I in the short-term redistribution and expansion of female labor were visible in most combatant countries during the second war. Eighty percent of the expansion of the British labor force between 1939 and 1943 consisted of women who had not maintained regular extradomestic paid work before the war. Their entry into war factories increased the labor force by 2.5 million. Some were directed to work under female conscription – a truly revolutionary measure. Most did so voluntarily. The result was to increase the proportion of the female population at work from 27 percent in 1939 to 37 percent in 1943. In the Soviet Union the participation rate of women also rose, but it did so from higher prewar levels. Women constituted 38 percent of the labor force in 1940 and 53 percent in 1942. Rosie the Riveter was a representative Russian figure: women comprised one-third of the Soviet Union's welders, one-third of its lathe operators, and two-fifths of its stevedores in 1942. Half the country's tractor drivers were women (Milward, 1977, pp. 219–20; Linz, 1988, pp. 11–37).

The trend in Germany was quite different. Despite the call to arms and the need to control an entire continent at the peak of German military fortunes, there was little difference between the number of women in the

German labor force in 1939 and in 1943. This can be explained in two ways. First, Nazi ideology stressed maternity (of the pure race) to a point that precluded the full exploitation of female labor. Second, POWs, enslaved civilians, forced expatriates, and voluntary migrants were employed in jobs that in other combatant countries were done by the indigenous female population (Milward, 1977, pp. 220–28).

The effects of the industrial mobilization of women in the World War II were complex and varied substantially in different European countries. But in general demobilization meant a return to the prewar sexual division of labor and a reiteration of the definition of a skilled job as one that was not done by a women. To an extent, postwar labor scarcity, particularly in countries with heavy war losses in male cohorts at working ages, softened or deflected this trend. But on the whole, the two postwar periods share this striking similarity: both were marked by a female retreat from industrial employment and a female advance into the service sector.

WAR, THE BIRTH RATE, AND THE POPULARITY OF MARRIAGE

Demographic adjustments to these upheavals were bound to be severe. A drop in the birth rate during World War I was inevitable, but some of the births deferred were registered in a brief baby boom in 1919–20. In some cases during and in all cases after World War II, the European birth rate rose and remained above prewar levels for two decades.

Nuptiality

Demographic and other evidence suggests that the source of this development was a change in patterns of nuptiality. In other words, the experience of total war surprisingly led not to a decline but rather to an increase in the popularity of marriage. This was not universally valid in the World War I period. There was no clear upward trend in nuptiality rates until the 1930s in Germany. In Britain, though, the change is apparent earlier. A greater proportion of the British population was marrying after the 1914–18 war than before it, and they were doing so at younger ages (Winter, 1985, p. 261).

It is likely that this change was not an effect of pronatalist campaigns but rather a reflection of social and demographic adjustments in the aftermath of war. In the French case, post-1918 nuptiality rates were stabilized through a shift in the age structure of marriage, such that women started to marry men the same age or younger than they were, because the men they would have married on prewar nuptiality patterns were dead. In addition, in-migration and a greater tendency to remarriage among widowers helped increase the pool of potential marriage partners for French women and thereby helped prevent a collapse in French marriage rates (Henry, 1966, pp. 272–332).

The effect of the Great War on the age structure of migration had important repercussions for European nuptiality patterns in general, and on British nuptiality in particular. The war brought to an end the period of open emigration to America and thereby trapped in Europe young unmarried males who dominated prewar emigration flows. This kept up the stock of potential husbands on the British side of the ocean. Political changes affecting migratory flows were therefore important in determining the extent to which the war would undermine marriage patterns. Here we find a clue to the mystery of why a war of unprecedented carnage did not occasion an increase in celibacy. In sum, the Great War had some positive and surprisingly few deleterious effects on the propensity of the population to marry and raise a family.

The contrast between Eastern and Western Europe during the World War II period was pronounced. Western Europeans (and their Allies) suffered substantial casualties in the war, but not on the scale of the Soviet Union. Consequently, we must distinguish Soviet demographic history from that of the West in this period. In the U.S.S.R. the war severely distorted the sex ratio, leading to increasing celibacy among some cohorts and ethnic intermarriage in the form of "Russification" (Anderson and Silver, 1988).

In Western Europe and in North America, Australia, and New Zealand, the impact of war on marriage patterns was fundamentally different. Indeed, one of the most striking features of the demographic history of Western Europe in the World War II period is a clear and abrupt rise in nuptiality. In effect, women entered married life earlier and in much greater numbers after 1945 than before 1939. Here British data indicate more general trends. Male nuptiality fluctuated radically in the war period, but the proportion of men "never marrying" – that is, not married before age 50 – in the 1950s and 1960s was not much higher than that of the 1920s and 1930s (see figure 14.1). The real change occurred with respect to women's marriage patterns.

In Britain there is a clear break in levels of female nuptiality in the World War II period: in the interwar years nearly 20 percent of women did not marry during their childbearing years; in the postwar period only about 5 percent were never married. Given the fact that marriage was much more universal and women entered it earlier in their childbearing lives, and given relatively good economic conditions, a rise of fertility was likely prior to the 1960s, when reliable contraception became available to all. Thus the baby boom was more than a sustained recovery of deferred births. It signified a change in women's attitudes toward marriage and the family.

This development, which occurred in several European and other countries, can be illustrated in other ways as well. The crude marriage rate rose in most European countries after World War II. But this change is not

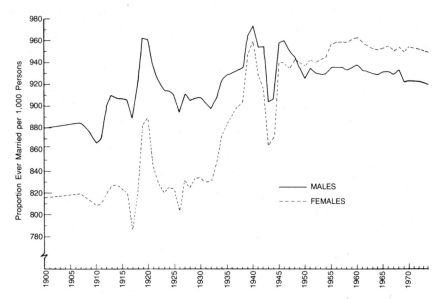

Figure 14.1 Proportion ever married by exact age 50, according to period gross nuptiality tables, England and Wales (Source: Farid, 1976, p. 149)

very significant in and of itself. The marriage rate is only a very rough indicator of nuptiality patterns. Because population totals during wartime and the completeness of registration under turbulent conditions fluctuated substantially, these data must be treated with caution.

Of greater usefulness are long-term data on the timing of marriage (Hajnal, 1953–4, pp. 111–28). One valuable way of measuring this phenomenon is to study proportions single at different ages. A glance at table 14.1 will show that in parts of Europe and in the United States, the proportions single under age 30 declined substantially in the World War II period. For example, in Britain in 1931, 42 percent of all women in the 25–9 age group were still unmarried. Two decades later, only 22 percent were unmarried. Whatever the level of the crude marriage rate, British women were marrying earlier after World War II than before it. The same clear divide occurs in the history of American nuptiality in this period; the proportion still single in the 25–9 age group in 1951 is exactly half that in 1930.

The scale and the suddenness of the change were unprecedented. The Swedish case illustrates this point well. Throughout the nineteenth century, roughly 50 percent of Swedish women aged 25–9 were unmarried. But in the World War II period, a precipitate decline in celibacy in this age group took place. Whereas 49 percent of Swedish women aged 25–9 were single in 1935, only 30 percent were single in 1945. Similar trends occurred in the

Table 14.1 Proportions single at specified ages in several countries during
the World War II period

		Ages men			Ages women		
		20–24	25–9	45–9	20–24	25–9	45–9
France	1936	0.79	0.35	0.10*	0.49	0.23	0.13*
	1949	0.81	0.39	0.12*	0.54	0.22	0.11*
Britain	1931	0.86	0.41	0.12	0.74	0.42	0.17
	1951	0.77	0.35	0.10	0.53	0.22	0.16
Netherlands	1930	0.90	0.49	0.11	0.75	0.38	0.15
	1951	0.89	0.48	0.09	0.71	0.31	0.13
Sweden	1930	0.94	0.67	0.17	0.80	0.52	0.23
	1945	0.87	0.52	0.17	0.64	0.30	0.21
Switzerland	1930	0.93	0.60	0.14	0.82	0.48	0.19
	1950	0.86	0.50	0.13	0.66	0.31	0.19
United States	1930	0.71	0.37	0.11[†]	0.46	0.22	0.09[†]
	1951	0.52	0.20	0.08[†]	0.31	0.11	0.07[†]

* 40–49
† 45–54
Source: Hajnal, 1953, table 3

Netherlands and Switzerland, while in France prewar nuptiality patterns
survived the war intact. Proportions single in France were already lower than
elsewhere in Europe in the late nineteenth century; hence the shift toward
younger marriages that occurred elsewhere in Europe during World War II
period did not occur in France (Hajnal, 1953, pp. 83–4, tables 2 and 3).
French "exceptionalism" is still the rule in modern demographic history,
just as it is in the history of eighteenth century fertility decline.[3]

Using the standard demographic unit I_m as a a fertility-weighted summary
measure of propensity to marry, we can see as well the substantial change in
nuptiality patterns in the decades before and after World War II (see table
14.2). The absence of full data for 1940 makes precise comparison impossible, but taken together with the statistics in table 14.1, it is apparent that the
institution of marriage went through a substantial revival in this period. In
1930 the I_m for England and Wales stood at about 0.5 (of the Hutterite
experience used as a standard of "natural" fertility) (Henry, 1961b, pp. 1–
11); by 1960 the figure was 0.7. A similarly impressive increase in Scottish I_m
occurred over this interval of time, and less marked, though parallel, trends
can be noted for other European countries.

Table 14.2 Nuptiality (I_m)* for several European countries, 1910–60

	1910	1920	1930	1940	1950	1960
Belgium	0.502	0.477	0.577	–	0.605	0.697
England and Wales	0.472	0.485	0.507	–	–	0.703
France	0.605	0.541	0.616	–	–	0.645
Germany	0.523	–	0.527	–	–	0.686
Italy	0.535	0.497	0.515	0.522	0.539	0.581
Netherlands	0.475	0.488	0.506	–	–	0.636
Portugal	0.488	0.468	0.486	0.495	0.524	0.561
Scotland	0.390	0.403	0.419	–	–	0.658
Switzerland	0.459	0.413	0.417	0.471	0.517	0.564

$$* \ I_m = \frac{\Sigma m(i) \, F(i)}{\Sigma w(i) \, F(i)}$$

where for each age group (i) m(i) is the number of married women, w(i) is the total number of women, and F(i) is the age-specific marital fertility rate for Hutterite women married in the years 1921–30.

Source: Watkins, 1981, table 1

Thus various data reflect what John Hajnal has called end of the "European marriage pattern," dating from at least the eighteenth century, under which Europeans tended to marry late and a substantial proportion of women never married at all (Hajnal, 1965, pp. 101–46). These two key features of the demographic history of Western Europe vanished in the years before and after World War II. Such changes occurred in countries directly involved in the war, as well as in those that remained neutral. Clearly, long-term social and economic developments as well as short-term factors were involved in this remarkable departure from previous demographic patterns.

Divorce

It is worthwhile to note that divorce rates also rose substantially after the two world wars. This is hardly surprising given the existential gap between the men who went away and the women they left behind. The heady days following the outbreak of war twice produced a rash of marriages, which on occasion were regretted when the time came to treat them as serious long-term enterprises rather than as ephemeral emotional gestures. Even those who had been married well before 1914 or 1939 found that restoring marriages after a separation of years (which to some seemed like decades) was always difficult and frequently impossible. Legal and administrative changes in a number of countries helped expedite proceedings in both postwar periods.

Table 14.3   Frequency of divorce (per 100,000 married couples) in selected
countries, 1906–35

	1906–15	*1916–25*	*1926–35*
Germany	126	216	288
Austria	56	394	460
Belgium	72	215	128
Denmark	152	229	318
Finland	49	91	178
France	151	283*	211
Hungary	152	290	225
Norway	106	145	181
Netherlands	94	145	184
England and Wales	10	28	43
Sweden	71	134	193
Switzerland	249	292	361
Canada	4	26	50
United States	485	687	720
Japan	701	460	401
Australia	71	117	150
New Zealand	108	263	217

* 1921–5

Source: *Statistique internationale du mouvement de la population*, 1931–5, table 3.J

It was inevitable, therefore, that divorce rates rose substantially after 1918
and 1945, enabling us to conclude that more people were getting into and out
of marriage after the two world wars than before them (Winter, 1986).

The scale of the change that occurred during and after World War I can
be seen in table 14.3. For example, in prewar Austria there were only about
50 divorces per 100,000 couples. In the war period that number increased by
a factor of eight and continued to rise in the 1920s. The same ascending
curve of divorce can be seen in countries as disparate as New Zealand and
Hungary, suggesting that both long-term social and legal causes, as well as
short-term developments, were responsible for the rise in dissolution of
marriages in the World War I period.

The same mix of causes was responsible for the surge in divorce during
and after World War II. Here again the steepness of the trend is apparent.
In Britain the divorce rate rose by a factor of five during World War II and
stayed as high or higher in the late 1940s (Rowntree and Carrier, 1956–7,
p. 210). But it is important to note that more divorce did not mean more
celibacy but rather a rearrangement of marriages at a time when the
"marriage boom" was under way.

Conclusion

It would be foolish to deny that there were some straightforward material explanations for these changes, which I have outlined elsewhere (Winter, 1986). Any account of nuptiality in this period must take note of labor-market and social-policy shifts that made marriage and childrearing more attractive. But it would be wise to abjure strictly economic interpretations of trends in nuptiality and fertility in this – or in any other – period. Scholars in this field have increasingly come to see that purely economic factors can "explain" fertility fluctuations in only the most general way.

Consequently, we need to begin with the assumption that women's attitudes were at the heart of fertility trends in this period, and that such attitudes embodied more than a reflex reaction to economic conditions. We know that the female cohorts producing the larger families of the postwar period were born in the 1920s and 1930s. Having lived through World War II either as children, adolescents, or young adults, a substantial proportion of these women, *for a variety of reasons*, came to see early marriage and relatively large families in a more favorable way than did their mothers' generation. In the remainder of this essay I consider some of the social forces that led women to modify their attitudes and behavior in this fundamental way.

FAMILY LIFE IN THE AFTERMATH OF WAR

Images of Women in Wartime

The celebration of masculine virtues is perhaps inevitable in wartime, as the evidence of popular culture in the visual arts suggests. What is less well known is the reiteration and deepening in wartime of traditional stereotypes of women. These stereotypes present women in many poses, but not as people with active (extradomestic) working and (party) political lives. Let us consider three standard images of women repeated time and again in wartime art: as passive victims or nurturing and grieving mothers; as prostitutes; or as mythological creatures.

The first image has a long religious history behind it and expresses aspects of popular Protestantism and Catholicism, which present women as the carriers of a stoic faith or as silent witnesses of the unavoidable sufferings of this world. The second pose is also time-honored but took on a patriotic form in some World War I lithographs. One popular example is of a French prostitute seducing Wilhelm II and Franz Joseph while a smiling French soldier steals around to surprise and rout the enemy. To add insult to injury, as it were, the caption to this slightly scurrilous bit of adolescent humor was "Your 42 cm guns look all right, but when the time comes, they never seem to work."[4] This example could be repeated hundreds of times and suggests the extent to which images of women became cruder and more blatantly misogynist as the war went on. Much propaganda dwelled lovingly and luridly on the sexual aspect of atrocity stories, virtually all of which were totally fictitious.

Prewar artists frequently portrayed women as vain, silly, and unproductive. In contrast, cartoons and caricatures in the popular press in wartime France elevated women to the level of political symbol. They stood for everything an invaded nation needed: force, courage, and consolation. The image of Marianne was a standard feature of wartime poster art, the epitome of republican virtues in neoclassical robes, striding forward to confront the enemies of France. She is an allegorical rather than a party political figure; she encompasses ideals, not real power. In Marianne Left and Right iconography met (Agulhon, 1980, pp. 9–20, 1989; Warner, 1985) in celebration of womanly virtues that departed from the crude misogyny of prewar and wartime caricature. But only for a time: the older conventions were restored after the war in the popular press (Wautier, 1981; Delatour, 1965; Agulhon, 1976, pp. 143–52).

In effect, the representation of women in wartime was timeless, reiterating very old images in a period when families had to make do without men and when women took on a range of responsibilities in their place. The message they bear is clear: women are meant for maternity and the sexual comfort of men.

This popular art also offered a celebration of "traditional" family life, rescued from the mundane by its patriotic function. Indeed, through the medium of the graphic arts, family life was glorified as the embodiment of the virtues for which the men in uniform were risking their lives. In the 1914–18 war this propaganda took the form of posters and postcards, many of which broadcast a blatantly pronatalist message. In France production of these postcards was a major industry and clearly responded to popular taste. These advertisements for maternity were anything but subtle. Children emerging from roses (girls) and cabbages (boys) remind a couple, "On your honeymoon, don't forget about us" (Huss, 1988).

During World War II the broadcasting of sexual stereotypes was more aggressive. Nazi propaganda had no doubt about gender roles and the "true" nature of women. It also spent much time glorying in the difference between virility and decadence, between Aryan masculinity and Jewish femininity. The Allies did not directly repeat these images but still managed to portray the war as a sexual struggle. In addition, classic posters presented women in the usual pin-up form or as empty-headed gossips – "Careless talk costs lives" – or as Mata Haris playing on the weaknesses of men – "Keep mum, she's not so dumb." Whether or not these were male responses to sexual fears or expressions of sexual hatred, as one scholar has suggested (Gubar, 1987), they helped to perpetuate a view of women as inferior, primarily sexual, and occasionally dangerous. The only place where both women and their men could be safe is, therefore, in the confines of the family.

Social Policy, Women, and the Family

The barrage of images about women's nature and women's realm that appeared in popular art was not engineered by some controlling or influential groups intent on putting women back in the home after the upheaval of war. The social pressures in this direction were much more subtle and much more pervasive, but they were indeed strongly reinforced by the nature of government policy during and after the war in several countries.

Fears of depopulation certainly antedated both world wars, but during and after both conflicts a positive effort was made to encourage what were seen as family values and to reduce the economic burden of childbearing. The formulation of family policy was an attempt to coordinate and realize these objectives.

For conservatives, the defense of the family came naturally. For socialists and social democrats, family policy was an important expression of patriotism and one that could demonstrate national solidarity at a time of national peril. It is hardly surprising, therefore, that major steps were taken in the provision of antenatal and childcare during both world wars (Winter, 1985, chap. 6; Titmuss, 1950).[5] After 1945 population policy by and large became family policy. This entailed a plan to help equalize the costs of child care, in recognition of the essential service parents rendered to the nation (Winter, 1989).

A wide array of groups kept up the pressure on postwar governments to ensure that they would turn this rhetoric into practical proposals. One of the most famous was the French Alliance Nationale pour l'Accroissement de la Population, founded in 1896. Its activists managed to carry on a vigorous pronatalist and antifeminist policy whichever way the political winds were blowing. The group's spokesmen were influential figures in the formulation of the Family Code of 1939, made their peace with Vichy and its German masters, and helped restate family policy under the Fourth Republic after the Liberation.

This body held clearly conservative views about the proper role of women. Domesticity was their national duty, and any assertion of equality under the law, in political life or at work, was to be resisted. The alliance consisted of notables from all walks of life and clearly expressed centrist views on these issues. Its members tirelessly worked for a family vote as an alternative to votes for women. Consider this message of the alliance's president in early 1945, when the decision to give women the vote had already been taken: "If women's suffrage is passed without representation of the family, the influence of fathers and mothers, of those who in giving the country her defenders, her producers and her inheritors, assuring its life now and in perpetuity, will wane, especially if the age of voting will be reduced to 18." Celibates and the childless would come to dominate the electorate and thereby "govern against the family" (Toulemon, 1945, p. 2). This frame of mind, not at all restricted to the political Right, in which women were "overfeminized," in Denise Riley's phrase (1987), gave to social policy in the aftermath of the two world wars its characteristically patriarchal form.

The Inner Migration

War in Europe in this century has both torn families apart and increased social, economic, and political pressures leading to a revival of domesticity. The politics of the family thus symbolized and gave practical form to a broad body of opinion that, during and after World War II, considered the strengthening of hearth and home the core of social reconstruction.

One way of looking at the demographic data on the rise in nuptiality and fertility in this period is to suggest that most young women of marital age agreed. That is to say, the revival in the popularity of marriage, the decrease in the age at first marriage, and the increase in the total fertility rate in the period surrounding the 1939–45 war represented a real response of ordinary women to the political and social disturbances through which they lived.

It is not my intention to reduce demographic change to a response, crude or otherwise, to political change. There were clearly many pathways to higher fertility in post-1945 Europe, just as there were many pathways to fertility decline in the 1870–1940 period. The revival of nuptiality also took place in Sweden and Switzerland after the 1940s, suggesting that it is unwise to place too much emphasis on military participation in the unfolding of complex social and economic processes (Coale and Watkins, 1986, chap. 2).

But it would be equally foolish to ignore the upheaval of war in the overall history of demographic change in Europe in World War II period. Evidence in support of this contention was visible during the war itself. French scholars have disputed the reasons why the birth rate rose under the Nazi occupation. Could it not be that couples saw marriage and raising children as a kind of inner migration, a withdrawal from a disturbed and disturbing public realm to the supposedly simpler and more certain rewards of the private realm?[5] Even among those who did not know the humiliations of invasion and defeat, similar reactions may be discerned. The stress of a struggle for survival, the tensions of separation and loss of loved ones, the anxiety of waiting, hoping, and struggling against despair – these were experiences most Europeans shared, to a greater or lesser degree, in the two world wars. The reaction against this dark phase of European history took many forms. The post-1945 revival of family life was one of them. It is this fact demographic historians must recognize if they wish to make sense of the complex history of the family and fertility decline in twentieth-century Europe.

NOTES

1 Thanks are due in particular to Joanna Bourke, Martine Segalen, and Louise Tilly for helpful comments and suggestions.
2 Male labor in textiles dropped from 400,000 in 1913 to 98,000 in 1918 and reached only 233,000 in 1920. The female labor force in textiles also declined, but not as precipitately. For the same pattern in Britain, see Kirkaldy (1921), table 8.
3 So is Irish exceptionalism. I am grateful to Dr. Joanna Bourke for her help on this and other points.
4 Thanks are due to Mme Cecille Couttin of the Bibliotheque de la Documentation Internationale Comparée at the Hotel des Invalides in Paris for allowing me access to an invaluable collection of popular lithographs. Of course, legal provision and full services are entirely different phenomena; the gains of 1945 were much more substantial than those of 1918.
5 I say "couples" for lack of evidence about differences in fathers' and mothers' attitudes toward family life. Such differences, frequently asserted and almost certainly significant, are still to be substantiated.

15

Safety in Numbers: Social Welfare Legislation and Fertility Decline in Western Europe

Lynn Hollen Lees

> The government under which...the citizens do most increase and multiply is infallibly the best. Similarly, the government under which a people diminishes in number and wastes away is the worst.
>
> – J.-J. Rousseau, *The Social Contract*

Around 1800 Western European states spent most of their money on guns, roads, and bureaucrats. Building up their armies, transport systems, and civil-service sectors plus financing old debts accounted for almost all of state budgets. In contrast, investments in human capital were tiny. In England in 1802, under 0.1 percent of all government revenues went toward education or science, and the French central government in 1820 alotted only 2.3 percent of its budget to public health, pensions, housing, or education. Yet if we look ahead to the 1970s, we find priorities reversed: human capital investments replaced guns and government as the preferred purchase. Social welfare programs and education now account for well over half of government expenditures in Germany, and Sweden and are almost as high in the United Kingdom (Mitchell and Deane, 1962, p. 396; Flora et al., 1983, 2:382). Meanwhile, defense spending and investments in infrastructures have shrunk to relative insignificance.

This shift began after 1820, when public education and then state social insurance plans spread rapidly and widely throughout Western Europe. By World War I, 12 countries offered workmen's compensation benefits, 10 had begun health insurance programs, and several had introduced old-age

I wish to thank Andrew Lees, Paul Hohenberg, Stefano Fenoaltea, Peter Lindert, Hilton Root, and members of the European Fertility Decline conference for comments on an earlier draft of this essay.

pensions and unemployment insurance. During the 1920s and 1930s these plans were broadened to cover new risks and new groups, while additional states began similar programs. Within 70 years of the first state social security plans in the German empire, most countries in Western Europe offered their citizens comprehensive insurance against major risks of the labor market and to improve their health (Flora and Heidenheimer, 1981, pp. 49, 54). How can this new willlingness to invest in citizens' welfare be explained?

The major theories for the rise of the welfare state fall within either a pluralist or a neo-Marxist tradition, both of which – despite significant differences – share a basic emphasis on economic and political variables. The former place the welfare state within a "modernization" story: welfare policies become part of the adaptation of nations to changing economic, political, and ideological conditions. In short, economic growth plus the rise of mass democracies provided the resources, as well as the political impetus, for redistributing wealth at a national level. A variety of scholars work within this tradition. Peter Flora and Arnold Heidenheimer see the welfare state "as an answer to basic and long-term developmental processes," focusing on the demands for socioeconomic equality and security arising out of mass democracy and the modernizing economy (1981, p. 8). Gaston Rimlinger notes that although differing political conditions produced welfare legislation, the basic impetus for change arose from industrialization, class relations, and the growing acceptance of liberal ideas and consititutional practices (1971, pp. 8–9). Even studies that avoid an explicit modernization model usually stress a combination of political and economic imperatives that prompted bureaucrats and politicians to enact social security measures (Dawson, 1912, pp. 1, 10).

While rejecting major elements of pluralist arguments, analysts of social security systems from the political Left also base their arguments on economic and political variables. Neo-Marxist explanations of the welfare state link capitalist development to a growing need for regulation of the labor force, both to dampen class conflict and to regulate labor supplies (Offe, 1972; Diven and Cloward, 1971). According to this version as well as the pluralist one, economic development produced both the resources and the need for social welfare policies, while the capitalists' political agendas and power permitted their use of the state for their own purposes.

Neither of these explanatory strategies is as useful as their exponents would have us believe. Analysts of the welfare state working within these traditions find it hard to explain why countries like Denmark, Sweden, Austria, and Norway, which experienced relatively late and limited industrial growth in the nineteenth century, were among the first states to pass social security measures, and those whose analyses draw on modernization theory find it difficult to account for the early German adoption of insurance laws. Deviant cases abound. Why should French politicians, when faced with a slow-growing and incompletely industrialized economy, have agreed to limited responsibility for and funding of old-age pensions several decades before a British government followed suit? Indeed, Jens Alber has shown that the states of Western Europe introduced their early social security laws at widely varying stages of industrial and urban growth, and he rejects functional arguments tying the emergence of state welfare measures to economic development (1982, p. 133).

In this essay I link the story of the welfare state to other variables – population structures, theories of human capital, and an awareness of demographic changes. The story of state subsidies for social needs is incomplete without attention to demography. The linkage between demography and welfare spending is not a new idea. Thomas Malthus feared that poor relief payments encouraged early marriages and high fertility, while proponents of pronatalist policies in the nineteenth and twentieth centuries sought to raise birth rates through state grants to mothers and families. Such arguments have become an integral part of the "new home economics." Gary Becker, for example, in *A Treatise on the Family*, links fertility levels to the net costs of childrearing: welfare programs – for example, family allowances – encourage higher fertility by reducing the price of children (1981). Becker's work and that of other neoclassical economists focus, however, on the realm of individual choice, not on the level of societies or cultures – that is, on the macro level. Arguments made on this level include those of J. C. Caldwell, who has discussed institutional effects on fertility, concentrating on public schooling (1982). In a similar vein, many demographers have asserted a direct connection between old-age insurance and fertility decline, arguing that security in old age is an important motivation for fertility and that the provision of alternative sources of support influences demographic decisions (Nugent, 1985). All of these arguments treat fertility as a *response* to public social policies; I wish, however, to reverse this argument and to emphasize how on the national level policy decisions about social investments were tied to attitudes about the size and health of populations.

During the nineteenth century, national governments in Western and central Europe were faced with a series of similar, partly demographic, partly political challenges. Demographic growth produced rapidly expanding populations, everywhere except in France. Yet structures to control and to protect these new citizens seemed in decay. Urban migration made cities threatening to physical health and was thought to undermine political loyalty. Meanwhile, democratic revolutions demonstrated the power of nations-in-arms and increased the lure of liberal political theories among the middle classes and of socialist ideas among some workers and intellectual. Although political power remained in the hands of social elites, legislatures debated government policies while periodic increases in the suffrage expanded workers' influence on representatives. Governments of all political persuasions were faced with a dilemma: how to maintain a strong population both willing and able to defend the state.

Early in the nineteenth century, when the voting power of adults was not an issue and when the numbers of younger age cohorts were expanding most rapidly, governments responded to this dilemma by expanding national spending on education. During the last quarter of the nineteenth century, as birth rates declined and the public became concerned with high mortality and disability, politicians from a variety of parties argued that increased social investment in the citizenry was required for a healthy state. Governments approved both pronatalist measures and social insurance plans. In this essay I examine the changing linkages between demography and social policy from the late 1700s to the mid 1900s.

DEMOGRAPHY AND EARLY INVESTMENT IN EDUCATION

During the early and mid-eighteenth century, men interested in political arithmetic proposed that a nation's strength was directly related to the number of its citizens and to their health. Moreover, wise and effective governments were those that promoted population growth, according to Rousseau, David Hume, and Leibnitz. This easy acceptance of population growth faded, however, during the later eighteenth century in both Great Britain and the German states as the size of populations exploded. Thomas Malthus's theories, which linked rapid population growth to poverty, gained wide acceptance, and German intellectuals saw rising crime rates, begging, and disorder as the outcome of rising fertility and lowered mortality (Schleunes, 1989, p. 19; Porter, 1986, p. 20).

Among the remedies sought to counter the problems posed by demographic growth was education. Malthus advocated public schools to teach citizens the true cause of their misery and to encourage them to adopt self-restraint and later marriage. In the 1780s influential Swiss reformer J. H. Pestalozzi explained how education could lead to moral improvement among the peasants, thereby decreasing the incidence of threatening social problems. Meanwhile, publicists and philanthropic noblemen in Prussia touted schools as an appropriate response to growing beggary and banditry. The notion that education could alter the behavior of citizens and thereby improve the society was widespread (Porter, 1986, p. 26; Schleunes, 1989, pp. 26–7).

When states began to invest in public education, the new policies were often defended in terms of their ability to secure existing governments against the threat of political and social disorder posed by large, undisciplined populations. The Bavarian government in 1771 mandated compulsory education in state-run schools. Heinrich Braun, the Benedictine theologian who designed the plan, told the elector, "The better educated people are, the more moral they will be and the more amenable to obeying good laws and leaders" (quoted in Schleunes, 1989, p. 33). Early Prussian education schemes were implemented by social elites during a period following military defeat when that state was threatened by disintegration. Reformers like Wilhelm von Humboldt thought schools were needed to educate Prussians to the idea of the nation and to common sentiments. More conservative politicians, whose ideas dominated in the 1820s, backed schools designed to keep each group of citizens in its proper social position. Yet they too accepted the notion that education was necessary for the health of the state. In France after 1789, regimes of all political persuasions saw salvation for the state in the education of good citizens. Education minister François Guizot claimed in 1833 that universal primary education was "one of the greatest guarantees of order and social stability" and saw it as productive of "unity" within the French nation (quoted in Maynes, 1985a, p. 55, 1985b, p. 49).

Public commitments to primary education began slowly in the German states during the later eighteenth century, in France during the Revolution, and in Great Britain during the early 1830s against a background of demographic growth and political turmoil. In each of these cases, educational reformers – relatively isolated from direct expressions of popular wants and needs – were wary of unruly, potentially disloyal populations. They chose primary education as their first target for investment in the growing human capital of the nation, at a time when molding the minds of new citizens seemed more needful than improving their living conditions.

THE CHANGING AGE STRUCTURE OF EUROPEAN POPULATIONS

The demographic context of social policy shifted during the later nineteenth century. Social statisticians showered bureaucrats with demographic facts, newly available from censuses, state statistical offices, insurance societies, and medical reports. The messages they spread were profoundly unsettling to political elites because they portrayed populations under siege from diseases and declining birth rates.

Between the mid-nineteenth and mid-twentieth centuries, decreases in mortality and fertility shifted substantially the relative numbers of adults and children in European populations. Just before the late nineteenth-century declines in birth rates, children under age 15 constituted approximately one-third of national populations, while in the early 1950s they comprised only one-fifth to a quarter of the citizenry. Meanwhile, between 1850 and 1950 the proportion of those age 60 or over approximately doubled in much of Europe, rising from averages of 7–8 percent to about 16 percent of the total

Table 15.1   Age distributions of English and Welsh populations, 1851–1971
(proportion per 10,000 population)

Age (years)	1851	1871	1891	1911	1931	1951	1971
0–4	1,310	1,349	1,225	1,069	748	850	801
5–9	1,167	1,189	1,171	1,025	832	723	830
10–14	1,067	1,065	1,111	970	803	643	744
15–19	980	958	1,017	925	860	618	680
20–24	930	903	912	880	875	669	765
25–9	820	782	810	854	840	750	655
30–34	712	685	699	798	765	704	589
35–9	607	589	614	724	702	759	572
40–44	540	540	533	619	667	769	602
45–9	446	463	461	534	639	725	643
50–54	395	415	400	444	596	646	594
55–9	294	315	305	354	518	554	610
60–64	268	274	266	283	415	490	583
65–9	183	194	197	224	318	418	492
70–74	140	142	144	153	218	326	365
75$^+$	141	136	132	144	206	358	475

Source: Flora, ed., 1983, 2:138

population around 1950 (Mitchell, 1975, pp. 29–55; Flora et al., 1987, 2: 111–39). Ansley Coale has shown that fertility rather than mortality is the "dominant force" in shaping age cohort sizes. Using stable age distributions for females and a variety of fertility and mortality schedules, he has demonstrated that fertility declines quickly swell the proportion of the population between the ages of 15 and 40 (1965, pp. 252, 262). Large decreases in fertility produce a substantial restructuring of a population over the long run. Such changes could be seen earliest in France, whose national fertility transition by the measures of the Princeton University European Fertility Project began around 1827 and then underwent a second marked decline around 1870 (Coale and Watkins, 1986, p. 38). In most of the rest of Europe, the proportion of people up to age 9 increased until 1880–1900. The effects of the demographic transition on age distribution can easily be seen in tables 15.1 and 15.2. Among the French, the proportion of children in the population was already declining by 1851, while the proportion of people over 60 rose by 20 percent between 1851 and 1871. In England, where fertility decline occurred later, the proportion of children decreased after 1871, when the age cohort between 15 and 40 began to grow. Unlike the French case, the proportion over 60 remained roughly stable until after World War I.

Table 15.2   Age distributions of the French population, 1851–1968 (proportion per 10,000 population)

Age (years)	1851	1872	1891	1911	1931	1954	1968
0–4	928	928	871	886	872	874	700
5–9	921	905	880	848	857	893	843
10–14	879	870	872	842	566	862	827
15–19	880	844	876	813	741	673	851
20–24	832	879	860	791	821	713	762
25–9	801	721	766	784	847	738	579
30–34	756	704	712	760	793	762	625
35–9	718	688	667	715	677	419	676
40–44	659	645	630	655	651	694	670
45–9	586	608	602	616	626	705	622
50–54	578	547	537	553	604	685	397
55–9	439	495	471	481	547	586	567
60–64	367	416	422	421	464	485	538
65–9	278	305	333	346	382	427	476
70–74	195	232	245	250	277	343	360
75$^+$	174	204	250	240	276	443	507

Source: Flora, ed., 1983, 2:120–21

A secondary effect of demographic change needs to be recognized. George Alter and James Riley argue that declining mortality produces rising rates of illness and disability. As death rates decline, a population includes more people with higher susceptibilities to various diseases. Therefore the incidence of morbidity in a population rises. This seems to have been the case in England, where from the 1860s to at least the later 1890s age-specific morbidity rates increased among the members of Friendly Societies – custodians of workers' privately subscribed insurance funds, to which about half of the employed males in Britain subscribed by 1890 – during a period when mortality rates among members decreased (Alter and Riley, 1989, p. 25; Gilbert, 1966, pp. 171–2). Not only were British Friendly Society members at greater risk of being sick in the later nineteenth century, but the incidence of chronic illnesses among them rose and, on average, the time a member spent out of work with each sickness episode lengthened for each age group within the Friendly Societies (Riley, 1989, pp. 164–72).

The policy implications of fertility decline combined with rising disability were particularly acute because of issues raised by urban growth and urban poverty. Intensive urbanization seemed to threaten the demographic health of the nation because city dwellers were the earliest to contracept and to decrease family size. Because urban death rates and urban rates of contagious diseases remained relatively high, cities in much of continental Europe continued to rely on immigrants to renew and to expand their populations, but these migrants got sick and died more quickly and produced fewer children than did their rural counterparts. In the towns, the effect of the fertility decline was accentuated, while that of the mortality decrease was muted. Cities brought to public attention the question of social reproduction. Who would people the cities of the future? What should governments do to avert possible demographic disaster? In a Europe threatened by war and obsessed by imperialist rivalries, these questions, whose answers affected future military strength, called for creative answers.

Public awareness of these demographic shifts was accentuated in the later nineteenth century, when statistical reports attracted widespread attention. In France prominent politicians, demographers, and doctors publicly reviewed census results and articulated fears of demographic decline. After France's defeat in the Franco-Prussian War, many commentators defined the German threat in demographic terms. In England the Registrar-General's reports, in combination with compulsory birth registration, brought to public attention a decline in the birth rate after 1872. Later, when Charles Booth's research on poverty, first published in the 1890s, identified 30 percent of London's population as living at or below the poverty line, the magnitude of the urban social problem was made explicit within a context that detailed the ravages of disease, high mortality, and low wages (Booth, 1902). Both children and adults were clearly at risk in an environment whose threats were largely beyond their control. Government health inquiries carried out after the turn of the century directed attention to high infant and child mortality rates, as well as to the circumstances of early childhood deprivation. In Germany, demographers and economists such as Georg von Mayr, Adolf Weber, and Felix Theilhaber linked low urban birth rates to a dismal view of the German future; the proponents of theories of demographic decline waxed eloquent after the 1891 census revealed an absolute decline in the share of the rural population (Lees, 1985, pp. 145–6).

Around 1900 European policy-makers were surrounded by a furor created by public health reports and demographers' projections; few were unaware of declining birth rates, high incidences of diseases, and of the consequent threats posed for military strength and national efficiency. They began to design policies they hoped would reverse fertility decline and improve the health of survivors. They in fact had a double problem – a perceived need to encourage reproduction and a growing concern for an unhealthy, economically insecure adult population whose ability to pressure states was increasing because of mass political parties and trade unions. By the late nineteenth century, the aim of increasing national strength and efficiency seemed to dictate social investment and planning in areas other than education. Slowly, most states developed both pronatalist policies and social insurance.

INVESTMENT IN REPRODUCTION

An awareness of declining birth rates led politicians and social reformers to consider subsidizing reproduction as well as children's health. Through increased provision of medical care, as well as other resources for mothers and infants, children were to be protected and families were to be encouraged to reproduce. In several European states, the fear of population decline prompted pronatalist policies between the 1870s and the 1930s.

The earliest and clearest linkages of pronatalism to state welfare legislation were made in France, where fertility decline began at least half a century earlier than in other European countries. By the late 1860s, not only the French Academy of Medicine but also the legislature had discussed fears of slow population growth. In fact, the implications of social policy for population growth became a standard topic in parliamentary debates over the next several decades (Spengler, 1979, pp. 112, 117–25). Some of the earliest French welfare allocations were designed to improve infant care through payments to crèches. By the early years of the Third Republic, the French state also regulated wet nurses and funded departmental grants to unmarried mothers who kept and nursed their babies (Klaus, 1986, pp. 246, 262, 271–2). Maternity leaves, which were discussed seriously since the mid 1880s, had the support of obstetricians, demographers, pronatalist groups, and charities, on the grounds that they would lower infant mortality, helping thereby to "repopulate" France. "France lost one army corps a year to preventable infant disease," concluded a 1901 study of infant mortality (McDougall, 1983, pp. 80, 93, 95); maternal and infant welfare measures seemed the remedy. When statisticians counted more coffins that cradles, the French state responded with schemes to promote maternal and infant health, agreeing in 1913 to finance maternity leaves.

The demographic losses of World War I intensified pressures in France for pronatalist policies. Criminal penalties for both abortion and distributing birth-control information were reenacted in the 1920s. In an effort to use the carrot rather than the stick, French civil servants were given family allowances, which soon spread to other sectors and industries, until they were made universal in 1932 (Glass, 1940, pp. 101–7). Most commonly, French mothers received monthly grants via postal orders for every child under age 14.

In great Britain fears of population decline and children's health mounted throughout the 1880s, when medical studies of slum populations advanced theories of physical decline. Doctors and anthropologists popularized images of city dwellers as short feeble, squinting, impotent, and neurotic – a "dying race" (Cantlie, 1885; Fothergill, 1889). In combination with the obvious growth of cities and declines in birth rates, these images of degeneration prompted cries of protest and demands for change through improvements in public health. Pronatalists joined forces with eugenicists and social reformers, such as Seebohm Rowntree, to support campaigns for the breeding of a stronger, more fit set of Anglo-Saxons. Starting in the 1880s, charities throughout England set up free food services for children, and town councils assigned local medical officers of health to schools. Voluntarist measures, quite in keeping with strong English resistance to state bureaucracies, began pronatalist activities. Central government action took place only after military recruitment difficulties during the Boer War intensified concern for workers' physical fitness, but it remained limited both in size and in budgetary commitment. The Liberal party, which came to power in 1906 with a large agenda of social welfare proposals, enacted legislation designed to improve childrens' and mothers' health throughout the country. The provision of free school meals and medical inspections both in school and at home by medical officers of health was the first step; a state maternity benefit, provided in the 1911 National Insurance Act, was the second (Gilbert, 1966, pp. 102–7, 117, 349). Overall, however, most English pronatalist welfare measures came from private sources until after World War II, when the state provided child allowances (Kohler et al., 1982, p. 153).

Fears of population decline grew throughout Europe after World War I, producing increased support for pronatalist programs. The combination of war losses with continued decline in birth rates alarmed politicians and intellectuals in much of Western Europe. Georges Clemenceau warned in 1919 that "if France turns her back upon large families...France will be lost because there will be no more Frenchmen" (quoted in Teitelbaum and Winter, 1985, p. 35). In a 1927 speech Mussolini warned that "with a falling population, one does not create an empire but becomes a colony" (quoted in Glass, 1940, p. 220). In Germany continued concern for the demographic effects of urbanization intensified the problem posed by fertility decline. Articles such as "The Metropolis as the Mass Grave of the People" appeared in the popular press, while Nazi writers condemned both low birth rates and the conditions that produced them (Lees, 1985, p. 280). Both Mussolini's and Hitler's governments tried a combination of repressive measures and economic incentives to raise birth rates. Fascist policies to increase population size included prohibition of abortion and, in Italy, of the manufacture, advertisement, and sale of birth-control devices. Financial methods were also tried: bachelors were taxed more heavily than married men, while low-interest loans were offered to newlyweds and were partially canceled after the birth of children. Explicit welfare provisions in Italy included pre- and post-natal clinics, free layettes and food for mothers and their newborns, care for unmarried mothers, confinement grants, prohibitions on women working one month before and one month after childbirth, and, by the 1930s, family allowances. Meanwhile, the Fascist Union of Large Families and celebrations such as "Mother and Child Day" were designed to encourage happy, frequent reproduction (Glass, 1940, pp. 230–60). German policies were quite similar, although they included fewer elaborate measures to benefit new mothers and greater investment in children as they entered school (Glass, 1940, pp. 287–99; Kälvemark, 1980, p. 36).

Fertility decline in Sweden also prompted discussion there of pronatalist legislation. During the later 1930s, the Swedish state adopted a policy of limited financial support for parenthood, designed to encourage childbirth within a framework of individual choice. During the early 1930s, Conservative, Agrarian, and National Socialist parties called for various tax breaks and grants to encourage fertility among their favorite sectors of the population, but nothing was done until Gunnar and Alva Myrdal brought the problem of population decline or, as they described it, "family crisis" to the notice of Social Democrats. Soon thereafter the Swedish government decided to provide marriage loans, maternity benefits for poor women, and job security for women during pregnancy and childbirth (Myrdal, 1945; Kälvemark, 1980, pp. 51–8).

Pronatalism became a characteristic element of state social policies in Europe between the 1870s and the 1940s, whatever the political complexion of the party in power. Although they used different strategies, Liberals, Conservatives, Social Democrats and Fascists responded to declining birth rates with a variety of proposals to subsidize reproduction and children's health. Most of their efforts proved ineffective, however – perhaps because propaganda and repressive legislation were ignored, while subsidies proved far from generous. Maternal welfare and infant care, even if accepted by governments as laudable goals, were less politically compelling than the claims of adult male workers, whose organizations and voting power increased throughout Europe during the later nineteenth and early twentieth centuries, the period when the first wave of social security legislation was passed.

THE ADOPTION OF PENSIONS AND SOCIAL INSURANCE

Patterns of state investment in citizen's welfare shifted dramatically between 1880 and 1920 as governments undertook a series of new commitments to the disabled, the unemployed, the sick, and elderly. State subsidies for the elderly came earliest in France, where legislators began discussions of a pension plan during the 1840s and established small, voluntary savings funds, the Caisse nationale des Retraites pour la Vieillesse, during the early 1850s. Access to the fund was widened in the 1890s, when the state increased its subsidy and its monitoring of employer pension plans. The French example attracted attention in other parts of Europe, particularly in Germany, where the government adopted compulsory, contributory pensions for wage earners in 1889. Other states soon followed. By 1914 subsidized pensions or old-age insurance had been enacted in Britain, Belgium, Denmark, Italy, the Netherlands, and Sweden (Hatzfeld, 1971, pp. 56–8; Flora, ed., 1983, 1:454).

Both parliamentary democracies and more autocratic, monarchical regimes shifted their welfare policies in similar directions, although the adoption of old-age insurance was not a simple case of the diffusion of an appealing idea. British politicians expressly rejected the German model of pension legislation, and most other European countries that enacted pensions by the early twentieth century preferred some sort of voluntary program to the German compulsory one (Hennock, 1987, p. 2). Each national form arose within a particular set of political circumstances with a unique combination of pressure groups. Nevertheless, a common thread was awareness of demographic problems and issues of workers' poverty, sickness, and injury. A look at two rather different cases – that of the German empire and of Great Britain – shows how demographic issues shaped pension debates.

At the behest of Otto von Bismarck, the German Reichstag passed the earliest comprehensive insurance programs within a decade of the foundation of the empire. Historians have generally explained German social insurance as the result of Bismarck's dual wish to fight socialism and to tie workers to the state (Ritter, 1986; Born, 1957; Wehler, 1969). Yet this interpretation neglects both the contributions of industrialists to the development of the early insurance programs and the background of demographic change. Indeed, Bismarck did direct ministers to draw up plans for accident, health, and old-age insurance, but he did not actively intervene in the planning. The choice of time was largely his, but the legislation was written by K. H. von Boetticher, state secretary in the Ministry of the Interior. Representatives of the iron, steel, and mining industries, who had organized effective pressure groups worked with Boetticher before the bill was sent to the Reichstag to be shaped into legislation. These groups had not only strongly supported the bills for accident and health insurance but had lobbied with Bismarck for these measures and supplied him with arguments and data to use against opponents in the civil service (Mommsen, 1981, pp. 76, 140–43).

Ample precedents existed in Prussia for state regulation of workers' social insurance. According to state decree, miners as well as various sorts of artisans belonged to groups that provided payments for illness, accidents, disability, and, in a few cases, old age. Moreover, the larger firms in German heavy industry had compulsory accident insurance and pension programs, whose funds were under company control. By the 1880s these paternalist programs had proven inadequate. High migration rates combined with rapid reorganization of the German economy meant that most workers were not covered by an insurance plan. Those excluded had to be supported in times of need by local poor rates – a situation opposed by local officials and resented by workers. Moreover, rising disability rates from occupational diseases, well documented in factory-inspector and physician reports, increased charges on the funds. Among miners and other insured workers the average age of those taking up disability pensions declined steadily from the late 1860s to 1900. Workers put in fewer and fewer years in the labor force before they were deemed unfit to continue. Employers whose insurance costs were rising had every reason to champion the extension of the funds and the widening of their financial bases. In fact, an industrialist, Count von Stumm-Halberg, was one of the first to suggest adoption of a national compulsory old-age and disability pension program. At least part of the support for state-funded pensions came from local officials and industrialists who wanted to change current methods of financing the elderly and the disabled – groups whose demographic weight was increasing as both fertility and mortality rates shifted (Ritter, 1983, pp. 38–9; Tenfelde, 1977, pp. 286–8).

In Britain the political context for the enacting of the earliest forms of social insurance differed markedly from the German case; yet there were parallel pressures being exerted by demographic changes and a similar concern for rising disability rates. During the last quarter of the nineteenth century, extensions of the suffrage brought workers into the House of Commons, while the growth of socialist parties, trade unions, and Friendly Societies expanded the number of pressure groups on the Left calling for social reforms. At roughly the same time, statistics provided new information on the scope of social problems, particularly urban poverty and pauperism among the elderly. Many voices spoke for change, albeit in different tones. Between 1890 and 1910 knowledge of social demography was translated into politically effective terms, triggering action.

Large-scale discussion of old-age pensions began in Great Britain around 1880. Canon Blackley, an Anglican clergyman, proposed that young workers be required to purchase annuities, which would give them a pension at age 70, and he wrote commentaries on the German pension program for *Contemporary Review*. Soon after, the National Providence League organized to agitate for universal, compulsory retirement insurance. By the early 1890s, when government reports showed that 30 percent of the population over 65 was dependent on the Poor Law for support, Joseph Chamberlain and others took up the cause. The National Committee of Organized Labour (NCOL) for Promoting Old Age Pensions, which became an effective lobbying group, had the backing of Charles Booth, the most prominent social statistician in Britain of his generation, and Booth marshalled the weight of numbers to bolster the pension case (Booth, 1892). Supported by the Trades Union Congress, the Co-Operative Movement, the Independent Labour party, and the Labour Representation Committee, the NCOL lobbied effectively for pensions (Hennock, 1987, pp. 117–25). Nevertheless, members of Britain's Friendly societies feared losing their power and initially blocked reform. They, however, were slowly being bankrupted by the joint effects among their members of declining adult mortality and rising morbidity, which helped to produce a large increase in claims for support. Politically unable to raise rates or to change the rules of eligibilty, leaders of the Friendly Societies slowly dropped their opposition to the idea of state-funded pensions, finally realizing how their interest would be served by the change. Their funds could be used for workers under 70, while the state would support those at higher ages (Gilbert, 1966, pp. 170–76, 220–21). By the time the Liberals came to power in 1906, a variety of politicians had been won over to the cause. The examples of Germany, Denmark, and New Zealand could be cited as successful precedents, and Herbert Asquith's government successfully piloted pension legislation through the Parliament.

The stories of German and British welfare legislation have many parallels in other parts of Europe. Between 1900 and 1920 old-age pensions were introduced in several countries, most notably Sweden and the Netherlands, where coverage was compulsory. The stronger monarchies generally preceded parliamentary regimes in the drive to enact welfare measures, but political systems with relatively powerful legislatures quickly made social commitments similar to those of their monarchical neighbors.

The timing of this legislative innovation is instructive. While not tightly correlated with either economic development or the coming to power of socialists and radicals, social welfare legislation was enacted in a time of growing demographic awareness and sharpening threats from workers' organizations to existing distributions of political power. The depression of the 1880s and early 1890s intensified levels of morbidity and infant mortality, while imperial rivalries and increasingly contentious workers' groups gave administrators ample reason to decide that social spending was necessary for the welfare of the polity as well as for that of the individual.

The practical impact of welfare legislation was limited, however, in most of Europe until after World war I. Most programs were designed as insurance plans to benefit male industrial workers, the group most politically threatening to national regimes. Not only did legislation usually ignore women and men employed in agriculture and service jobs, but small firms and sometimes entire trades were excluded from coverage. Moreover, except in Germany and Austria, membership was not compulsory. Only a small minority of citizens in northwestern Europe were covered by the new legislation before World War I (Kohler et al., 1982; Alber, 1982). During the years immediately following the onset of fertility decline, social programs were more symbolic than effective. In any case, the cost to central governments at this time was negligible, because the majority of the new laws called for financing solely by employers and the workers themselves. Money was to be shifted from capitalist to proletarian and from active to inactive workers, but not from the entire range of wealthier taxpayers to the poor. Redistribution was not an intended aim of this legislation.

During the twentieth century, both the financing and the social impact of state insurance plans shifted. In the 1920s and 1930s political, demographic, and economic events combined to increase the cost and the coverage of social

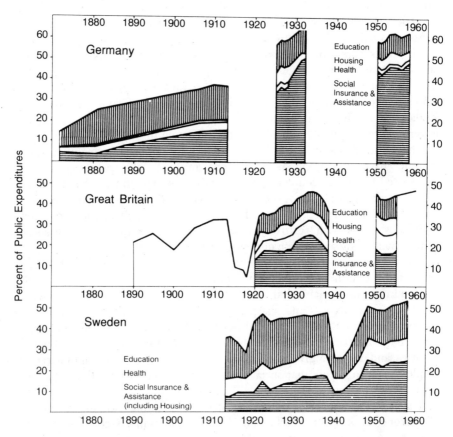

Figure 15.1   The development of public expenditures in Germany, Great Britain, and Sweden

security measures. Wars cut into the proportions of healthy, adult males. As a result, disabled veterans and war widows needed pensions. The unemployed mounted in numbers. Both conservative and radical regimes reacted similarly: in search of votes and popular support, they spent more money on housing, public health, and welfare, expanding benefits to new sections of the population.

The adult population slowly became the major target of social spending. In Belgium in 1900, 9 percent of the labor force belonged to state pension plans, but the proportion reached 51 percent by 1930: in France between these two dates the proportion of workers insured increased from 8 to 36 percent (Flora, ed., 1983, 1:460). Health insurance, which covered 22 percent of the German and around 15 percent of the Danish and Austrian labor forces in 1895 and fewer elsewhere, was available by 1930 to more than half the employed population in Austria, Denmark, Germany, Norway, Switzerland, and Great Britain (Flora, ed., 1983, 1:460). Scandinavia and Britain moved most quickly toward universal provision of pensions and health insurance, but the rest of Europe was not far behind. Under these conditions, the relative share of national budgets devoted to social security, health, and housing increased rapidly.

Greater coverage and greater total cost went hand in hand, of course. As social security plans expanded in size, more tax money was diverted into them, until by the 1920s government spending on social insurance in Western Europe generally exceeded payments for education (see figure 15.1). Under the pressures of mass unemployment and wartime demographic losses, insurance funds had to be partially subsidized out of general revenues, and this pattern of income transfer persisted in the long run. After 1914 the flow of government social expenditure therefore shifted more toward social insurance and away from education as direct entitlements for adults and the elderly increased.

The rise of the welfare state therefore is a story intertwined with that of population growth and change. Politicians and bureaucrats increased social expenditures in line with their perceptions of the population – its needs and deficiencies. The earliest targets of spending were children under age 14, a group growing fast in size and potentially threatening to social stability as it aged. This allocation of resources was unstable, however, as social statisticians compiled more information on the demographic consequences of urbanization, as well as on fertility and mortality decline. Fears of a falling birth rate produced pronatalist policies, while concern for public health and national efficiency encouraged interest in social insurance among politicians, bureaucrats, industrialists, workers, and reformers. The specific coalitions of groups and parties responsible for social insurance varied in each national setting, but the net effect was quite similar. Within a few decades, most of the states in Western, central, and northern Europe enacted far-reaching social insurance plans that increased investment in human capital. The simultaneity of this shift in both national expenditure patterns and demographic rates was not an accident; the political commitments to social insurance and to pronatalism arose within milieux aware of demographic problems and attempting to compensate for them.

Moments in Time: A Historian's Context of Declining Fertility

David Levine

In the statistics of declining fertility, depicting the transformation from provincial cultures in 1870 to the boundaries of nation-states by 1930, we have evidence of an immense social movement. Like the Industrial Revolution, urbanization, the doubling of life expectancy, the institutionalization of society, the politicization of war, and the militarization of the world economy, the transformation of reproductive patterns was part of a massive shift in the nature of social relations. The effects of this revolution are visible in the statistics of fertility as well as in the reconstruction of gender and the newly reconstituted life cycle, with its sequential age-graded roles and activities, providing the framework within which we need to locate the making of the modern family. And, furthermore, the causal arrows also flowed in the other direction: changing forms of behavior modified social systems.

Social change was experienced by thinking people who reflected on it and in consequence changed their behavior. Change and continuity are not rigid categories so much as interacting polarities in the same field of force. Models of historical change cannot be predicated on the simple reproduction of social systems; they must be flexible enough to comprehend both replication and mutation within the same frame of reference. It is in the process of reproduction that history transforms order and is itself reordered: "The great challenge to an historical anthropology is not merely to know how events are ordered by culture, but how, in the process, the culture is reordered. How does the reproduction of a structure become its transformation?" (Sahlins, 1981, p. 5). By rendering problematic "the reproduction of a structure," Marshall Sahlins's point has also been emphasized by Anthony Giddens: "The seed of change is present...in every act which contributes toward the reproduction of any 'ordered' form of social life" (1976, p. 102).

We might extend the points concerning social reproduction made by Sahlins and Giddens: social transformation might be understood as a continuum of product-moments resulting in the constant recombination of historical forces – biological, cultural, and material. Perhaps another way of conceptualizing the problem of social reproduction might be helpful. The paradigmatic metaphor that suggests itself to me is drawn from molecular biology: division and recombination, mutation and evolution. The "biological clock" is attuned to its system of information coding: cell divisions recombine inherited characteristics while mutations emerge on those rare occasions when this coding system goes amiss; the "evolutionary success" of each mutation depends on the context in which it occurs. Many mutations are called, few are chosen.

Since 1870 the "stopping" pattern of fertility has become the primary method of fertility centrol. Before this time the "starting" and "spacing" patterns had been employed, albeit with varying degrees of success, as regulatory strategies. In the third quarter of the nineteenth century "stopping" was exceptional; four generations later this pattern had become hegemonic (Lesthaeghe, 1980). The transformation of marital fertility has been both rapid and complete. The difference between marital-fertility practices in 1870 and those prevalent today represents a dramatic change in lived experience. The publications of Princeton University's European Fertility Project have voluminously documented this transformation in reproductive behavior in the project's treasure trove of statistics for 700 regional units – *départements*, counties, and provinces – and have analyzed this huge data set according to several standardized measures.

This immense, coordinated effort has served to transform our appreciation of the fertility decline even though most of the results have been negative in the sense that neither industrialization nor urbanization nor even nationality seem to count for as much – taken individually or together – as the seeming homogeneity of the process itself. To say the least, this is an interesting finding, but it is hardly the last word on the subject. On simple methodological grounds, for example, doubts can be raised about this seeming homogeneity because of the sheer size of the standardized units used. Such doubts are enhanced when it is acknowledged that "the decline in fertility so distinctly evident at the end of the nineteenth century in national and provincial level statistics shows considerable variation on the village level" (Knodel, 1986).

In giving pride of place to aggregate-level statistics in mapping the transition to lower fertility, the Princeton project has chosen to privilege large-group behavior at the expense of familial experience. One is bound to ask whether couples or regions, as it were, had babies. The method of analysis employed by the European Fertility Project's answer is that regions had babies. Parenting decisions regarding family-formation strategies reflected the commonality of group norms over and against individual interpretations of those norms. However, local population studies – using the micro-level method of family reconstitution – suggest that aggregation homogenizes large-scale data sets so that variations on a common theme are systematically downplayed. It is therefore not surprising that John Knodel's comparison of regional and national statistics with village-level data produced such contradictory results. Ernest Benz's social history has provided evidence that distinctive "demographic footprints" distinguished three of Knodel's contiguous villages from each other. In addition, *within* these villages a recomposition of age-specific fertility – that is, a new "spacing" strategy – occurred in the period prior to the fertility decline (Benz, 1988). Other studies have suggested that occupational characteristics, both *between* groups and over time, may have had small but cumulatively significant implications (Levine 1987, 1989). It seems to have been the case that the maintenance of high fertility rates was symptomatic of neither "traditionalism" nor "irrationality"; nor was it just the continuation of inherited behavior in changing circumstances. Rather, it reflected a peculiar relationship between production and reproduction that was first provoked and then rendered anachronistic by the impact of industrial capitalism on the proletariat. Between 1750 and 1843 the European proletariat doubled, rising from 58.4 to 70.8 percent of the population; this proportion hardly changed between 1843 and 1900, when the proletarian component rose to 200 million in a total population of 285 million (C. Tilly, 1984, pp. 32–4).

How were private decisions concerning family size coordinated with social processes? It is instructive to contrast the social-scientific mode of explanation with the historian's narrative. In the social-scientific mode, experience is chopped up into little parts, and each one is considered in its own right. To be sure, something is gained in precision, but much more is lost as complexity (or what social statisticians like to call "intercollinearity") is reduced to a series of disconnected parts. For the historian, it is the very act of connection that sets the parts in motion – an act of connection that takes place in time and space. For this reason, above all, when something happens and how it happens and in what context it happens are central in explaining what has happened. The fertility decline occurred in a period of massive migration, urbanization, proletarianization, and industrialization. It was a century that not only lurched through nationalism and imperialism into two world wars but also developed state-directed welfare systems protecting – and controlling – its citizens from "the cradle to the grave." No one's life was exempt from these massive processes, yet the thrust of recent explanations of the historical context of declining fertility has been, in fact, to disconnect public and private behavior. This is not to say that attempts have not been made to correlate aggregated measures of marital fertility with aggregated measures of social life so much as to say that the very act of correlation has been construed in a way that is prejudicial to the seamlessness of historical experience.

Another point regarding the seeming homogeneity of the fertility decline must be made: by giving this demographic process a central position in its own explanation, precision with reference to one part is achieved at the expense of an understanding of its relationship to the whole, and vice versa. Insofar as rational decision-making was linked with other changes in social experience, I would want to situate it in the changing structures of daily life and, thus, to connect biological reproduction with social reproduction. There is a very deep methodological gulf between the method of explanation used by the social statistician and that used by the historian. It pivots on divergent understandings of causality in historical time. I would not propose to substitute a single narrative in place of the aggregated analyses of large-scale units; my goal is more modest. I want to indicate a different direction for students of the historical context of declining fertility – a direction based on the multiple paths across which the transitional generations traveled. This way of seeing suggests not one but many fertility declines.

Was there one or were there many fertility declines? This line of inquiry immediately seems to break apart a logjam in the literature that has rather single-mindedly sought a magic key to unlock the puzzle. If there were many fertility declines then historians' concern with when something happens, how it happens, and in what context it happens takes on a pointed relevance. The issue is subtly transformed from a search for the master combination that will make all the tumblers in the historical lock fall simultaneously to the discovery of many smaller combinations. For the social historian, this line of inquiry provides the possibility of locating the context of declining fertility in the historically contingent blend of multiple levels of decision-making. Such multiplicity draws our attention not only to the separate motivations of those countless couples who each made individual decisions to "stop" but also to the larger social processes that provided the changing social framework within which novel decisions were made and then enacted. This duality is akin to Anthony Giddens's "double hermeneutic," encompassing both structural change *and* subjective agency (1976, p. 162). It is also what Marx had in mind when he wrote in *The Eighteenth Brumaire of Louis Bonaparte* that

Men [*sic*] make their own history, but they do not make it just as they please; they do not make it under circumstances chosen by themselves, but under circumstances directly encountered, given and transmitted from the past. The tradition of all dead generations weighs like a nightmare on the brain of the living. And just when they seem engaged in revolutionising themselves and things, in creating something that has never yet existed, precisely in such periods of revolutionary crisis they anxiously conjure up the spirits of the past to their service and borrow from them names, battle cries and costumes in order to present the new scene of world history in this time-honored disguise and this borrowed language. (1959 [1852], p. 320)

Thus the reproduction of a structure becomes its transformation. The social construction of decision-making connects the private behavior of individuals to the wider networks of intersecting and overlapping relationships in which everyone is enmeshed. For the historian, the issue is not the hierarchical ordering of relationships so much as their concatenation that provides the point of entry for analysis.

Central to any historical description is the *timing* of interaction. The historical conjunction of forces can be expected to be profoundly differentiated owing to its sensitivity to initial conditions. The same set of social forces does not necessarily produce the same set of responses. The precise impact between individual motivation and social determination is necessarily unpredictable and therefore unique. For this reason, the social-scientific mode of explanation has difficulty with historical contingency, which is the actual choice made from a portfolio of possible choices. If we raise the order of magnitude to accommodate multiple contingencies in mass societies, then clearly it is nearly impossible to provide a satisfactory set of statistical correlations to predict the changing pattern of private behavior with any precision. And, as historical researchers begin to explore the fertility decline, the realm of private behavior is found to be ripe with diversity. The historian's characteristic concern for change *and* continuity is indeed well-placed. The real question, then, is, How do we hold both change *and* continuity within a single field of vision?

Perhaps the most satisfactory method of analyzing historical time derives from the concept of uneven development, which has been used to study the symbiotic existence of "modern" productive routines in "traditional" social structures. Ernest Mandel argues that "to reduce economic history to a series of 'stages' or to the successive appearance of 'categories' is to make it excessively mechanical, to the point of rendering it unrecognizable. But to eliminate from historical study any allusion to successive stages of economic organization and any reference to the progressive appearance of these 'categories' is to make it merely incomprehensible" (1962, vol. 1, p. 91). By jettisoning a literal-minded belief in revolutionary change and substituting a more complex evolutionary pattern of social development, it becomes apparent that social "modernization" has led to curious hybridizations in which "modern" features are found to be combined unevenly with "traditional" ones (Roxburgh, 1988). How do these two characteristics interact? The optic provided by the concept of uneven development draws us back to the ways that apparently unpredictable outcomes emerge from unstable systems that will themselves provide the starting point for further development (Gleick, 1987). Timing, then, creates a field of forces joining the individual and the social, which is irreducibly contingent. In historical time, events are not iterated; they are unique. When we deal with social events in historical time it might be arguable that we have something close to an iterated system, but such an analogy is misleading precisely because it provides no place for the agency of individuals who choose their own response from a portfolio of alternatives (Alter, 1988, p. 61). In historical time these portfolios are never quite the same for any individual.

A myriad of factors combine unevenly to render micro-level social experience chaotic in the face of macro-level systemic order. The interface between the micro and macro level is contingent because of the role played by human agency. So the best that historians can hope to do is to specify the various combinations in which the individual and the social confront one another. To describe their individual responses to each historically decisive moment is impossible; we simply cannot plumb such depths. Thus we are left on the horns of a dilemma: on the one side, it is quite clearly apparent that large-scale aggregation results in spurious specificity while, on the other side, small-scale analyses are inevitably incomplete because we do not possess data detailed enough to probe the plethora of individual decisions that were unevenly combined to transform reproductive behavior. Our goal, then, must necessarily be more modest. In place of the explanations for declining fertility forwarded by social scientists using large-scale aggregations, we would like to begin a quite different project by situating individual decisions in contingent, historical time.

We might next consider several dimensions of timing: the spatial, the temporal, the material, the political, and the familial. Like any schema, this division is artificial; it stops a dynamic process and considers the parts at the expense of the whole. This is inevitable in any approach that decomposes the monolith of historical time and substitutes something rather more manageable. This exercise might indeed be more germane to human experience than the spurious specificity implied by the statistical manipulation of large-scale aggregations. It faces some of the concerns noted above regarding both the nuanced complexity of individual agency as well as the contingent circumstances in which individuals exist in historical time. Yet, like any intellectual artifice, it simplifies in order to comprehend complexity; and if the whole is, in fact, rather more than the sum of whatever parts we put together, then we must acknowledge that the parts themselves are important not only in their own right but also because their configuration is part of the internal architecture of the whole. Let us, then, look more closely at these five dimensions of historical time.

Spatial timing can be separated into two levels: the global and the local. It can be argued that the modern era is to be distinguished from its predecessor, the early modern period, in the vertical integration of continental, regional, community, and family space. The nineteenth century witnessed the final stage of this process of transformation – a moment of congealment, rather like ice forming on the surface of a lake. Indeed, as Robert Muchembled writes, "One model of society replaced another." He goes on to describe that world we have lost as "a 'polysegmentary' society...a social system composed of many subgroups: clans, lineages, families, and kinship relationships, age groups, corporations, guilds, fraternities and confraternities, parishes and neighborhoods, village or urban communities, and so on. The reality of existence and the organization of power were situated at the level of these subgroups and of their organization. In short, France was made up of thousands, even hundreds of thousands of politico-domestic units that overlapped and that reached their greatest cohesion in the framework of the village and of the urban *quartier*, rather than in that of an entire city or town, a region or a province" (1985, p. 313). This model of society, while still existing vestigially in the interstices of modern society, came under acute attack in the era of the demographic transition. This was not a spurious correlation. It is crucial.

The immense growth and influence of the nation-state was achieved at the cost of lesser sovereignties. In the era of declining fertility national differences became more important than regional or local ones. The Princeton statistics, reanalyzed by Susan Watkins, disclose how linguistic boundaries and demographic frontiers were redrawn as unified national cultures superseded the polyphonic world we have lost (1991). Spatially, Europe was redrawn; the patchwork of horizontal bonds – Muchembled's "thousands, even hundreds of thousands of politico-domestic units" – were reconstituted and replaced by a small number of vertically integrated nation-states. As late as "1863, according to official figures, 8,381 of France's 37,510 communes spoke no French: about a quarter of the country's population," whereas for the generation that manned the trenches in the Great War, French was the mother tongue for French nationals (Weber, 1976, pp. 67, 77). In Italy, too, the shift to a single national language has paralleled the fertility decline: in 1861, for example, only 2.5 percent spoke Italian, the rest lived in a "forest of dialect" (de Mauro, 1972, p. 43). Even Belgium, which seems to afford an exception, was not immune to the process of centralization except insofar as the recognized status of two languages meant that there was a dualistic structure instead of a unitary one (Lesthaeghe, 1977).

Temporal timing, too, can be understood in a variety of ways: as the narrative of real-time chronology, in terms of social stages or phases, and in relation to other events so that history itself might be a variable of some importance. Historical causation is not infrequently considered in relation to either contingent situations or deep, subterranean contradictions. What is at issue in the delineation of a popular movement like the fertility decline is the compounded nature of decision-making as well as the immensely complicated articulation of change itself. In explaining the fertility decline we have to make sense of a myriad of individuals who decided to change their observable, measurable behavior. And, secondarily, in explaining the fertility decline we have also to make sense of what forces set these individual decisions in motion. How and why was the fertility decline connected to the deep changes in the mode of production and the contours of everyday life? In the framework just set forth we are asking two rather different kinds of questions and are quite probably seeking two quite different kinds of answers. Confusion on this point litters the debate on the historical context of declining fertility. The best way to approach this point is by reference to the indeterminacy of individual behavior. However, even if individual behavior was indeterminate it nonetheless seems clear that the point at issue is the penumbra of uncertainty at the interface of the individual and the social – or, to put it in other terms, conjuncture and structure. It has become increasingly popular in "traditional" historical circles to eschew theory – be it grand or small – and to reconcile the job of the historian to the task of narrative. This resignation is understandable but regrettable. It narrows the scope of historical inquiry while leaving the connections between process and experience unattended. It is precisely this interaction of choice and circumstance that lies at the heart of the problem. Not only was the fertility decline within "the calculus of conscious choice," but it also took place within historical circumstances.

Each decision to restrict fertility was an act of conscious calculation to start stopping; without specifying how each decision was made we cannot make sense of the actor's conscious choices because we do not know from which alternatives they could or would choose. How can we then resolve this quandary and get out of this predicament? In a certain sense, of course, it is quite impossible unless we can embark on a collective biography based on individual-level data beyond anything we possess. In another sense, however, research based on sampling procedures can reduce the task enormously even if there will inevitably remain a problem of "confidence." By deconstructing the unitary fertility decline and looking at many fertility declines, bound together in the long term but each acting independently in the short term, we can begin to reconstruct the portfolio of viable choices within which the "calculus of conscious choice" operated. While doing so it is salient to remember that just as subatomic activity is both indeterminate and unpredictable so, too, is the explication of individual behavior.

Material timing subsumes technical and economic change in production routines and products themselves and is, in this way, connected with consumerism. Capitalism is not a thing but a process; capital is continuously reproducing itself and the social relations associated with accumulation. Similarly, technological change continuously changed the frontiers of what was humanly possible in the age-old quest to master the material world. Moreover, change built up its own momentum. The quantum leap afforded by the substitution of inanimate, inorganic energy for natural energy was the equivalent of creating an industrial reserve army of slaves. This metaphor, suggested by Emile Levasseur at the end of the nineteenth century, relates to the French economy between the 1840s and the 1880s, when the augmentation to the labor force was the equivalent of 98 million new "hands" – or, as he put it in a rather more pointed manner, "deux esclaves et demi par habitant de France" (1892, vol. 3, 74). France brought up the rear among the leading industrial economies – behind England, Germany, and the American colossus. Just imagine the combined size of this industrial reserve army of slaves! With the aid of a revolutionary technological break from the age-old dependence on animate sources of energy, capitalism was successful in providing a growing population with both basic necessities and more consumer goods of seemingly unimaginable variety. Everyone living today in an advanced capitalist society benefits from this form of industrial slavery, although, to be sure, such benefits have been divided unequally, and the trickle-down effect has been hardly immediate. But there can be no doubt that more people living in advanced industrial societies now have more – and live longer and healthier lives – than did their predecessors.

Triumphant industrial capitalism has quite clearly changed the human social situation from generalized want to generalized need. This point connects the timing of capitalist industrialization to the experience of social change. For if it is not credible to question the absolute impact of capitalism, it is germane to point out its uneven development and the discriminatory impression made on people living within its sway. Moreover, this impression has itself differentiated individuals – not only from one another but also within themselves – as bearers of labor power and as consumers. The apparent uniformity suggested by a cursory reference to "capitalism" dissolves on inspection, and one sees not structure but fragmentation at the interface of the individual and the social. And, as has been insisted throughout this postscript, chaotically fragmented experience was itself indeterminately structured by historical forces in the sense that only certain choices were possible. The demographic implications of this change were recognized by Thorstein Veblen, who argued that "the low birthrate of the classes upon whom the requirements of reputable expenditure fall...is probably the most effectual of the Malthusian prudential checks" (1967 [1899], p. 113). Moreover, as James Wickham has argued about proletarian family life in Weimar Frankfurt, "The ideology of the respectable family, nucleated and domesticated, was the private property of neither left nor right" (1983, p. 333). Both parents – the respectable husband and the Malthusian wife – decided together to control their fertility in order to enhance their domestic respectability and to improve the life chances of their children. In place of the economically useful child, the modernization of the family has substituted the emotionally priceless one (or two) (Zelizer, 1985, p. 333).

Political timing considers the public processes of state formation, class formation, and military confrontation with the private processes of family formation. We might begin a discussion linking our theme of uneven development and the fertility decline with an obvious point: political power is about the ability to exercise choice. It was not distributed equally, and its distribution was not stable. Political power existed in constitutional frameworks of widely differing types, which were the subject of local, national, and international contestation. Public life was not only punctuated by debates and contests but was riven with factions – sometimes representing ideological or religious viewpoints and sometimes regional or sectional grievances. The nineteenth century was an age of revolution, an age of the bourgeoisie, and an age of empire: new groups crowded the stage of demanding a share in the constituted processes of decision-making. Pluralism of interest contested with the singularity of vision demanded by nationalism and ideology to yield yet another kind of chaotic order set in motion by the contingency of each succeeding product-moment. Public life, then, divided men (and, in a quite different way, women, insofar as their lives were less "public") against one another even while creating and recreating communities, real and imagined. Vertical unification and horizontal diversity were a crucial part of the contested terrain of class formation and state formation. It would probably be untrue to say that no two people followed the same path across that ground; there was less homogeneity of experience than the spurious specificity of large-scale abstraction might imply.

To generalize from the macro-political clock's fearful symmetry to the micro-chronometer of lived experience betrays a blind leap of faith. But can one say more? Muchembled's contrast between "polysegmentary" social formations of the ancien régime and the goal-oriented national consciousness inculcated by the modern state offers that possibility. At the center of this "civilizing offensive," the study of which has been described as "a scholarly no-man's land, adjacent to the historical imperium," one finds a "modernizing missionary morality" thriving on the power derived from knowledge and the knowledge derived from power (Mitzman, 1987). Communication – systematic and tightly controlled – has given the modern state the opportunity to put into practice the goals of its absolutist predecessor, on whose foundations many of its civilizing initiatives were founded. Much of this battle has been fought on the terrain of culture and education; nowhere has this struggle been more intense than in the sphere of languange, which "is less a prior determinant of nationality than part of a complex process of cultural innovation, involving hard ideological labour, careful propaganda and a creative imagination: dictionaries and elementary primers are among the earliest and most important cultural artefacts of a national tradition" (Eley, 1981, p. 91). But whereas subordination in the premodern world was formal – in the sense that "consent" was externalized in public declarations of submission while being internalized in the private thoughts and deeds of the minority composing the "political nation" – the aim of the modern world has been to make it real by forming its citizens in its own image.

This power/knowledge matrix has provided the arena within which the state's power of domination in the exercise of choice has been contested by a kaleidoscope of alliances, associations, cabals, caucuses, clans, circles, cliques, coalitions, combinations, coteries, disciples, divisions, factions, federations, fraternities, minorities, movements, partnerships, parties, sects, societies, and so on. Quantum leaps in communication during the nineteenth century combined with a complete overhaul in educational organization to manufacture radically new forms of consent. Both advances derived from the same impulse in the politics of knowledge, an impulse whose "logic is perfectly clear, the aims decipherable, and yet it is often the case that no one is there

to have invented them, and few who can be said to have formulated them."
The politics of knowledge is one side of a coin; the advance of bureaucratic
administration is the other. The impact of this politics of knowledge, like all
deployments of power, is concerned with "mobile and transitory points of
resistance, producing cleavages in a society that shift about, fracturing
unities and effecting regroupings, furrowing across individuals themselves,
cutting them up and remolding them, marking off irreducible regions in
them, in their bodies and minds" (Foucault, 1980, p. 95).

The hallmark of this new knowledge politics was the state's enhanced
power to police and invigilate, discipline and punish, and reward. The
growth of a state apparatus concerned with "human capital" speaks very
much to this point. Indeed, it provides the glue that joins "the public" and
"the private," the social and the individual. We can locate its beginnings in
the statistical study of social relations in which "the flow of information
about the lower classes [w]as the countermovement of the flow of domination
from the top of the social structure to the bottom....[S]ocial domination
increasingly required accurate information flowing upward to social and
political leaders" (Leclerc, 1979, p. 196 [cited in Lynch, 1988]). The key
sites of this new disciplinary program were the public school and the private
family. Faced with recalcitrance and outright resistance, social disciplinarians
sought recourse to the courts and argued that it was both a social and an
individual good to break up immoral family units (Donzelot, 1979).

In the school – with its hidden curriculum favoring obedience and rote
learning as its gendered differentiation of the fit and proper concerns for the
"education" of boys/men as opposed to girls/women – control over the socialization of the young was wrested from the family and the community in
order to be made into an exercise in administration, categorization, and
subordination. Compliance with the rule of law in modern societies is a
reflection of the way in which "a gentle empire of moral habits" (Dupin,
1827, vol. 1, pp. 101–2 [cited in Lynch, 1988]) exercises suzerainty over the
everyday life of citizens. This project of moralization was the political terrain
on which compulsory education was erected. Edmond Holmes, a Victorian
school inspector, recollected, "For me they were so many examinees and as
they all belonged to the 'lower orders' and as (according to the belief in
which I had been allowed to grow up) the lower orders were congenitally
inferior to the 'upper classes' I took little or no interest in my examinees
either as individuals or as human beings, and have never tried to explore
their hidden depths. Indeed, the idea of their having hidden depths was
foreign to my way of thinking, and had it ever presented itself to my mind I
should probably have dismissed it with a disdainful smile" (1920, p. 64).
With the benefit of hindsight, Holmes was to regret the moralizing pedagogy
provided to the "examinees" in the state's compulsory schools. It was, he
came to understand, "in the highest degree anti-education": the average
14-year-old would have been subjected to 2,000 "scripture lessons" and

3,000 "reading lessons" in the course of her or his "acutely de-vitalizing" schooling (1920, pp. 144, 146, 41). School leavers – the product of a moralized family and a moralized pedagogy – were given a "certificate" and sent away to enter the labor market.

The reproduction of "human capital" draws this discussion to the final dimension of contingent, historical time so as to consider intimate inter-actions structured by gender, age, the life cycle, and family life itself. Let us approach *familial timing* in a roundabout way. The reproduction of "human capital" connects human agency with the macro processes of manufactur-ing consent. A Manchester woman's 1945 observation weaves together several threads into something like a whole cloth: "People wish to have a small family on account of public opinion which has now hardened into custom. It is customary – and has been so during the last twenty-five years or so – to have two children and no more if you can avoid it. A family of five or six children loses in prestige and, some think, in respectability. It is on behalf of their children that parents feel this most keenly" (*Mass Observation*, 1945, pp. 74–5). She captures, first, the temporality of change ("during the last twenty-five years or so" – i.e., since the end of World War I); second, the reconstruction of mentalities that have "now hardened into custom"; third, the interpenetration of the public and the private, neatly encapsulated by the use of those notoriously elastic terms "public opinion" and "respectability"; fourth, "on behalf of their children" joins the sentimentalization of child-hood together with the exigencies of human-capital formation; and, fifth, it is both "parents" – the respectable husband and his Malthusian wife – who decide together to control their fertility.

Fertility control was possible without the active involvement of *both* husbands and wives – the widespread prevalence of abortion stands in testi-mony to the studied indifference of men – but the sentimentalization of the family made it more likely that methods of control would come within the parameters of conjugal agreement. Because most of the decline in marital fertility was the product of two ancient practices – abstinence and coitus interruptus – it is clearly important to pay attention to the changing temper of communication between husbands and wives. Cultural forces, especially the "regendering" of the marital union, both narrowed the scope of family life and intensified its internal dynamics. It is in this sense that the texture of intimate relationships was not just important in its own right but also of crucial significance in reconstructing attitudes toward fertility. This is not simply a matter of acknowledging yet another *independent* variable so much as one of shifting our focus toward the culture of fertility. The importance of this point comes through forcefully in another vignette: after World War I the "old type of [Cockney] working-class mother" who accepted what was seemingly inevitable – a brutal husband, 15 pregnancies, and a home perpetually in pawn – was not reproducing herself. A Rotherhithe woman said that "the young ones will never put up with what what we did" (A.

Martin, 1919, p. 553). Why? Why were "the young ones" able to take hold of their reproductive lives when their mothers did not? Answering this question makes it both obvious and imperative to connect the public with the private, the social with the familial. If we can understand the way that that proletarian mother's daughter differed from her we can begin to do justice to the splintering impact of family time on the multifaceted experience of large-scale social processes. If we cannot begin to do justice to their individuality, then our explanations desiccate the lived experience of that mother and her daughter. They will have lost their historical personality, their agency sacrificed to an abstract determination.

This example forces us to recognize that, in the end, individual experience is intractably problematic. The social-scientific mechanism of standardization is itself no more than a series of images that must be surveyed whole. Freeze frames significantly enhance our visualization of moments in time, but those moments exists serially, in historical time. In arguing against overreliance on the Princeton method of large-scale aggregation, I am in a sense caught on the other horn of the dilemma – that is, to focus on the indeterminacy of individual actions is rather like the sound of one hand clapping. We must, therefore, connect the aggregate and the individual, and I think that we can do so by reference to Anthony Giddens's concept of "reflexive monitoring" in which "agency and structure *presuppose one another*" (1979, p. 53). In closing, then, I would argue that we might visualize the operation of "reflexive monitoring" not only in relation to the individual decisions of Europeans but also to the complex processes of social reproduction that were recombined in modern European history.

Bibliography

Accampo, Elinor. 1988. *Industrialization, Family Life, and Class Relations: Saint Chamond, 1815–1914.* Berkeley and Los Angeles: University of California Press.

Acorn, George [pseud.]. 1911. *One of the Multitude.* London: Heinemann.

Agulhon, Maurice. 1976. Un usage de la femme au XIXe siècle: l'allégorie de la République. *Romantisme*, 13–14, 143–52.

—. 1980. La Place des symboles dans l'histoire, d'après l'exemple de la République française. *Bulletin de la Société d'histoire moderne*, 7, 9–20.

—. 1981. *Marianne into Battle.* Cambridge: Cambridge University Press.

—. 1989. *Marianne au pouvoir: L'Imagerie et la symbolique republicaines de 1880 à 1914.* Paris: Flammarion.

Alber, Jens. 1982. *Vom Armenhaus zum Wohlfahrtsstaat: Analysen zur Entwicklung der Sozialversicherung in Westeuropa.* Frankfurt: Campus Verlag.

Alter, George. 1988. *Family and the Female Life Course: The Women of Verviers, Belgium, 1849–1880.* Madison: University of Wisconsin Press.

Alter, George, and James C. Riley. 1989. Frailty, sickness, and death: models of morbidity and mortality in historical populations. *Population Studies*, 43, 25–45.

Anderson, Barbara. 1980. *Internal Migration during Modernization in Late Nineteenth-Century Russia.* Princeton: Princeton University Press.

Anderson, Barbara A., and Brian D. Silver. 1988. Demographic consequences of World War II on the non-Russian Nationalities of the USSR. In S. Linz, ed., *The Impact of World War II on the Soviet Union.* Lanham, Md.: Rowman and Allanheld.

Anderson, Benedict. 1983. *Imagined Communities.* London: Verso.

Anderson, Eugene, and Pauline R. Anderson. 1967. *Political Institutions and Social Change in Continental Europe in the Nineteenth Century.* Berkeley: University of California Press.

Anderson, Michael. 1985. The emergence of the modern life cycle in Britain. *Social History*, 10, 69–87.

—. 1990. The social implications of demographic change. *Cambridge Social History of Britain, 1750–1950*, vol. 2. Cambridge: Cambridge University Press.

Anderson, Peter. 1983. The reproductive role of the human breast. *Current Anthropology*, 24, 25–45.

Anderton, Douglas L., and Lee L. Bean. 1985. Birth spacing and fertility limitation: a behavioral analysis of a nineteenth century frontier population. *Demography*, 22, 169–83.

Arceri, Margherita. 1973. La natalità nei comuni siciliani dal 1861 al 1961. *Collana di Studi Demografici*, 6. Palermo: University of Palermo, Institute of Demographic Sciences.

Ardigo, Achille. 1964. *Emancipazione femminile e urbaneismo.* Brescia: Morcelliana.

Ariès, Philippe. 1960. Interprétation pour une histoire des mentalités. In Hélène Bergues et al., *La Prévention des naissances dans la famille: Ses origines dans les temps moderne.* National Institute of Demographic Studies, Research and Documents, Monograph no. 35. Paris: Presses universitaires de France. Reprinted as An interpretation to be used for a history of mentalities. In Orest and Patricia Ranum, eds., *Popular Attitudes toward Birth Control in Pre-Industrial France and England.* New York: Harper & Row, 1972.

Armengaud, André. 1976. Population in Europe, 1700–1914. In Carlo Cipolla, ed., *The Fontana Economic History of Europe,* vol. 3. New York: Barnes & Noble.

Armstrong, William A. 1972. The use of information about occupation. In E. Anthony Wrigley, ed., *Nineteenth Century Society: Essays in the Use of Quantitative Methods for the Study of Social Data.* Cambridge: Cambridge University Press.

—. 1989. Rural population growth, mobility and the changing social structure. In George E. Mingay, ed., *The Agrarian History of England and Wales, 1750–1850,* vol. 6. Cambridge: Cambridge University Press.

Ascoli, G. 1910. Italian language. *Encyclopaedia Brittanica,* vol. 14, 11th ed. New York: Encyclopaedia Brittanica Co.

Bade, Klaus. 1980. German emigration to the United States and continental immigration to Germany, 1879–1929. *Central European History*, 13, 348–77.

Baines, Dudley. 1985. *Migration in a Mature Economy: Emigration and Seasonal Migration in England and Wales, 1861–1900.* Cambridge: Cambridge University Press.

Bairoch, Paul. 1976. *Commerce extérieur et development économique de l'Europe au XIXᵉ siècle.* The Hague: Mouton.

Balbo, Laura. 1976. *Stato di famiglia.* Milan: Etàs libri.

Ballestrero, Maria Vittoria. 1979. *Dalla tutela alla parità.* Bologna: Il Mulino.

Banks, James A. 1954. *Prosperity and Parenthood: A Study of Family Planning among the Victorian Middle Classes.* London: Routledge & Kegan Paul.

—. 1978. The social structure of nineteenth century England as seen through the census. In Richard Lawton, ed., *The Census and Social Structure: An Interpretative Guide to Nineteenth Century Censuses for England and Wales.* London: Frank Cass.

—. 1981. *Victorian Values: Secularism and the Size of Families.* London: Routledge & Kegan Paul.

Banks, Joseph A., and Olive Banks. 1964. *Feminism and Family Planning.* Liverpool: Liverpool University Press.

Barbagli, Marzio. 1982. *Educating for Unemployment: Politics, Labor Markets, and the School System: Italy, 1959–1973.* New York: Columbia University Press.

—. 1988. *Sotto lo stesso tetto: Mutamenti della famiglia in Italia dal XV al XX secolo.* Bologna: Il Mulino.

Bardet, Jean-Pierre, 1983. *Rouen aux XVIIe et XVIIIe siècles: Les Mutations d'un espace sociale*, vol. 1. Paris: Société d'Edition d'Enseignement Supérieur.

Bardet, Jean-Pierre, and Jacques Dupâguier. 1986. Contraception: les Français les premiers, mais pourquoi? In Dénatalité, l'antériorité française, 1800–1914, *Communications*, 44, 3–33.

Barthes, Roland. 1975. *Mythologies*. London: Paladin Press.

Barnsby, George J. 1971. Chartism and the miners' strike of 1842 in the Black Country. *Bulletin of the Society for the Study of Labour History*, 23, 33–5.

Becker, Gary S. 1981. *A Treatise on the Family*. Cambridge: Harvard University Press.

Becker, Gary S., and H. Gregg Lewis. 1973. On the interaction between the quantity and quality of children. *Journal of Political Economy*, 81, S279–88.

Becker, Jean-Jacques. 1986. *The Great War and the French People*. Leamington Spa: Berg.

Beer, William R. 1980. *The Unexpected Rebellion: Ethnic Activism in Contemporary France*. New York: New York University Press.

Bell, Daniel. 1975. Ethnicity and social change. In Nathan Glazer and Daniel P. Moynihan, eds., *Ethnicity: Theory and Experience*. Cambridge: Harvard University Press.

Bellettini, Andrea. 1972. Alcuni risultati di una ricerca sulla fecondità delle donne coniugate in una popolazione urbana. In *Atti della XXVII riunione scientifica della Società italiana di statistica*. Palermo: University of Palermo.

Benz, Ernest. 1988. Fertility in three Baden villages, 1650–1900. Ph.d. diss., University of Toronto.

Berdoe, Edward. 1891. Slum-mothers and death-clubs. A Vindication. *The Nineteenth Century*, 57, 560–63.

Berkner, Lutz. 1973. Family, social structure, and rural industry: a comparative study of the Waldviertel and the Pays de Caux in the eighteenth century. Ph.d. diss. Harvard University.

Berkner, Lutz, and Franklin Mendels. 1976. Inheritance systems, family structure and demographic patterns in Western Europe, 1700–1900. In Charles Tilly, ed., *Historical Studies in Changing Fertility*. Princeton: Princeton University Press.

Berlanstein, Lenard. 1980. Illegitimacy, concubinage and proletarianization in a French town, 1760–1914. *Journal of Family History*, 5, 360–74.

—. 1984. *The Working People of Paris, 1871–1914*. Baltimore: Johns Hopkins University Press.

Berry, B. Midi, and Roger S. Schofield. 1971. Age of baptism in preindustrial England. *Population Studies*, 25, 453–63.

Bertoni Jovine, Dina. 1963. *L'alienazione dell'infanzia*. Rome: Editori Riuniti.

Bielli, Carla; Antonia Pinnelli; and Angela Russo. 1973. *Fecondità e lavoro della donna in quattro zone tipiche italiane*. Rome: University of Rome Demographic Institute.

Bielli, Carla, et al., 1975. *Fecondità e lavoro della donna in ambiente urbano*. Rome: University of Rome Demographic Institute.

Bimbi, Franca. 1985. La doppia presenza: diffusione di un modello e trasformazioni dell'identità. In Franca Bimbi and Flavia Pristinger, eds., *Profili sovrapposti*. Milan: Franco Angeli.

Blacker, Carlos P. 1924. Birth control. *Guy's Hospital Gazette*, 460, 564.

342   *Bibliography*

—. 1926. *Birth Control and the State: A Plea and Forecast*. London: E. P. Dutton.

Blagg, Helen, 1910. *Statistical Analysis of Infant Mortality and Its Causes in the United Kingdom*. London: P. S. King.

Bland, Lucy, 1986. Marriage laid bare: middle-class women and marital sex, c. 1880–1914. In Jane Lewis, ed., *Labour and Love: Women's Experience of Home and Family, 1850–1940*. Oxford: Basil Blackwell.

Blanqui, Adolphe. 1849. Des classes ouvrières en France pendant l'année 1848. In *Petits Traités publiés par l'Academie des sciences morales et politiques*. Paris: Firmin Didot.

Blok, Anton. 1966. Land reform in a west Sicilian latifondo village: the persistence of a feudal structure. *Anthropological Quarterly*, 39, 1–16.

Blom, Ida. 1980. *Barnebegrensning-synd eller sunn fornuft*. Bergen: Universitetsforlaget.

Bogue, Donald J. 1969. *Principles of Demography*. New York: John Wiley & Sons.

Bongaarts, John. 1980. Does malnutrition affect fecundity? A summary of evidence. *Science*, 208, 564–9.

Bongaarts, John, and Jane Menken. 1983. The supply of children: a critical essay. In Rodolfo A. Bulatao and Ronald D. Lee, eds., *Determinants of Fertility in Developing Countries*. New York: Academic Press.

Booth, Charles. 1892. *Pauperism: A Picture and the Endowment of Old Age*. London: Macmillan & Co.

—. 1902. *Life and Labour of the People of London*. 5 vols. London: Macmillan & Co.

—. 1969. *Life and Labour of the People of London. First Series: Poverty*. 1902. New York: Augustus M. Kelley.

Borchardt, Lothar. 1984. The impact of the war economy on the civilian population of Germany during the First and Second World Wars. In W. Deist, ed., *The German Military in the Era of Total War*. Leamington Spa: Berg.

Born, Karl E. 1957. *Staat und Sozialpolitik seit Bismarcks Sturz: ein Beitrag zur Geschichte der Innenpolitischen Entwicklung des Deutschen Reiches, 1890–1914*. Wiesbaden: F. Steiner.

Borruso, Vincenzo. 1966. *Pratiche abortive e controllo delle nascite in Sicilia*. Palermo: Libri Siciliani.

Boswell, John. 1988. *The Kindness of Strangers: The Abandonment of Children in Western Europe From Late Antiquity to the Renaissance*. New York: Pantheon.

Bouce, Paul-Gabriel. 1988. Imagination, pregnant women, and monsters in eighteenth century England and France. In George S. Rousseau and Roy Porter, eds., *Sexual Underworlds of the Enlightenment*. Chapel Hill: University of North Carolina Press.

Bourdieu, Pierre. 1962. Cèlibat et condition paysanne. *Etudes rurales*, 5–6, 132–5.

Boydston, Jeanne. 1990. *Home and Work: Work, Wages and the Ideology of Labor in the Early Republic*. New York: Oxford University Press.

Branca, Patricia. 1975. *Silent Sisterhood: Middle-Class Women in the Victorian Home*. London: Croom Helm.

—. 1978. *Women in Europe since 1750*. London: Croom Helm.

Brancato, Francesco. 1977. Dall 'Unità ai Fasci dei Lavoratori. In *Storia della Sicilia*, vol. 8. Naples: Società editrice Storia di Napoli e della Sicilia.

Brand, John. 1877. *Observations on Popular Antiquities*. London: Chatto & Windus.

Braudel, Fernand. 1982. *The Wheels of Commerce*. New York: Harper & Row.

—. 1984. *The Perspective of the World. New York: Harper & Row.*

Braun, Rudolf. 1978. Early industrialization and demographic change in the canton of Zurich. In Charles Tilly, ed., *Historical Studies of Changing Fertility*. Princeton: Princeton University Press.

Breed, Mary, and Edith How-Martyn. 1930. *The Birth Control Movement in England*. London: J. Bale.

Brettell, Caroline. 1986. *Men Who Migrate, Women Who Wait: Population and History in a Portuguese Village*. Princeton: Princeton University Press.

Briant, Keith. 1972. *Marie Stopes: A Biography*. New York: Norton.

Britain and Her Birth-Rate. 1945. London: Murray.

Brookes, Barbara. 1983. The illegal operation, abortion 1919–1939. In London Feminist History Group, *The Sexual Dynamics of History*. London: Pluto Press.

—. 1986. Women and reproduction, c. 1860–1939. In Jane Lewis, ed., *Labour and Love, Women's Experience of Home and Family, 1850–1940*. Oxford: Basil Blackwell.

—. 1988. *Abortion in England, 1900–1967*. London: Routledge.

Browne, F. W. Stella. 1922. Abortion. In *Report on the Fifth International Neo-Malthusian and Birth Control Conference*. London: Heinemann.

Brumberg, Joan Jacobs. 1988. *Fasting Girls: The Emergence of Anorexia Nervosa as a Modern Disease*. Cambridge: Harvard University Press.

Bull, Thomas. 1837. *Hints to Mothers, for the Management of Health during the Period of Pregnancy and the Lying-in Room*. London: Longman.

Burgoyne, Jacqueline. 1987. Change, gender, and the life course. In Gaynor Cohen, ed., *Social Change and the Life Course*. London: Tavistock.

Burnett, John, ed. 1984a. *Destiny Obscure: Autobiographies of Childhood, Education and Family from the 1820s to the 1920s*. Harmondsworth: Penguin.

Burnett, John, ed. 1984b. *Useful Toil: Autobiographies of Working People from the 1820s to the 1920s*. New York: Penguin Books.

Burrit, Elihu. 1869. *Walks in the Black Country and Its Green Borderland*. London: Sampson, Low, and Marston.

Busfield, Joan. 1974. Ideologies and reproduction. In M. P. M. Richards, ed., *The Integration of a Child into a Social World*. Cambridge: Cambridge University Press.

—. 1987. Parenting and parenthood. In Gaynor Cohen, ed., *Social Change and the Life Course*. London: Tavistock.

Busfield, Joan, and Michael Paddon. 1977. *Thinking about Children: Sociology and Fertility in Post-War Britain*. Cambridge: Cambridge University Press.

Cacioppo, Maria. 1982. Condizioni di vita familiare negli anni cinquanta. *Memoria*, 6, 84–90.

Calabrese, Omar. 1975. *Carosello o dell 'educazione serale*. Firenze: Sansoni.

Caldwell, John C. 1980. Mass education as a determinant of the timing of fertility decline. *Population and Development Review*, 6, 225–55.

—. 1982. *Theory of Fertility Decline*. New York: Academic Press.

Caldwell, John, C.; P. H. Reddy; and Pat Caldwell. 1988. *The Causes of Demographic Change: Experimental Research in South India*. Madison: University of Wisconsin Press.

Callaway, Helen. 1978. "The most essentially female function of all": giving birth. In Shirley Ardener, ed., *Defining Females: The Nature of Women in Society*. London: Croom Helm.

Campbell, Janet. 1917. *Report on the Physical Welfare of Mothers and Children: England and Wales.* Liverpool: Carnegie U. K. Trust.

——. 1924. *Maternal Mortality.* London: His Majesty's Stationery Office.

Cancian, Francesca. 1987. *Love in America: Gender and Self-Development.* Cambridge: Cambridge University Press.

Cantlie, James. 1885. *Degeneration among Londoners.* London: Leadenhall Press.

Cardia, Carlo. 1975. *Il diritto di famiglia in Italia.* Rome: Editori Riuniti.

Carlsson, Gosta. 1966. The decline of fertility: innovation or adjustment process? *Population Studies,* 20, 149–74.

Caruso-Rasa, G. 1966. *La questione siciliana degli zolfi.* 1896. Turin: Fratelli Bocca Editori.

Casterline, John, et al., 1984. The proximate determinants of fertility. *WFS Comparative Studies.* Voorburg, Netherlands: International Statistical Institute.

Cavanagh, F. 1906. The responsibility of a maternity nurse. *Nursing Times,* March 10, 196–7.

Challinor, Raymond, and Brian Ripley. 1968. *The Miners' Association: A Trade Union in the Age of the Chartists.* London: Lawrence & Wishart.

Chamberlàin, Mary, and Ruth Richardson. 1983. Life and death. *Oral History,* 11, 31–43.

Charles, Enid. 1932. *The Practice of Birth Control: An Analysis of the Birth-Control Experiences of Nine Hundred Women.* London: Williams & Norgate.

Chatelain, Abel. 1977. *Les Migrants temporaires en France de 1800 à 1914.* Lille: Université de Lille III.

Chaunu, Pierre. 1973. Reflections sur la démographie normande. In *Sur la population française au XVIIIᵉ et XIXᵉ siècles.* Paris: Société de démographie historique.

Chayanov, Alexander V. 1966. *The Theory of Peasant Economy.* 1925. Homewood, Ill.: Irwin.

Chesnais, Jean Claude. 1986. *La transition démographique.* Paris: Presses universitaires de France.

Chevasse, P. H. 1832. *Advice to a Wife on the Management of Her Own Health.* London.

Child, Mrs. 1837. *The Family Nurse, a Companion of the Frugal Housewife.* London: Bentley.

Chinn, Carl. 1988. *They Worked All Their Lives: Women of the Urban Poor in England, 1880–1939.* Manchester: Manchester University Press.

Ciucci, Luciano, and Anna De Sarno Prignano. 1974. L'Influence de l'éducation sur la fécondité en Italie. *Genus,* 30, 121–33.

Clark, David. 1982. *Between Pulpit and Pew: Folk Religion in a North Yorkshire Fishing Village.* Cambridge: Cambridge University Press.

Clark, Peter, and Paul Slack. 1976. *English Towns in Transition, 1500–1700.* London: Oxford University Press.

Clark, Peter, and David Souden. 1982. Rural-urban migration and its impact in early modern England. In *Proceedings of the Eighth International Economic History Congress, B8,* Budapest.

Coale, Ansley J. 1965. Birth rates, death rates, and rates of growth in human population. In Mindel C. Sheps and Jeanne C. Ridley, eds., *Public Health and Population Change: Current Research Issues.* Pittsburgh: University of Pittsburgh Press.

—. 1973. The demographic transition reconsidered. In International Union for the Scientific Study of Population, *International Population Conference, Liège*. Liège: IUSSP.

Coale, Ansley J., and Paul Demeny. 1966. *Regional Model Life Tables and Stable Populations*. Princeton: Princeton University Press.

Coale, Ansley J., and Roy Treadway. 1986. A summary of the changing distribution of overall fertility, marital fertility, and the proportion married in the provinces of Europe. In Ansley J. Coale and Susan Cotts Watkins, eds., *The Decline of Fertility in Europe*. Princeton: Princeton University Press.

Coale, Ansley J., and T. James Trussell. 1974. Model fertility schedules: variations in the age structure of childbearing in human populations. *Population Index*, 40, 185–258.

Coale, Ansley J., and Susan Cotts Watkins, eds. 1986. *The Decline of Fertility in Europe*. Princeton: Princeton University Press.

Comas d'Argemir, Dolorès. 1987. Rural crisis and the reproduction of family systems: celibacy as a problem in the Aragonese Pyrenees. *Sociologia Ruralis*, 27, 263–77.

Conquest, John. 1848. *Letters to a Mother, on the Management of Herself and Her Children in Health and Disease*. London: Longman.

Corbin, Alain. 1975. *Archaïsme et modernité en Limousin au XIXᵉ siècle*. Paris: Marcel Rivière.

Corleo, Simone. 1871. *Storia della enfiteusi dei tereni ecclesiastici di Sicilia*. Palermo: Stabilimento Tipografico Lao.

Cornelisen, Ann. 1977. *Women of the Shadows*. New York: Vintage Books.

Corsi, Pietro. 1936. *La tutela della maternità e dell'infanzia in Italia*. Rome: Società editrice di Novissima.

Corsini, Carlo. 1967. Fecondità completa delle fiorentine secondo il censimento del 1961. In *Atti della XXV riunione scientifica della Società italiana di statistica*. Bologna.

Cottereau, Alain. 1986. The distinctiveness of working-class cultures in France, 1848–1900. In Ira Katznelson and Aristide R. Zolberg, eds., *Working-Class Formation: Nineteenth-Century Patterns in Western Europe and the United States*. Princeton: Princeton University Press.

Courgeau, Daniel. 1970. *Les Champs migratoires en France*. National Institute of Demographic Studies, Monograph no. 58. Paris: Presses universitaires de France.

Court, W. H. B. 1938. *The Rise of Midland Industries, 1600–1838*. London: Oxford University Press.

Coveney, Peter. 1957. *Poor Monkey: The Child in Literature*. London: Rockliff.

Crew, David. 1979. *Town on the Ruhr: A Social History of Bochum, 1860–1914*. New York: Columbia University Press.

Crooke, George F. 1898. Fatal case of acute poisoning by lead combined in diachylon. *Lancet.*, 2, 255–6.

Cullen, Michael J. 1975. *The Statistical Movement in Early Victorian Britain: The Foundations of Empirical Social Research*. New York: Barnes & Noble.

Currie, C. R. J. 1979. Agriculture, 1793–1875. In M. V. Greenshade and D. A. Johnson, eds., *A History of the County of Staffordshire*, vol. 7. London: Oxford University Press.

Dantec, François. 1964. *Foyers rayonnants: Fécondité et éducation. Amour mutuel. Régulation chrétienne des naissances. Guide moral de l'amour chrétien.* Quimper: Direction des oeuvres.

D'Apice, Carmela. 1981. *L'arcipelago dei consumi.* Bari: De Donato.

Dauzat, Albert. 1927. *Les Patois.* Paris: Librairie Delagrave.

David, Paul A., and Warren C. Sanderson. 1976. Contraceptive technology and fertility control in America: from facts to theories. Memorandum 202, Center for Research in Economic Growth, Stanford University.

Davidoff, Leonore. 1973. *The Best Circles: Society, Etiquette and the Season.* London: Croom Helm.

Davidoff, Leonore, and Catherine Hall. 1987. *Family Fortunes: Men and Women of the English Middle Class, 1780–1850.* Chicago: University of Chicago Press.

Davies, Margaret Llewelyn, ed. 1978. *Maternity: Letters from Working Women.* 1915. London: Virago Press.

Davies, V. L., and H. Hyde. *Dudley and the Black Country.* N.p.: Dudley Public Library, 1970.

Davin, Anna. 1978. Imperialism and motherhood. *History Workshop*, 5, 6–66.

—. Forthcoming. *"Little Women": The Childhood of Working-Class Girls in Late Nineteenth-Century London.* London: Routledge.

Davis, John. 1969. Honour and politics in Pisticci. *Proceedings of the Royal Anthropological Institute of Great Britain and Ireland*, 69–81.

Davis, Kingsley, and Judith Blake. 1955. Social structure and fertility: an analytical framework. *Economic Development and Cultural Change*, 4, 235.

Davis, Natalie. 1983. *The Return of Martin Guerre.* Cambridge: Harvard University Press.

Dawson, William H. 1912. *Social Insurance in Germany, 1883–1911: Its History, Operation, Results.* London: T. Fisher Unwin.

De Brandt, Alexandre. 1901. *Droits et coutumes des populations de la France en matière successorale.* Paris: Librairie de la société du recueil général des lois et des lettres.

De Grand, Alexander. 1976. Women under Italian Fascism. *Historical Journal*, 19, 947–68.

Delatour, Yvette. 1965. Les Effets de la guerre sur la situation de la Française d'après la presse feminine, 1914–1918. Diplome d'études supérieures d'histoire, University of Paris, I.

Della Peruta, Franco. 1979. Infanzia e famiglia nella prima metà dell'Ottocento. *Studi storici*, 3, 473–91.

De Mauro, T. *Storia linguistica d'Italia unità.* Bari: 1972.

Demeny, Paul. 1968. Early fertility decline in Austria-Hungary: a lesson in demographic transition. *Daedalus*, 97, 502–22.

Demos, John, 1982. *Entertaining Satan: Witchcraft and the culture of Early New England.* New York: Oxford University Press.

Dennis, Norman; F. Henriques; and C. Slaughter. 1956. *Coal Is Our Life.* London: Tavistock.

De Stefano, Francesco, and Francesco Luigi Oddo. 1963. *Storia della Sicilia dal 1860 al 1910.* Bari: Laterza.

Detragiache, Denise, 1980. Un aspect de la politique démographique de l'Italie fasciste: la répression de l'avortement. *Mélanges de l'Ecole française de Rome: Moyen Age – Temps Modernes*, 92, 691–731.

Devun, M. 1944. L'Utilisation des rivières du Pilat par l'industrie. *Revue de géographie alpine*, 32, 241–305.

Di Cori, Paola. 1979. Storia, sentimenti, solidarietà nelle organizzazioni femminili cattoliche dall'età giolittiana al fascismo. *Nuova DWF*, 10–11, 80–125.

Di Giorgio, Micaela. 1979. Metodi e tempi di una educazione sentimentale: la gioventù femminile cattolica negli anni venti. *Nuova DWF*, 10–11.

Di Leonardo, Micaela. 1987. The female world of cards and holidays: women, families, and the work of kinship. *Signs*, 12, 440–53.

Dingwall, Robert W. J. 1977. Collectivism, regionalism and feminism: health visiting and British social policy, 1850–1975. *Journal of Social Policy*, 6, 291–315.

Donnison, Jean. 1977. *Midwives and Medical Men: A History of Inter-Professional Rivalries and Women's Rights.* New York: Shocken.

Donzelot, Jacques. 1979. *The Policing of Families.* New York: Pantheon.

Douglas, Ann. 1977. *The Feminization of American Culture.* New York: Knopf.

Du Châtellier, Armand. 1835–7. *Recherches statistiques sur le département du Finistère.* Nantes: Imprimerie de Mellinet.

Duesenberry, James. 1960. Comment on "An economic analysis of fertility" by Gary S. Becker, in *Demographic and Economic Change in Developed Countries.* Universities-National Bureau Conference Series. Princeton: Princeton University Press.

Dupâquier, Jacques. 1972. De l'animal à l'homme: le mécanisme auto-régulateur des populations traditionnelles. *Revue de l'Institut de sociologie, Université libre de Bruxelles*, 2, 177–211.

—. 1986. Combien d'avortements en France avant 1914? *Communications*, 44, 87–106.

Dupeux, Georges. 1973. Immigration urbaine et secteurs économiques: l'exemple de Bordeaux au debut du xxᵉ siècle. *Annales du Midi*, 85, 209–20.

Dupin, Charles. 1827. *Les Forces productives et commerciales de la France.* 2 vols. Paris: Bachelier.

Dwork, Deborah. 1987. *War Is Good for Babies and Other Young Children: A History of the Infant and Child Welfare Movement in England, 1898–1918.* London: Tavistock.

Dyhouse, Carol. 1978. Working-class mothers and infant mortality in England, 1895–1914. *Journal of Social History*, 12, 248–67.

Easterlin, Richard A. 1978. The economics and sociology of fertility: a Synthesis. In Charles Tilly, ed., *Historical Studies of Changing Fertility.* Princeton: Princeton University Press.

Easterlin, Richard A., and Eileen M. Crimmins. 1985. *The Fertility Revolution.* Chicago: University of Chicago Press.

Eccles, Audrey. 1982. *Obstetrics and Gynecology in Tudor and Stuart England.* Kent, Ohio: Kent State University Press.

Elderton, Ethel M. 1914. *Report on the English Birthrate.* London: Cambridge University Press.

Eldred, John. 1955. *I Love the Brooks.* London: Skeffington & Son.

Eley, Geoff. 1981. Nationalism and social history. *Social History* 6, 83–107.

Ellis, Havelock. 1910. *Studies in the Psychology of Sex.* Philadelphia: F. A. Davis.

Elrington, C. R. 1964. Local government and public services. In R. B. Pugh, ed., *A History of the County of Warwick.* London: Oxford University Press.

348   Bibliography

Elschenbroich, Donata. 1977. *Kinder werden nicht geboren.* Frankfurt/Main: Pada-gogisch Extra-Buchverlag.

Engel, Sigmund. 1912. *The Elements of Child Protection.* London: George Allen.

England and Wales. 1923. *Census of England and Wales: 1911.* Vol. 13, Fertility of marriage, part 2. London: His Majesty's Stationary Office.

Eversley, D. E. C. 1964. Industry and trade, 1500–1850. In R. B. Pugh, ed., *A History of the Country of Warwick.* London: Oxford University Press.

Ewen, Elizabeth. 1985. *Immigrant Women in the Land of Dollars: Life and Culture on the Lower East Side, 1890–1925.* New York: Monthly Review Press.

Eyler, John M. 1976. Mortality statistics and Victorian health policy: program and criticism. *Bulletin of the History of Medicine,* 50, 335–55.

Eyles, Margaret Leona. 1922. *The Woman in the Little House.* London: Grant Richards.

Fabbri, Sergio. 1934. *L'Opera nazionale per la protezione della maternità e dell' infanzia.* Verona: Mondadori.

Fairchilds, Cissie. 1984. *Domestic Enemies: Servants and Their Masters in Old Regime France.* Baltimore: Johns Hopkins University Press.

Farid, S. M. 1976. Cohort nuptiality in England and Wales. *Population Studies* 30, 149.

Faure, Olivier. 1986. Les Hôpitaux des villes industrielles de la region stéphanoise au XIXᵉ siècle. *Bulletin du Centre d'histoire économique et sociale de la région lyonnaise* nos. 3–4, 61–83.

Federici, Nora. 1984. *Procreazione, famiglia, lavoro della donna.* Turin: Loescher.

Ferguson, Sheila. 1977. Labour women and the social services. In Lucy Middleton, ed., *Women in the Labour Movement: The British Experience.* London: Croom Helm.

Festy, Patrick. 1979. *La Fécondité des pays occidentaux de 1870 à 1970.* Paris: Presses universitaires de France.

Fildes, Valerie A. 1986. *Breasts, Bottles and Babies.* Edinburgh: Edinburgh University Press.

Fine, Agnès. 1978. La Limitation des naissances dans le sud-ouest de la France. *Annales du Midi,* 90, 155–84.

Fishman, Joshua A. 1977. Language and ethnicity. In Howard Giles, ed., *Language, Ethnicity and Intergroup Relations.* New York: Academic Press.

Fitch, Nancy. 1986. "Les Petits parisiens en province": the silent revolution in the Allier, 1860–1900. *Journal of Family History,* 11, 131–55.

Flecken, Margarete. 1981. *Arbeiterkinder im 19. Jahrhundert.* Weinheim/Basel: Beltz.

Flinn, Michael W. 1984. *The History of the British Coal Industry, 1700–1830: The Industrial Revolution.* 2 vols. Oxford: Clarendon Press.

Flora, Peter, ed. 1983. *State, Economy, and Society in Western Europe, 1815–1975.* 2 vols. Chicago: St. James Press.

Flora, Peter, and Arnold J. Heidenheimer, eds. 1981. *The Development of Welfare States in Europe and America.* New Brunswick, N.J.: Transaction Books.

Folk-Lore. 1938. 49, 224.

Fothergill, John M. 1889. *The Town Dweller: His Needs and Wants.* London: A. K. Lewis.

Foucault, Michel. 1980. *The History of Sexuality, vol. 1, An Introduction.* New York: Vintage.

France. Ministère du Travail et de la Prévoyance Sociale. 1912. *Statistique generale de la France: Statistique des familles en 1906.* Paris: Imprimerie nationale.

Franchini, Silvia. 1986. L'istruzione femminile in Italia dopo l'Unità: Percorsi di una ricerca sugli educandati pubblici di elite. *Passato e Presente,* 10, 53–94.

Frere, Margaret. 1903. The charitable work of a local manager in a board school. *Charity Organisation Review,* n.s., 75, 120–34.

Frey, Michel. 1978. Du mariage et du concubinage dans les classes populaires à Paris (1846–1847). *Annales: Economies, Sociétés, Civilisations,* 33, 803–29.

Frijhoff, Willem, ed. 1983. *L'Offre de l'école.* Paris: INRP.

Gabaccia, Donna. 1984. *From Sicily to Elizabeth Street: Housing and Social Change among Italian Immigrants, 1880–1930.* Albany: State University of New York Press.

—. 1988. *Militants and Migrants: Rural Sicilians Become American Workers.* New Brunswick: Rutgers University Press.

Gachon, Lucien. 1933. *Les Populations rurales de Puy-de-Dome: Mémoires de l'Academie des sciences, belles lettres, et arts de Clermont Ferrand,* vol. 33. Clermont-Ferrand: Bussac.

Gaiotti De Biase, Paola. 1957. *Le donne oggi.* Rome: Le Cinque Lune.

—. 1979. *Questione femminile e femminismo nella vita della Republica.* Brescia: Morcelliana.

Galoppini, Angela. 1981. *Il lungo viaggio verso la parità.* Bologna: Zanichelli.

Garden, Maurice. 1982. Le Bilan démographique des villes: un système complexe. In *Annales de démographie historique.* Paris and The Hague: Mouton.

Garrier, Gilbert. 1973. *Paysans de Beaujolais et du Lyonnais.* Grenoble: Presses universitaires de Grenoble.

Gaunt, David. 1977. Pre-industrial economy and population structure. *Scandinavian Journal of History,* 2, 183–210.

Gebhard, Paul H., et al., 1958. *Pregnancy, Birth, and Abortion.* New York: Harper.

Geertz, Clifford. 1971. The integrative revolution: primordial sentiments and civil politics in the new states. In Jason L. Finkle and Richard W. Gable, eds. *Political Development and Social Change,* 2d ed. New York: John Wiley & Sons.

Gellner, Ernest A. 1983. *Nations and Nationalism.* Ithaca: Cornell University Press.

Gestrich, Andreas. 1986. *Traditionelle Jugendkultur und Industrialisierung.* Göttingen: Vandenhoeck & Ruprecht.

Giarrizzo, Giuseppe. 1976. La Sicilia e la crisi agraria. In Giuseppe Giarrizzo et al., eds. *I Fasci siciliani,* vol. 1. Bari: De Donato.

Giddens, Anthony. 1976. *New Rules of Sociological Method: A Positive Critique of Interpretive Sociologies.* London: Hutchinson.

—. 1979. *Central Problems in Social Theory: Action, Structure and Contradiction in Social Analysis.* Berkeley and Los Angeles: University of California Press.

Gilbert, Bentley B. 1965. Health and politics: the British Physical Deterioration Report of 1904. *Bulletin of the History of Medicine.,* 39, 143–53.

—. 1966. *The Evolution of National Insurance in Britain: The Origins of the Welfare State.* London: Michael Joseph.

Gillis, John. 1974. *Youth and History.* New York: Academic Press.

—. 1985. *For Better, for Worse: British Marriages, 1600 to the Present.* New York: Oxford University Press.

—. 1989. Ritualization of middle-class family life in nineteenth century Britain. *International Journal of Politics, Culture and Society,* 3, 213–35.

350 *Bibliography*

Ginsborg, Paul. 1989. *Storia d'Italia dal dopoguerra ad oggi.* Turin: Einaudi.

Gittins, Diana. 1982. *Fair Sex: Family Size and Structure, 1900–1939.* London: Hutchinson.

Giuffrida, Romualdo. 1969. Dal 1819 al 1860. In Domenico Demarco et al., eds., *Centocinquanta Anni della Camera di commercio di Palermo: 1819–1969.* Palermo: Camera di commercio industria artigianlo e agricoltura.

—. 1973. *Aspetti dell'economia siciliana nell'ottocento.* Palermo: Sellario.

—. 1977. Investimenti di capitali straniero in Sicilia nella prima metà dell '800. In *Storia della Sicilia*, vol. 9. Naples: Società editrice Storia di Napoli e della Sicilia.

—. *Politica ed economia nella Sicilia dell'ottocento.* Palermo: Sellerio.

Giuntella, Maria Christina. 1988. Virtù e immagini della donna nei settori femminili. In *Chiesa e progetto educativo nel secondo dopoguerra, 1945–1958.* Brescia: Morcelliana.

Giura, Vincenzo. 1973. *La questione degli zolfi siciliani, 1838–1841.* Geneva: Librairie Droz.

—. 1977. L'industria zolfiera siciliana nei secoli XIX e XX. In *Storia della Sicilia*, vol. 9. Naples: Società editrice Storia di Napoli e della Sicilia.

Glass, David V. 1940. *Population Policies and Movements in Europe.* Oxford: Clarendon Press.

—. 1967. *Population Policies and Movements in Europe.* London: Frank Cass.

Glass, David V., and Eugene Grebenik. 1954. *The Trend and Pattern of Fertility in Great Britain.* London: Her Majesty's Stationery Office.

Gleik, James. 1987. *Chaos: Making a New Science.* New York: Penguin.

Gordon, David. 1985. *Merchants and Capitalists: Industrialization and Provincial Politics in Mid-Nineteenth-Century France.* University: University of Alabama Press.

Gordon, Linda. 1988. *Heroes of Their Own Lives: The Politics and History of Family Violence, Boston 1880–1960.* New York: Penguin Books.

Gordon, Peter. 1974. *The Victorian School Manager: A Study in the Management of Education, 1800–1902.* London: Woburn Press.

Goubert, Pierre. 1960. *Beauvais et le Beauvaisis de 1600 à 1730* Paris: SEVPEN.

Gould, J. D. 1980. European inter-continental emigration. The road home: return migration from the U.S.A. *Journal of European Economic History*, 9, 41–112.

Grabill, Wilson H.; Clyde Kiser; and Pascal K. Whelpton. 1958. *The Fertility of American Women.* New York: Wiley.

Grafteaux, Serge. 1985. *Mémé Santerre: a French Woman of the People.* New York: Schocken Books.

Graham, Stephen. 1980. *1900 Public Use Sample: User's Handbook* Seattle: University of Washington. Center for Studies in Demography and Ecology.

Granovetter, Mark. 1985. Economic action and social structure: the problem of embeddedness. *American Journal of Sociology* 91, 481–510.

Grant, Clara. [1930.] *Farthing Bundles.* London: Fern Street Settlement.

Gras, Louis Joseph. 1904. *Essai sur l'histoire de la quincaillerie et petite metallurgie.* Saint-Etienne: Theolier.

—. 1922. *Histoire économique générale des mines de la Loire*, 2 vols. Saint-Etienne: Theolier.

Grew, Raymond. 1984. The nineteenth century European state. In Charles Bright and Susan Harding, eds., *State-Making and Social Movements.* Ann Arbor: University of Michigan Press.

Griffin, C. P. 1971. Chartism and the miners in the early 1840s: a critical note. *Bulletin of the Society for the Study of Labour History*, 22, 21–5.

Gubar, Susan. 1987. "This is my rifle, this is my gun": World War II and the blitz on women. In M. R. Higgonet et al., eds., *Behind the Lines: Gender and the Two World Wars*. New Haven: Yale University Press.

Guidetti Serra, Bianca. 1977. *Compagne*. Turin: Einaudi.

Guignet, Philippe. 1977. *Mines, manufactures et ouvriers du Valenciennois au XVIIᵉ siècle*. New York: Arno Press.

Guillaume, Pierre. 1966. *La Compagnie des mines de la Loire, 1846–1854*. Paris: Presses universitaires de France.

Guillaumin, Emile. 1983. *The Life of a Simple Man*. Hanover, N.H.: University Press of New England.

Gullickson, Gay. 1986. *Spinners and Weavers of Auffay: Rural Industry and Sexual Division of Labor in a French Village, 1750–1850*. Cambridge: Cambridge University Press.

Gutmann, Myron. 1988. *Toward the Modern Economy: Early Industry in Europe, 1500–1800*. New York: Knopf.

Gutmann, Myron, and René Leboutte. 1984. Rethinking proto-industrialization and the family. *Journal of Interdisciplinary History*, 14, 587–607.

Habakkuk, H. J. 1955. Family structures and economic change in nineteenth century Europe. *Journal of Economic History*, 15, 1–13.

Haines, Michael R. 1979. *Fertility and Occupation: Population Patterns in Industrialization*. New York: Academic Press.

—. 1985. Inequality and childhood mortality: a comparison of England and Wales, 1911, and the United States, 1900. *Journal of Economic History*, 45, 885–912.

—. 1989. Social class differentials during fertility decline: England and Wales revisited. *Population Studies*, 43, 305–23.

Hajnal, John. 1953. The marriage boom. *Population Index*, 19, 80–101.

—. 1953–4. Age at marriage and proportion marrying. *Population Studies*, 7, 111–28.

—. 1965. European marriage patterns in perspective. In David V. Glass and D. E. C. Eversley, eds., *Population in History*. London: Edward Arnold.

—. 1982. Two kinds of pre-industrial household formation system. *Population and Development Review*, 8, 449–94.

—. 1983. Two kinds of pre-industrial household formation. In Richard Wall, ed., *Family Forms in Historic Europe*. Cambridge: Cambridge University Press.

Haley, Bruce. 1978. *The Healthy Body and Victorian Culture*. Cambridge: Harvard University Press.

Hall, Arthur, and W. B. Ransom. 1906. Plumbism from the ingestion of diachylon as an abortifacient. *Lancet*, 1, 511.

Hall, Ruth. 1977. *Marie Stopes: A Biography*. London: Deutsch.

—, ed. 1978. *Dear Dr. Stopes: Sex in the 1930s*. London: Penguin.

—, ed. 1981. *Dear Dr. Stopes, Sex in the 1920s*. Harmondsworth: Penguin.

Hanagan, Michael. 1986. Agriculture and industry in the nineteenth century Stéphanois: household employment patterns and the rise of a permanent proletariat. In Michael Hanagan and Charles Stephenson, eds., *Proletarians and Protest: The Roots of Class Formation in an Industrializing World*. Westport, Conn.: Greenwood Press.

—. 1989a. *Nascent Proletarians: Class Formation in Post-Revolutionary France.* Oxford: Basil Blackwell.

—. 1989b. Nascent proletarians: migration patterns and class formation in the stéphanois region: 1840–1880. In P. E. Ogden and P. E. White, eds., *Migrants in Modern France: Population Mobility in the Later Nineteenth and Twentieth Centuries.* London: Unwin Hyman.

Hannan, Michael T. 1979. The dynamics of ethnic boundaries in modern states. In John W. Meyer and Michael T. Hannan, eds., *National Development and the World System.* Chicago: University of Chicago Press.

Hatzfeld, Henri. 1971. *Du pauperisme à la sécurité sociale: Essai sur les origines de la sécurité sociale en France, 1850–1940.* Paris: Armand Colin.

Heather-Bigg, Ada. 1894. The wife's contribution to the family income. *Economic Journal,* 4, 51–8.

Helias, Pierre-Jakez. 1978. *The Horse of Pride.* New Haven: Yale University Press.

Hennock, E. P. 1987. *British Social Reform and German Precedents: The Case of Social Insurance, 1880–1914.* Oxford: Clarendon Press.

Henry, Louis. 1961a. La Fécondité naturelle: observations – theorie – resultats. *Population,* 16, 625–36.

—. 1961b. Some data on natural fertility. *Eugenics Quarterly,* 6, 81–91; 7, 1–11.

—. 1966. Perturbations de la nuptialité résultant de la guerre 1914–1918. *Population,* 21, 272–332.

—. 1977. Current concepts and empirical results concerning natural fertility. In Henri Leridon and Jane Menken, eds., *Natural Fertility.* Liège: Ordina Editions.

Heywood, Colin. 1987. *Childhood in Nineteenth-Century France.* Cambridge: Cambridge University Press.

Higginbotham, Ann Rowell. 1985. The unmarried mother and her child in Victorian London, 1834–1914. Ph.d. diss., Indiana University.

Himes, Norman E. 1928. British birth control clinics. *Eugenics Review,* 20, 157–65.

—. 1936 and 1963. *Medical History of Contraception.* New York: Gamut Press.

Hirst, J. D. 1981. A failure "without parallel": the school medical service and the London County Council, 1907–1912. *Medical History,* 25, 281–300.

Hobsbawm, Eric. 1983. Mass-producing traditions: Europe 1870–1914. In Eric Hobsbawm and Terence Ranger, eds., *The Invention of Tradition.* Cambridge: Cambridge University Press.

—. 1987. *The Age of Empire, 1875–1914.* New York: Pantheon.

Hochstadt, Steve. 1981. Migration and industrialization in Germany, 1815–1977. *Social Science History,* 5, 445–68.

—. Socioeconomic determinants of mobility in nineteenth-century Germany. Mainz: Arbeitspapier, Institut fur Europaische Geschichte.

—. 1987. Temporary migration and rural social science history. Paper presented at the Annual Meeting of the Social Science History Association, New Orleans.

Hoerder, Dirk. 1985a. An introduction to labor migration in the Atlantic Economies, 1815–1914. In Dirk Hoerder, ed., *Labor Migration in the Atlantic Economies: The European and North American Working Classes during the Period of Industrialization.* Westport, Conn.: Greenwood Press.

—, ed. 1985b. *Labor Migration in the Atlantic Economies: The European and North Ameican Working Classes during the Period of Industrialization.* Westport, Conn.: Greenwood Press.

Hoggart, Richard. 1971. *The Uses of Literacy*. London: Chatto and Windus.

Hohenberg, Paul. 1972. Change in rural France in the period of industrialization, 1830–1914. *Journal of Economic History*, 32, 219–40.

—. 1974. Migration et fluctuations démographiques dans la France rurale, 1836–1901. *Annales: Economies, Sociétés, Civilizations*, 29, 461–97.

Holcombe, Lee. 1983. *Wives and Property: Reform of the Married Women's Property Law in Nineteenth-Century England*. Toronto: University of Toronto Press.

Holmes, Edmond. 1911. *What Is and What Might Be*. London: Constable.

—. 1920. *In Quest of an Ideal*. London: Constable.

Holtzman, Ellen M. 1982. The pursuit of married love: women's attitudes towards sexuality and marriage in Great Britain, 1918–1939. *Journal of Social History*, 16, 39–52.

Hope, Edward W. 1917. *Report on the Physical Welfare of Mothers and Children*. London: Carnegie U.K. Trust.

Hopkin, W. A. B., and John Hajnal. 1947. Analysis of births in England and Wales, 1939, by Father's Occupation. *Population Studies*, 1, 187–203, 275–300.

Houghton, Walter. 1957. *The Victorian Frame of Mind, 1830–1870*. New Haven: Yale University Press.

Houlbrooke, Ralph. 1984. *The English Family, 1450–1700*. New York: Longman.

Houston, Rabb, and K. D. M. Snell. 1984. Protoindustrialization? Cottage industry, social change, and Industrial Revolution. *Historical Journal*, 27, 473–92.

Hufton, Olwen. 1974. *The Poor of Eighteenth-Century France*. Oxford: Oxford University Press.

Humphries, Stephen. 1981. *Hooligans or Rebels? An Oral History of Working-Class Childhood and Youth, 1889–1939*. Oxford: Basil Blackwell.

Hunt, E. H. 1973. *Regional Wage Variations in Britain, 1850–1914*. Oxford: Clarendon Press.

Huss, Marie Monique. 1988. Pronatalism in wartime France: the Evidence of the picture postcard. In Richard Wall and J. M. Winter, eds., *The Upheaval of War, Family, Work, and Welfare in Europe, 1914–1918*. Cambridge: Cambridge University Press.

Illich, Ivan. 1982. *Gender*. New York: Pantheon.

Illick, Joseph. 1974. Childrearing in seventeenth century England and America. In Lloyd de Mause, ed., *The History of Childhood*. New York: Psychohistory Press.

INEA (Istituto Nazionale di Economia Agraria). 1947. *La distribuzione della proprietà fondiaria in Italia. Tavole statistiche, Sicilia*. Rome: Edizioni Italiane.

INED (Institut national d'études démographiques). 1931–5. *Statistique internationale du mouvement de la population*. Paris. INED.

Inglehart, Ronald. 1977. *The Silent Revolution*. Princeton: Princeton University Press.

Innes, John W. 1938. *Class Fertility Differentials in England and Wales, 1876–1934*. Princeton: Princeton University Press.

—. 1941. Class birth rates in England and Wales, 1921–1931. *Milbank Memorial Fund Quarterly*, 19, 72–96.

Jackson, James, Jr. 1980. Migration and urbanization in the Ruhr Valley, 1850–1900. Ph.d. diss., University of Minnesota.

Jackson, James, Jr., and Leslie Page Moch. 1989. Migration and the social history of modern Europe. *Historical Methods*, 22, 27–36.

Jackson, Margaret. 1983. Sexual liberation or social control: some aspects of the relationship between feminism and the social construction of sexual knowledge in the early twentieth century. *Women's Studies International Forum*, 6, 1–18.

Jeffreys, Sheila. 1985. *The Spinster and Her Enemies*. London: Pandora.

Jenkins, Alice. 1940. *Conscript Parenthood: The Problem of Secret Abortions*. London: George Standring.

Jones, Peter M. 1985. *Politics and Rural Society: The Southern Massif Central, c. 1750–1880*. Cambridge: Cambridge University Press.

Jordanova, Ludmilla. 1980. Natural facts: a historical perspective on science and sexuality. In Carol P. MacCormack and Marilyn Strathern, eds., *Nature, Culture, and Gender*. Cambridge: Cambridge University Press.

—. 1986. Naturalizing the family: literature and bio-medical sciences in the late eighteenth century. In Ludmilla Jordanova, ed., *Languages of Nature: Critical Essays on Science and Literature*. London: Free Association Press.

Jones, Elise F. 1982. Socio-economic differentials in achieved fertility. In *Comparative Studies: ECE Analyses of WFS Surveys in Europe and USA*. Geneva: Population Activities Unit, United Nations Economic Commission for Europe.

Kaelble, Hartmut. 1981. Abweichung oder Konvergenz? Soziale Mobilitat in Frankreich und Deutschland wahrend des 19. und 20. Jahrhunderts. In Gerhard A. Ritter and Rudolf Vierhaus, eds., *Aspekte der historischen Forschung in Frankreich und Deutschland*. Göttingen: Vandenhoeck & Ruprecht.

Kälvemark, Ann-Sophie. 1980. *More Children of Better Quality? Aspects of Swedish Population Policy in the 1930's*. Uppsala: Almquist & Wiksell International.

Kanthack, Emilia. 1907. *The Preservation of Infant Life: A Guide for Health Visitors. Six Lectures to the Voluntary Health Visitors in the Borough of St. Pancras*. London: H. K. Lewis.

Katznelson, Ira, and Aristide R. Zolberg, eds. 1986. *Working-Class Formation*. Princeton: Princeton University Press.

Katznelson, Ira, and Margaret Weir. 1985. *Schooling for All: Class, Race, and the Decline of the Democratic Ideal*. New York: Basic Books.

Kelsall, R. K. 1967. *Population*. London: Longmans, Green & Co.

Kennedy, David. 1970. *Birth Control in America: The Career of Margaret Sanger*. New Haven: Yale University Press.

Keown, John. 1988. *Abortion, Doctors and the Law: Some Aspects of the Legal Regulation of Abortion in England from 1803 to 1982*. Cambridge: Cambridge University Press.

Kerr, James, ed. 1916. *The Care of the School Child: Lectures Delivered under the Auspices of the National League for Physical Education and Improvement, May to July 1916*. London: The National League.

Kerr, Madeleine. 1958. *The People of Ship Street*. London: Routledge & Kegan Paul.

Kertzer, David, and Dennis Hogan. 1985. On the move: migration in an Italian community, 1865–1921. *Social Science History*, 9, 1–23.

Kintner, Hallie. 1985. Trends and regional differences in breastfeeding in Germany from 1871 to 1937. *Journal of Family History*, 10, 163–82.

Kirkaldy, Adam W. 1921. *British Labour Replacement and Conciliation, 1914–1921*. London: I. Pitman.

Kisch, Herbert. 1981. The textile industries in Silesia and the Rhineland: a comparative study in industrialization. In Peter Kriedte et al., *Industrialization before Industrialization*. Cambridge: Cambridge University Press.

Kiser, Claude V. 1933. Trends in the fertility of social classes from 1900 to 1910. *Human Biology*, 5, 256–73.

Klaus, Alisa C. 1986. Babies all the rage: the movement to prevent infant mortality in the United States and France, 1890–1920. Ph.D. diss. University of Pennsylvania.

Klein, Josephine. 1965. *Samples from English Culture*. London: Routledge & Kegan Paul.

Knight, Patricia. 1977. Women and abortion in Victorian and Edwardian England. *History Workshop Journal*, 4, 56–68.

Knodel, John. 1968. Law, marriage and illegitimacy in nineteenth-century Germany. *Population Studies*, 22, 297–318.

—. 1974. *The Decline of Fertility in Germany, 1871–1939*. Princeton: Princeton University Press.

—. 1977a. Family limitation and the fertility transition: evidence from the age patterns of fertility in Europe and Asia. *Population Studies*, 31, 219–49.

—. 1977b. Town and country in Nineteenth-Century Germany: a review of urban-rural differentials in demographic behavior. *Social Science History*, 1, 356–82.

—. 1986. The demographic transition in German villages. In Ansley J. Coale and Susan Cotts Watkins, eds., *The Decline of Fertility in Europe*. Princeton: Princeton University Press.

—. 1988. *Demographic Behavior in the Past*. New York: Cambridge University Press.

Knodel, John; Aphichat Chamratrithirong; and Nibhon Debavalya. 1987. *Thailand's Reproductive Revolution*. Madison: University of Wisconsin Press.

Knodel, John, and Mary Jo Maynes. 1976. Urban and rural marriage patterns in imperial Germany. *Journal of Family History*, 1, 129–68.

Knodel, John, and Edward Shorter. 1976. The reliability of family reconstitution data in German village genealogies (Ortsippenbucher). In *Annales de démographie historique*. Paris and The Hague: Mouton.

Knodel, John, and Etienne van de Walle. 1967. Breast feeding, fertility and infant morality: an analysis of some early German data. *Population Studies*, 21, 109–31.

—. 1979. Lessons from the past: policy implications of historical fertility studies. *Population and Development Review*, 5, 217–45.

—. 1986. Lessons from the past: policy implications of historical fertility studies. In Ansley J. Coale and Susan Cotts Watkins, *The Decline of Fertility in Europe*. Princeton: Princeton University Press.

Kohler, Peter A.; Hans F. Zacher; and Martin Partington, eds. 1982. *The Evolution of Social Insurance, 1881–1981*. London: Frances Pinter.

Kohli, Martin. 1986. Retirement and the moral economy: an historical interpretation of the German case. *Working Paper No. 3*. Berlin, Institut für Soziologie der Freien Universität.

Kriedte, Peter, et al. 1981. *Industrialization before Industrialization*. Cambridge: Cambridge University Press.

Kulischer, Eugene. 1948. *Europe on the Move: War and Population Changes, 1917–1947*. New York: Columbia University Press.

Kussmaul, Ann. 1981. *Servants in Husbandry in Early Modern England*. Cambridge: Cambridge University Press.

Landry, Adolphe. 1933. La Révolution démographique. In *Economic Essays in Honour of Gustav Cassel*. London: Allen & Unwin.

Large, Peter. 1985. Urban growth and agricultural change in the west Midlands during the seventeenth and eighteenth centuries. In Peter Clark, ed., *The Transformation of English Provincial Towns*. London: Hutchinson.

La Rosa, Salvatore. 1977. Transformazioni fondiarie, cooperazione, patti agrari. In *Storia della Sicilia*, vol. 9. Naples: Società editrice Storia di Napoli e della Sicilia.

Laslett, Peter. 1983. *The World We Have Lost: England before the Industrial Age. 1965*. New York: Scribners.

Lawton, Richard. 1958. Population movements in the west Midlands, 1841–1861. *Geography*, 43, 164–77.

Leasure, J. William. 1962. Factors involved in the decline of fertility in Spain, 1900–1950. Ph.d. diss., Princeton University.

Leboutte, René. 1983. L'Infanticide dans l'est de la Belgique aux XVIIIᵉ–XIXᵉ siècles: une realité. In *Annales de démographie historique*. Paris: Editions de l'Ecole des hautes études en sciences sociales.

Leclerc, Gerard. 1979. *L'Observation de l'homme: Une histoire des enquêtes sociales*. Paris: Seuil.

Ledbetter, Rosanna. 1976. *A History of the Malthusian League, 1877–1927*. Columbus: Ohio State University Press.

Lees, Andrew. 1985. *Cities Perceived: Urban Society in European and American Thought, 1820–1940*. New York: Columbia University Press.

Lehning, James R. 1983. Nuptiality and rural industry: families and labor in the French countryside. *Journal of Family History*, 8, 333–45.

Lejeune, Philippe. 1971. *L'Autobiographie en France*. Paris: A Colin.

—. 1975. *Le Pacte Autobiographique*. Paris: Seuil.

—. 1980. *Je est un autre*. Paris: Seuil.

Le Play, Frederic. 1855. *Les Ouvriers européens*. Paris: Imprimerie impériale.

Léridon, Henri. 1987. *La Seconde révolution contraceptive: La Régulation des naissances en France de 1950 à 1985*. National Institute of Demographic Studies, Research and Documents, Monograph no. 117. Paris: Presses universitaires de France.

Le Roy Ladurie, Emmanuel. 1972. Système de la coutume: structures familiales et coutumes d'héritage en France au XVIᵉ siècle. *Annales: Economies, Sociétés, Civilisations*, 27, 825–46.

Lesthaeghe, Ron J. 1977. *The Decline of Belgian Fertility, 1800–1970*. Princeton: Princeton University Press.

—. 1980. On the social control of human reproduction. *Population and Development Review*, 6, 527–48.

—. 1983. A century of demographic and cultural change in Western Europe: an exploration of underlying dimensions. *Population and Development Review*, 9, 411–35.

—. 1989. Motivation and legitimation: living conditions, social control and the reproductive regimes in Belgium and France from the 16th through the 19th century. Working Paper 2. Vrije Universiteit Brussel: Inter-university Programme in Demography.

Lesthaeghe, Ron J., and Dominique Meekers. 1986. Value changes and the dimensions of familism in the European community. *European Journal of Population*, 2, 225–68.

Lesthaeghe, Ron J., and Chris Wilson. 1986. Modes of production, secularization, and the pace of the fertility decline in Western Europe, 1870–1930. In Ansley J. Coale and Susan Cotts Watkins, eds., *The Decline of Fertility in Europe*. Princeton: Princeton University Press.

Leunbach, Jonathan H. 1930. *Birth Control, Abortion, and Sterilization*. London: Kegan Paul.

Levasseur, Emile. 1889–92. *La Population française*. 3 vols. Paris: Rousseau.

Levine, David. 1977. *Family Formation in an Age of Nascent Capitalism*. New York: Academic Press.

—. 1987. *Reproducing Families: The Political Economy of English Population History*. Cambridge: Cambridge University Press.

—. 1989. Recombinant family formation strategies. *Journal of Historical Sociology*, 2, 89–115.

Levy, Marion J., Jr. 1966. *Modernization and the Structure of Societies: A Setting for International Affairs*. Princeton: Princeton University Press.

Lewis, Jan, and Kenneth Lockridge. 1988. "Sally has been sick": pregnancy and family limitation among Virginia gentry women, 1780–1830. *Journal of Social History*, 22, 6–14.

Lewis, Jane. 1980. *The Politics of Motherhood: Child and Maternal Welfare in England, 1900–1939*. London: Croom Helm.

—. 1984. *Women in England, 1870–1950: Sexual Divisions and Social Change*. Sussex: Wheatsheaf Books; Bloomington: Indiana University Press.

—. 1986. The working-class wife and mother and state intervention, 1870–1918. In Jane Lewis, ed., *Labour and Love, Women's Experience of Home and Family, 1850–1940*. Oxford: Basil Blackwell.

Lewis, Judith Schneid. 1986. *In the Family Way: Childbearing in the British Aristocracy, 1760–1860*. New Brunswick: Rutgers University Press.

Lewis-Faning, E. 1949. Report on an enquiry into family limitation and its influence on human fertility during the past fifty years. In *Papers of the Royal Commission on Population*, vol. 1. London: His Majesty's Stationery Office.

Lieberson, Stanley; Guy Dalto; and Mary Ellen Marsden. 1981. The course of mother-tongue diversity in nations. In Stanley Lieberson, ed., *Language Diversity and Language Contact*. Stanford: Stanford University Press.

Liddington, Jill. 1984. *The Life and Times of a Respectable Rebel: Selina Cooper (1864–1946)*. London: Virago.

Linz, Susan A. 1988. World War II and Soviet Economic Growth. In Susan A. Linz, ed., *The Impact of World War II on the Soviet Union*. London: Rowman & Allenheld.

Lis, Caterina, and Hugo Soly. 1979. *Poverty and Capitalism in Pre-Industrial Europe*. Atlantic Highlands, N.J.: Humanities Press.

Livi-Bacci, Massimo. 1971. *A Century of Portuguese Fertility*. Princeton: Princeton University Press.

—. 1977. *A History of Italian Fertility during the Last Two Centuries*. Princeton: Princeton University Press. Translated into Italian as *Donna, fecondità, figli*. Bologna: Il Mulino, 1980.

—. 1986. Social group forerunners of fertility control in Europe. In Ansley J. Coale and Susan Cotts Watkins, eds., *The Decline of Fertility in Europe*. Princeton: Princeton University Press.

Livi-Bacci, Massimo, and Antonio Santini. 1969. *Tavole di fecondità della donna italiana secondo le generazioni di appartenza*. Firenze: Dipartimento Statistico-Matematico.

London County Council. 1910. *Annual Reports*, vol. 3, *Report of the London Medical Officer of Health (MOH) for 1910*.

Lorenzoni, Giovanni. 1910. *Inchiesta parlamentare sulle condizioni dei contadini nelle provincie meridionali e nella Sicilia*, vol. 6. Rome: Tipografia nazionale di Giovanni Bertero.

Lowe, Nigel. 1982. The legal status of fathers: past and present. In Margaret O'Brien and Lorna McKee, eds., *The Father Figure*. London: Tavistock.

Lucassen, Jan. 1987. *Migrant Labour in Europe, 1600–1900*. London: Croom Helm.

Luckmann, Thomas. 1967. *The Invisible Religion*. New York: Macmillan.

Luker, Kristin. 1975. *Taking Chances: Abortion and the Decision Not to Contracept*. Berkeley: University of California Press.

Luzzatto, Gino. 1968. *L'economia italiana dal 1861 al 1894*. Turin: Einaudi.

Luzzatto-Fegiz, Paolo. 1956. *Il volto sconosciuto dell'Italia*. Milan: Giuffrè.

Lynch, Katherine A. 1988. *Family, Class and Ideology in Early Industrial France*. Madison: University of Wisconsin Press.

McCleary, George F. 1933. *The Early History of the Infant Welfare Movement*. London: H. K. Lewis.

McCloskey, Donald N. 1981. *Enterprise and Trade in Victorian Britain*. London: Allen & Unwin.

McDougall, Mary L. 1983. Protecting infants: the French campaign for maternity leaves, 1890s–1913. *French Historical Studies*, 13, 79–105.

Macfarlane, Alan. 1970. *The Family Life of Ralph Josselin*. New York: Norton.

—. 1977. *Reconstructing Historical Communities*. New York: Cambridge University Press.

—. 1984. The myth of the peasantry: family and economy in a northern parish. In Richard M. Smith, ed., *Land, Kinship and Life-Cycle*. Cambridge: Cambridge University Press.

Mack Smith, Denis. 1959. *Italy: A Modern History*. Ann Arbor: University of Michigan Press.

—. 1968. *A History of Sicily: Modern Sicily after 1713*. London: Chatto & Windus.

McLaren, Angus. 1977. Women's work and the regulation of family size: the question of abortion in the nineteenth century. *History Workshop Journal*, 4, 70–81.

—. 1978. *Birth Control in Nineteenth Century England*. London: Croom Helm.

—. 1983. *Sexuality and Social Order: The Debate over the Fertility of Women and Workers in France, 1770–1920*. New York: Holmes & Meier.

—. 1984. *Reproductive Rituals: The Perception of Fertility in England from the Sixteenth Century to the Nineteenth Century*. London: Methuen.

McMillan, Margaret. 1919. *The Nursery School*. London: J. M. Dent.

—. [1909.] *The School Clinic Today. Health Centres and What They Mean to the People*. London: ILP.

McNeill, William H. 1986. *Polyethnicity and National Unity in World History*. Toronto: University of Toronto Press.

Mafai, Miriam, 1987. *Pane nero.* Milan: Rizzoli.

Maher, Vanessa. 1983. Un mestiere da raccontare: Sarte e sartine torinesi fra le due guerre. *Memoria,* 8, 52–71.

Malthus, Thomas Robert. 1959. *Population: The First Essay.* 1798. Ann Arbor: University of Michigan Press.

Mandel, Ernest. 1962. *Marxist Economic Theory.* 2 vols. London: Merlin.

Marchant, James, ed. 1917. *The Declining Birth Rate: Its Causes and Effects.* London: Chapman & Hall.

—. 1926. *Medical Views on Birth Control.* London: Hopkinson.

Martin, Anna. 1911. *The Married Working Woman: A Study.* London: National Union of Women's Suffrage Societies.

—. 1913. The mother and social reform: part II. *The Nineteenth Century and After,* 73, 1235–55.

—. 1918. The irresponsibility of the father: part I. *The Nineteenth Century and After,* 84, 1091–1103.

—. 1919. The irresponsibility of the father: part II. *The Nineteenth Century and After,* 85, 548–62.

—. 1919. The irresponsibility of the father: part III. *The Nineteenth Century and After,* 85, 956–70.

Martin, Emily. 1987. *The Woman in the Body: A Cultural Analysis of Reproduction.* Boston: Beacon Press.

Marx, Karl. 1959. *The Eighteenth Brumaire of Louis Bonaparte.* In Lewis S. Feuer, ed., *Marx and Engels: Basic Writings on Politics and Philosophy.* New York: Doubleday.

Marx, Karl, and Friederich Engels. 1967. *The Communist Manifesto.* 1848. Harmondsworth: Penguin Books.

Mason, Karen O., and A. M. Taj. 1987. Differences between women's and men's reproductive goals in developing countries. *Population and Development Review,* 13, 611–38.

Matras, Judah. 1973. *Population and Societies.* Englewood Cliffs, N.J.: Prentice-Hall.

Mauco, Georges. 1932. *Les Migrations ouvrières en France aux debuts du XIXe siècle.* Paris: Lesot.

Maynes, Mary Jo. 1985a. *Schooling for the People: Comparative Local Studies of Schooling History in France and Germany, 1750–1850.* New York: Holmes and Meier.

—. 1985b. *Schooling in Western Europe: a Social History.* Albany: State University of New York Press.

Maynes, Mary Jo, and Tom Taylor. 1990. Children in German history. In N. Ray Hiner and Joseph M. Hawes, eds., *Children in Comparative and Historical Perspective: An International Handbook.* Westport, Conn.: Greenwood Press.

Meldini, Piero. 1975. *Sposa e madre esemplare.* Rimini: Guaraldi.

Mendels, Franklin. 1972. Proto-industrialization: the first phase of the industrialization process. *Journal of Economic History,* 32, 241–61.

Merley, Jean. 1974. *La Haute-Loire: De la fin de l'Ancien Régime aux debuts de la Troisième Republique.* Le Puy: Cahiers de la Haute-Loire.

—. 1977. Eléments pour l'étude de la formation de la population stéphanoise a l'aube de la révolution industrielle. *Bulletin du Centre d'histoire économique et sociale de la Région lyonnaise,* 8, 261–75.

Merli, Stefano. 1972. *Proletariato di fabbrica e capitalismo industriale: Il caso italiano, 1800–1900*. Firenze: La nuova Italia.

Midlands Mining Commission. 1843. *First Report – South Staffordshire*. London: William Clowes & Son.

Mill, John Stuart. 1929. *On the Subjugation of Women*. 1869. London: Everyman.

Miller, John Hawkins. 1978. "Temple and sewer": childbirth, prudery and Victoria regina. In Anthony Wohl, ed., *The Victorian Family: Structure and Stresses*. London: Croom Helm.

Milward, Alan S. 1977. *War, Economy, and Society, 1939–1945*. Harmondsworth: Allen Lane.

Ministère de l'agriculture, du commerce, et des travaux publiques. 1867. *Enquête agricole*, vol. 9. Paris: Imprimerie impériale.

Ministry of Health, Great Britain. 1939. *Report of the Inter-Departmental Committee on Abortion*. London: His Majesty's Stationery Office.

Minor, Iris. 1979. Working-class women and matrimonial law reform, 1890–1914. In David E. Martin and David Rubinstein, eds. *Ideology and the Labor Movement*. London: Croom Helm.

Miraglia, Emanuele Navarro della. 1963 *La nana*. Rocca San Gasciano: Cappelli.

Mitchell, Brian R. 1975. *European Historical Statistics, 1750–1970*. New York: Columbia University Press.

Mitchell, Brian R., and Phyllis Deane. 1962. *Abstract of British Historical Statistics*. Cambridge: Cambridge University Press.

Mitzman, Arthur. 1987. The civilizing offensive: mentalities high culture and individual psyches. *Journal of Social History*, 20 663–88.

Moch, Leslie Page. 1983. *Paths to the City: Regional Migration in Nineteenth-Century France*. Beverly Hills, Calif.: Sage Publications.

—. 1986. The family and migration: news from the French. *Journal of Family History*, 11, 193–203.

—. 1988. An intersection of dramas: urbanization and the decline of fertility. Oral presentation, May 20–22, 1988, Ontario Institute for Studies in Education, Toronto.

Moeller, Robert. 1988. Women and the state in the Wirtschaftswunder: protecting mothers and the family in post–World War II West Germany. *Feminist Studies*, 14, 1–30.

Mohr, James. 1978. *Abortion in America*. New York: Oxford University Press.

Mollat, Michel. 1979. *Histoire de Rouen*. Toulouse: Privat.

Mommsen, Wolfgang J. 1981. *The Emergence of the Welfare State in Britain and Germany, 1850–1950*. London: Croom Helm.

Moore, Barrington. 1978. *Injustice*. London: Macmillan.

Moore, Michael J. 1977. Social work and social welfare: the organization of philanthropic resources in Britain, 1900–1914. *Journal of British Studies*, 16, 85–104.

Moore, Wilbert E. 1965. *The Impact of Industry*. Englewood Cliffs, N.J., Prentice-Hall.

—. 1979. *World Modernization: The Limits of Convergence*. New York: Elsevier.

Morokvasic, Mirjana. 1981. Sexuality and control of procreation. In Kate Young, Carol Wolkowitz, and Roslyn McCullagh, eds., *Of Marriage and the Market*. London: CSE Books.

Mosca, Gaetano. 1949. *Partiti e sindacati nella crisi del regime parlamentare*. Bari: Laterza.

Mosley, W. Henry, ed. 1978. *Nutrition and Reproduction*. New York: Plenum.

Muchembled, Robert. 1985. *Popular Culture and Elite Culture in France, 1400–1750.* Baton Rouge: Louisiana State University Press.

Müller, Detlef K., Fritz Ringer, and Brian Simon, eds. 1987. *The Rise of Modern Educational Systems.* Cambridge: Cambridge University Press.

Musso, Stefano. 1988. La famiglia operaia. In Piero Melograni and Lucetta Scaraffia, eds., *La famiglia italiana dall'Ottocento ad oggi.* Bari: Laterza.

Myrdal, Alva. 1945. *Nation and Family: The Swedish Experiment in Democratice Family and Population Policy.* London: Kegan Paul, Trench & Trubner.

Nagel, Joanne, and Susan Olzak. 1982. Ethnic mobilization in new and old states: an extension of the competition model. *Social Problems,* 30, 139–43.

National Association for the Promotion of Social Science. 1858. *Transactions, 1857.* London: John W. Parker & Son.

Neuman, Robert P. 1978. Working class birth control in Wilhelmine Germany. *Comparative Studies in Society and History,* 20, 408–28.

Newman, L. F. 1942. Some references to the couvade in literature. *Folk-Lore,* 53, 148–57.

Newsholme, Arthur. 1935. *Fifty Years in Public Health.* London: Allen & Unwin.

Niggemann, Heinz. 1981. *Emanzipation zwischen Sozialismus und Feminismus.* Wuppertal: Hammer.

Norway. 1935. Det Statistiske Centralbyra. *Folketellingen i Norge,* December 1, 1930. Niende hefte. Barnetallet i norske ekteskap. Oslo: I Kommisjon Hos H. Aschehoug & Co.

Notes and Queries. 1878. 5th ser. (205), 255–6.

Notes and Queries for Somerset and Dorset. 1943–6, 24, 277.

Notestein, Frank W. 1953. Economic problems of population change. In *Proceedings of the Eighth International Conference of Agricultural Economists.* London: Oxford University Press.

Nugent, Jeffrey B. 1985. The old-age security motive for fertility. *Population and Development Review,* 11, 75–97.

Oakley, Ann. 1984. *The Captured Womb: A History of the Medical Care of Pregnant Women.* Oxford: Basil Blackwell.

Obelkevich, James. 1976. *Religion and Rural Society: South Lindsey, 1825–1875.* Oxford: Clarendon Press.

O'Brien, Patrick K., and Caglar Keyder. 1978. *Economic Growth in Britain and France, 1780–1914: Two Paths to the Twentieth Century.* London: Allen & Unwin.

O'Brien, Patrick K., and Stanley L. Engerman. 1981. Changes in income and its distribution during the industrial revolution. In Roderick Floud and Donald McCloskey, eds., *The Economic History of Britain since 1700,* vol. 1. Cambridge: Cambridge University Press.

Offe, Claus. 1972. *Strukturprobleme des kapitalistischen Staates.* Frankfurt: Suhrkamp.

O'Grada, Cormack O. 1981. Agricultural decline, 1860–1914. In Roderick Floud and Donald McCloskey, eds., *The Economic History of Britain.* vol. 2. Cambridge: Cambridge University Press.

—. 1988. *Ireland before and after the Famine.* New York: St. Martin's Press.

Omran, A. R. 1981. Review of the evidence – an update. In A. R. Omran and C. C. Standley, eds., *Family Formation and Patterns of Health: Further Studies.* Geneva: World Health Organization.

Oren, Laura. 1973. The welfare of women in labouring families: England, 1860–1950. *Feminist Studies*, 1, 107–25.

Ortner, Sherry. 1978. *Sherpas through Their Rituals*. Chicago: University of Chicago. Press.

P. L. 1841. Du pauperisme et de la mendicité. *Société agricole et industrielle de l'Arrondissement de Saint-Étienne, Bulletin*, 18, 121–34.

Page, William, ed., 1908. *The Victoria History of the County of Stafford*, vol. 1. London: University of London Press.

Parkerson, Donald H. and Jo Ann Parkerson. 1988. "Fewer children of greater spiritual quality": religion and the decline of fertility in nineteenth century America. *Social Science History*, 12, 49–70.

Parisi, Giovanni. 1966. *Note sullo sviluppo dell'agricultura siciliana dal 1947 al 1964*. Palermo: Quaderni del Comitato regionale siciliano del PCI, no. 1.

Parsons, Anne. 1969. *Belief, Magic and Anomie*. New York: Free Press.

Parsons, Talcott. 1975. Some theoretical considerations on the nature and trends of change in ethnicity. In Nathan Glazer and Daniel Moynihan, eds., *Ethnicity: Theory and Experience*. Cambridge: Harvard University Press.

Passerini, Luisa. 1984. *Torino operaia e fascismo*, Bari: Laterza.

Pedersen, Susan. 1990. Gender, welfare, and citizenship in Britain during the Great War. *American Historical Review* 95, 983–1006.

Peel, John. 1963. The manufacture and retailing of contraceptives in England. *Population Studies*, 17, 113–25.

Pelham, R. A. 1952. The agricultural geography of Warwickshire during the Napoleonic Wars as revealed by the Acreage returns of 1801. *Transactions of the Birmingham Archaeological Society*, 68, 89–106.

—. 1963. The water-power crisis in Birmingham in the eighteenth century. *University of Birmingham Historical Journal*, 9, 64–91.

Perricone, Rosa Anna. 1975. La nuzialità nei comuni siciliani dal 1862 al 1961. In *Collana di Studi Demografici*, vol. 8. Palermo: Universtiy of Palermo, Institute of Demographic Sciences.

Petchesky, Rosalind Pollack. 1984. *Abortion and Woman's Choice: the State, Sexuality, and Reproductive Freedom*. New York: Longmans.

Petersen, William. 1969. *Population*, 2d ed. New York: Macmillan.

Peterson, M. Jeanne. 1989. *Family, Love, and Work in the Lives of Victorian Gentlewomen*. Bloomington: Indiana University Press.

Phayer, J. Michael. 1977. *Sexual Liberation and Religion in Nineteenth-Century Europe*. London: Croom Helm.

Phillips, Marion. [1910.] *The School Doctor and the Home: Results of an Inquiry into Medical Inspection and Treatment of School Children*. London: Women's Labour League of Central London.

Phillips, Roderick. 1988. *Putting Asunder: A History of Divorce in Western Society*. Cambridge: Cambridge University Press.

Piccone Stella, Simonetta. 1981. Crescere negli anni cinquanta. *Memoria*, 2, 9–35.

Pieroni Bortolotti, Franca. 1963. *Alle origini del movimento femminile in Italia*. Turin: Einaudi.

—. 1987. Osservazioni sull'occupazione femminile durante il fascismo. In Franca Pieroni Bortolotti, *Il movimento politico delle donne: Scritti inediti*, ed. Annarita Buttafuoco. Rome: Utopia.

Pillitteri, Francesco. 1981. *Credito e risparmio nella Sicilia dell'unificazione*. Palermo: Palumbo.

Pinchemel, Phillippe. 1969. *France: A Geographical Survey*. New York: Praeger.

Pitkin, Donald D. 1985. *The House That Giaccomo Built: History of an Italian Family, 1898–1978*. Cambridge: Cambridge University Press.

Piva, Italo, and Giuseppe Maddalena. 1982. La tutela delle lavoratrici madri nel periodo 1923–1943. In Maria Luisa Betri and Ada Gigli Marchetti, eds., *Salute e classi lavoratrici in Italia dall Unità al Fascismo*. Milan: F. Angeli.

Piven, Frances F., and Richard A. Cloward. 1971. *Regulating the Poor: The Function of Public Welfare*. New York: Pantheon.

Poitrineau, Abel. 1962. Aspects de l'émigration temporaire et saisonnière en Auvergne à la fin du XVIIIe siècle et au debut du XIXe siècle. *Revue d'histoire moderne et contemporaine*, 9, 5–50.

—. 1965. *La Vie rurale en Basse Auvergne au XVIIIe siècle*. Paris: Presses universitaires de France.

—. 1983. *Remues d'hommes: Les Migrations montagnardes en France, 17e–18e siècles*. Paris: Aubier.

—. 1985. *Les Espagnols de l'Auvergne et du Limousin du XVIIIe au XIXe siècle*. Aurillac: Malroux-Mazel.

Pollard, Sidney. 1981. *The Integration of the European Economy since 1845*. London: Allen & Unwin.

Pollock, Linda. 1983. *Forgotten Children: Parent-Child Relations from 1500 to 1900*. Cambridge: Cambridge University Press.

—, ed. 1987. *A Lasting Relationship: Parents and Children over Three Centuries*. Hanover, N.H.: University Press of New England.

Polson, Cyril J. 1963. *The Essentials of Forensic Medicine*. Oxford: Pergamon.

Polson, Cyril J., and Reginald N. Tattersall. 1959. *Clinical Toxicology*. London: English University Press.

Poovey, Mary. 1987. Scenes of an indelicate character: the "medical treatment" of victorian women. In Catherine Gallagher and Thomas Laqueur, eds., *The Making of the Modern Body: Sexuality and Society in the Nineteenth Century*. Berkeley: University of California Press.

Porter, Theodore M. 1986. *The Rise of Statistical Thinking, 1820–1900*. Princeton: Princeton University Press.

Pounds, N. J. G. 1985. *An Historical Geography of Europe, 1800–1914*. Cambridge: Cambridge University Press.

Poussou, Jean-Pierre. 1983. *Bordeaux et le sud-ouest au XVIIIe siècle*. Paris: Editions de l'Ecole des hautes études en sciences sociales.

Pralong, Jean, and Yves Delomier. 1983. *La Charité: De l'hospice a l'hôpital geriatrique: 300 ans de l'histoire hospitalière a Saint-Etienne*. Saint-Etienne: Henaff.

Preston, Samuel H.; Michael R. Haines; and Elsie Pamuk. 1981. Effects of industrialization and urbanization on mortality in developed countries. In International Union for the Scientific Study of Population, *International Population Conference, Manila*. Liège: IUSSP.

Price, Roger. 1975. The onset of labour shortage in nineteenth-century France. *Economic History Review*, 2d ser., 28, 260–79.

Prost, Antoine. 1986. Monuments aux morts. In Pierre Nora, ed., *Les Lieux de mémoire*, vol. 3. Paris: Gallimard.

—. 1988. Catholic conservatives, population and the family in twentieth century France. In Michael S. Teitelbaum and Jay M. Winter, eds., *Population and Resources in Western Intellectual Traditions*, a supplement to Population and Development Review, 14, 147–64.

Raphael, Dana. 1975. Matrescence, becoming a mother, a "new old" rite of passage. In Dana Raphael, ed., *Being Female: Reproduction, Power, and Change*. The Hague: Mouton.

Rathbone, Eleanor. 1986. *The Disinherited Family*. 1924. Bristol: Falling Wall Press.

Raybould, T. J. 1973. *The Economic Emergence of the Black Country: A Study of the Dudley Estate*. Newton Abbot: David Charles.

—. 1984. Aristocratic landowners and the Industrial Revolution: the Black Country experience, c. 1760–1840. *Midland History*, 9, 59–86.

Reeves, Magdalen S. Pember. 1913. *Round about a Pound a Week*. London: G. Bell.

Renda, Francesco. 1963. *L'emigrazione in Sicilia*. Palermo: Editore Sicilia al Lavoro.

Report of the Proceedings of the National Conference on Infantile Mortality. 1908. London: P. S. King.

Rice, Margery Spring. 1939. *Working-Class Wives: Their Health and Conditions*. London: Penguin.

Richman, Joel. 1982. Men's experiences of pregnancy and childbirth. In Lorna McKee and Margaret O'Brien, eds., *The Father Figure*. London: Tavistock.

Riley, Denise. 1987. Some peculiarities of social policy concerning women in wartime and postwar Britain. In M. R. Higgonet et al., eds., *Behind the Lines: Gender and the Two World Wars*. New Haven: Yale University Press.

Riley, James C. 1989. *Sickness, Recovery, and Death: A History and Forecast of Ill Health*. Iowa City: University of Iowa Press.

Riley, Madeline. 1968. *Brought to Bed*. South Brunswick, N.J., and New York: A. S. Barnes.

Rimlinger, Gaston V. 1971. *Welfare Policy and Industrialization in Europe, America, and Russia*. New York: John Wiley & Sons.

Ritter, Gerhard A. 1986. *Social Welfare in Germany and Britain: Origins and Development*. Leamington Spa and New York: Berg.

Robert, Jean-Louis. 1988. Women and work in France during the Great War. In Richard Wall and Jay M. Winter, eds., *The Upheaval of War: Family Work, and Welfare in Europe, 1914–1918*. Cambridge: Cambridge University Press.

Roberts, David. 1979. *Paternalism in Early Victorian England*. London: Croom Helm.

Roberts, Elizabeth. 1984. *A Woman's Place: An Oral History of Working-Class Women, 1890–1940*. Oxford: Basil Blackwell.

—. 1986. Women's strategies, 1890–1940. In Jane Lewis, ed., *Labour and Love: Women's Experience of Home and Family, 1850–1940*. Oxford: Basil Blackwell.

Rochefort, Renée 1961. *Le Travail en Sicile: Étude de géographie sociale*. Paris: Presses universitaires de France.

Rose, Nikolas. 1985. *The Psychological Complex: Psychology, Politics and Society in England, 1869–1939*. London: Routledge.

Rosoli, Gianfausto. 1985. Italian migration to European countries from political unification to World War I. In Dirk Hoerder, ed., *Labor Migration in the Atlantic Economies: The European and North American Working Classes during the Period of Industrialization*. Westport, Conn.: Greenwood Press.

Ross, Ellen. 1982. Fierce questions and taunts: married life in working-class London. *Feminist Studies*, 5, 575–602.

—. 1983. Survival networks: women's neighbourhood sharing in London before World War I. *History Workshop*, 15, 4–27.

—. 1992. *Love and Labor in Outcast London: Motherhood, 1870–1918*. New York: Oxford University Press.

Rowan, Caroline. 1985. Child welfare and the working-class family. In Mary Langan and Bill Schwarz, eds., *Crises in the British State, 1880–1930*. London: Hutchinson.

Rowbotham, Sheila. 1977. *A New World for Women: Stella Browne, Socialist Feminist*. London: Pluto.

Rowlands, Marie B. 1975. *Masters and Men in the West Midlands: Metalware Trades before the Industrial Revolution*. Manchester: Manchester University Press.

Rowntree, Griselda, and Norman H. Carrier. 1958. The resort to divorce in England and Wales, 1938–1957. *Population Studies*, 11, 188–233.

Rowntree, Griselda, and Rachel M. Pierce. 1961. Birth control in Britain, Paris I and II. *Population Studies*, 15, 3–31, 121–60.

Roxburgh, Ian. 1988. Modernization theory revisited. *Comparative Studies in Society and History*, 30, 753–61.

Royal Statistical Society. 1840. Contributions to the economical statistics of Birmingham. *Journal of the Royal Statistical Society*, 434–41.

Rubinstein, D. 1969. *School Attendance in London, 1870–1904*. New York. Augustus Kelley.

Ruggles, Steven. 1987. *Prolonged Connections: The Rise of the Extended Family in Nineteenth-Century England and America*. Wisconsin: University of Wisconsin Press.

Ruston, Peter. 1983. Purification or social contract? Ideologies of reproduction and churching women after childbirth. In Eva Gamarnikow, ed., *The Public and Private*. London: Heinemann.

Sabbatucci Severini, Patrizia, and Angelo Trento. 1975. Alcuni cenni sul mercato del lavoro durante il fascismo. *Quaderni storici*, 10, 550–78.

Sahlins, Marshall. 1981. *Historical Metaphors and Mythical Realities: Structure in the Early History of the Sandwich Islands Kingdom*. Ann Arbor, Mich.: University of Michigan Press.

Sallume, Xarifa, and Frank W. Notestein. 1932. Trends in the size of families completed prior to 1910 in various social classes. *American Journal of Sociology*, 37, 398–408.

Sanderson, Warren C. 1976. On Two Schools of the Economics of Fertility. *Population and Development Review*, 2, 469–77.

Sanger, Margaret. 1923. *The Pivot of Civilization*. London; Jonathan Cape.

—. 1928. *Motherhood in Bondage*. New York: Brentano's.

Saraceno, Chiara. 1979–80. La Famiglia operaia sotto il fascismo. *Annali della Fondazione Gian Giacomo Feltrinelli*, vol. 20, pp. 189–230. Milan: Feltrinelli.

—. 1981. Percorsi di vita femminile nella classe operaia: Tra famiglia e lavoro durante il fascismo. *Memoria*, 2, 64–75.

—. 1988. La famiglia: I paradossi della costruzione sociale del privato. In Philippe Ariès and Georges Duby, eds., *La vita privata: Il Novecento*, pp. 37–8. Bari: Laterza. Now translated as The Italian family: paradoxes of privacy. In eds.,

P. Ariès and G. Duby. *A History of Private Life: Riddles of Identity in Modern Times*, pp. 451–502. Cambridge: Harvard University Press, 1991.

——. 1990. Women, family and the law, 1750–1942. *Journal of Family History*, 15, no. 5, 427–42.

Sauer, R. 1978. Infanticide and abortion in nineteenth-century Britain. *Population Studies*, 32, 81–93.

Saunders, George R. 1981. Men and women in southern Europe: a review of some aspects of cultural complexity. *Journal of Psychoanalytic Anthropology*, 4, 435–66.

Scaraffia, Lucetta. 1988. Esserre uomo, essere donna. In Piero Melograni and Lucetta Scaraffia, eds., *La famiglia italiana dall'Ottocento ad oggi*. Bari: Laterza.

Schiaffino, Andrea. 1982. Un aspect mal connu de la démographie urbaine: L'Émigration. In *Annales de démographie historique*. Paris and The Hague: Mouton.

Schleunes, Karl A. 1989. *Schooling and Society: The Politics of Education in Prussia and Bavaria, 1750–1900*. Oxford: Berg.

Schlumbohm, Jürgen. 1983. *Kinderstuben: Wie Kinder zu Bauern, Burgern, Aristo-kraten wurdern, 1700–1850*. Munich: DTV.

——. 1980. "Traditional" collectivity and "modern" individuality: some questions and suggestions for the historical study of socialization. The examples of the German lower and upper bourgeoisies around 1800. *Social History*, 5, 71–103.

Schneider, Jane. 1980. Trousseau as treasure: some contradictions of late nineteenth century change in Sicily. In Eric Ross, ed., *Behind the Myth of Culture*. New York: Academic Press.

Schneider, Jane, and Peter Schneider. 1976. *Culture and Political Economy in Western Sicily*. New York: Academic Press.

——. 1984. Demographic transitions in a Sicilian rural town. *Journal of Family History*, 9, 245–72.

Schneider, Peter. 1986. Rural artisans and peasant mobilisation in the Socialist International: the Fasci Siciliani. *Journal of Peasant Studies*, 13, 63–81.

Schofield, Roger. 1970. Perinatal mortality in Hawkshead, Lancashire, 1571–1710. *Local Population Studies*, 10, 11–16.

——. 1986. Did mothers really die? Three centuries of maternal mortality in the "world we have lost." In Lloyd Bonfield et al., eds., *The World We Have Gained*. Oxford: Oxford University Press.

Schomerus, Heilwig. 1981. The family life-cycle: a study of factory workers in nine-teenth-century Württemberg. In Richard J. Evans and W. Robert Lee, eds. *The German Family*. London: Croom Helm.

Schwartz, Robert. 1988. *Policing the Poor in Eighteenth-Century France*. Chapel Hill: University of North Carolina Press.

Sciascia, Leonardo, and Rosario La Duca. 1974. *Palermo felicissima*. Palermo: Edizioni il Punto.

Scott, Joan Wallach. 1988. *Gender and the Politics of History*. New York: Columbia University Press.

Scott, John W. 1901–2. Notes on a case of lead poisoning from diachylon as an abor-tifacient. *Quarterly Medical Journal*, 10, 148–52.

Scrofani, Serafino. 1962. *Sicilia: utilizzazione del suolo nella storia, nei redditi, e nelle prospettive*. Palermo: Editori Stampatori Associati.

—. 1977. Gli ordinamenti colturali. In *Storia della Sicilia*, vol. 9. Società editrice Storia di Napoli e della Sicilia.

Segalen, Martine. 1983. *Love and Power in the Peasant Family*. Chicago: University of Chicago Press.

—. 1985. *Quinze générations de bas bretons: Parenté et sociéte dans le pays bigouden sud 1720–1980*. Paris: Presses universitaires de France.

—. 1987. Diversité des systémes d'héritage en Finistére: Le Cas contrasté du Pays Bigouden et du Pays Léonard. *Bulletin de la Société archéologique du Finistére*, 106, 171–90.

Sharlin, Allan. 1978. Natural decrease in early modern cities: a reconsideration. *Past and Present*, 79, 126–38.

—. 1986. Urban-rural differences in fertility in Europe during the demographic transition. In Ansley J. Coale and Susan Cotts Watkins, eds., *The Decline of Fertility in Europe*. Princeton: Princeton University Press.

Sheppard, Francis. 1971. *London, 1808–1870: The Infernal Wen*. London: Secker & Warburg.

Short, Roger V. 1976. Lactation, the central control of reproduction. In *Ciba Foundation Symposium*, n.s., 45. Amsterdam: Elsevier Excerpta Medica.

Shorter, Edward. 1977. *The Making of the Modern Family*. New York; Basic Books.

—. 1982. *A History of Women's Bodies*. New York: Basic Books.

Shorter, Edward; John Knodel; and Etienne van de Walle. 1971. The decline of non-marital fertility in Europe, 1880–1940. *Population Studies*, 25, 375–93.

Showalter, Elaine. 1987. *The Female Malady: Women, Madness and English Culture, 1830–1980*. New York: Penguin.

Sieder, Reinhard. 1988. Behind the lines: working-class family life in wartime Vienna: the evidence of oral history. In Richard Wall and Jay M. Winter, eds., *The Upheaval of War: Family, Work, and Welfare in Europe, 1914–1918*. Cambridge: Cambridge University Press.

Simmel, Georg. 1955. *Conflict and the Web of Group Affiliations*. New York: Free Press.

Simms, Madeleine. 1974. Midwives and abortion in the 1930s. *Midwife and Health Visitor*, 10, 114–16.

Simms, Madeleine, and Keith Hindell. 1971. *Abortion Law Reform Reformed*. London: Owen.

Simons, John. 1986. Culture, economy and reproduction in contemporary Europe. In David Coleman and Roger Schofield, eds., *The State of Population Theory*. Oxford: Basil Blackwell.

Skultans, Vieda. 1970. The symbolic significance of menstruation and the menopause. *Man*, n.s., 5, 639–51.

Smith, Anthony D. 1981. War and ethnicity: the role of warfare in the formation of self-images and cohesion of ethnic communities. *Ethnic and Racial Studies*, 4, 375–97.

—. 1986. *The Ethnic Origins of Nations*. Oxford: Basil Blackwell.

Smith, Dennis. 1982. *Conflict and Compromise: Class Formation in English Society, 1830–1914*. London: Routledge & Kegan Paul.

Smith, Richard M. 1981. Fertility, economy, and household formation in England over three centuries, *Population and Development Review*, 7, 595–622.

Smith-Rosenberg, Carol. 1985. *Disorderly Conduct: Visions of Gender in Victorian America*. New York: Knopf.

Snell, K. D. M. 1985. *Annals of the Labouring Poor: Social Change and Agrarian England, 1660–1900*. Cambridge: Cambridge University Press.

Società Umanitaria. 1963. *L'emancipazione femminile: Un secolo di discussioni, 1861– 1961*. Florence: Sansoni.

Soliday, Gerald. 1974. *A Community in Conflict: Frankfurt Society in the Seventeenth and Early Eighteenth Centuries*. Hanover, N. H.: University Press of New England.

Soloway, Richard A. 1982a. *Birth Control and the Population Question in England, 1877–1930*. Chapel Hill: University of North Carolina Press.

—. 1982b. Counting the Degenerates: the statistics of race deterioration in Edwardian England. *Journal of Contemporary History*, 17, 137–64.

Somogyi, Stefano. 1974. La dinamica demografica delle provincie siciliane, 1861– 1971. In *Collana di Studi Demografici*, vol. 5. Palermo: University of Palermo, Institute of Demographic Science.

Souden, David. 1984a. Migrants and the population structure of later seventeenth-century provincial cities and market towns. In Peter Clark, ed., *The Transformation of English Provincial Towns, 1600–1800*. London: Hutchinson.

—. 1984b. Movers and stayers in family reconstitution populations, 1660–1780. *Local Population Studies* 33, 11–28.

Spaulding, Thomas Alfred. [1900.] *The World of the London School Board*. London: P. S. King.

Spengler, Joseph J. 1979. *France Faces Depopulation: Postlude Edition, 1936–1976*. Durham: Duke University Press.

Spree, Reinhard. 1981. *Soziale Ungleichheit vor Krankheit und Tod*. Göttingen: Vandenhoeck & Ruprecht.

Stephens, Meic. 1976. *Linguistic Minorities in Western Europe*. Llandysul, Dyfed, Wales: Gomer Press.

Stevenson, T. H. C. 1920. The fertility of various social classes in England and Wales from the middle of the nineteenth century to 1911. *Journal of the Royal Statistical Society*, 83, 401–44.

Stewart, Mary Lynn. 1987. Ethics in conflict: labor inspectors and working women, 1892–1914. Paper presented at the annual meeting of the Social Science History Association, New Orleans.

Stopes, Marie Carmichael. 1918a. *Married Love*. London: A. C. Fifield.

—. 1918b. *Wise Parenthood*. London: A. C. Fifield.

—. 1922. *Early days of Birth Control*. London: Putnam.

—. 1923a. *Contraception (Birth Control): Its Theory, History and Practice*. London: John Bale.

—. 1923b. *A Letter to Working Mothers*. London: Mothers' Clinic for Constructive Birth Control.

—. 1925. *"The First Five Thousand," Being the First Report of the First Birth Control Clinic in the British Empire*. London: John Bale.

—. 1928a. *Enduring Passion*. London: Putnam.

—. 1928b. *Radiant Motherhood*. London: Putnam.

—, ed. 1929. *Mother England*. London: John Bale, Sons and Danielsson.

—. 1930. *Preliminary Notes...from 10,000 Cases Attending the Pioneer Mothers' Clinic, London*. London: Mothers' Clinic for Constructive Birth Control.

—, ed. 1930. *Mother England, a Contemporary History*, 2d ed. London: Bale & Danielsson.

—. 1935. *Marriage in My Time*. London: Rich & Cowan.

Sturgess, R. W. 1971. Landownership, mining and urban development in nineteenth-century Staffordshire. In J. T. Ward and R. G. Wilson, eds., *Land and Industry: The Landed Estate and the Industrial Revolution*. Newton Abbott: David & Charles.

Suitor, J. Jill. 1981. Husbands' participation in childbirth: a nineteenth century phenomenon. *Journal of Family History*, 6, 275–93.

Summers, Anne. 1979. A home from home: women's philanthropic work in the nineteenth century. In Sandra Burman, ed., *Fit Work for Women*. London: Croom Helm.

Sutter, Jean. 1958. Evolution de la distance separante le domicile des futurs époux (Loir-et-Cher, 1870–1954; Finistère, 1911–1953). *Population*, 3, no. 2, 227–58.

Sutter, Jean, and Leon Tabah. 1955. L'Évolution des isolats de deux départements français: Loir-et-Cher, Finistère. *Population*, 10, no. 4, 645–74.

SVIMEZ. 1964. *Statistiche sul mezzogiorno d'Italia*. Rome: Associazione per lo sviluppo dell'industria nel Mezzogiorno.

Swaan, Abram de. 1988. *In Care of the State: Health Care, Education and Welfare in Europe and the USA in the Modern Era*. Cambridge. Polity Press.

Szreter, Simon R. S. 1984. The genesis of the Registrar-General's social classification of occupations. *British Journal of Sociology*, 35, 522–46.

Tadmor, Naomi. 1989. "Family" and "friend" in *Pamela*: a case study in the history of family in eighteenth century England. *Social History*, 14, 289–306.

Tarde, Gabriel. 1969. *On Communication and Social Influence*. 1898. Chicago and London: University of Chicago Press.

Tarle, Eugène. 1936. La Grande coalition des mineurs de Rive-de-Gier en 1844. *Revue Historique*, 177, 149–78.

Taylor, A. J. 1960. The sub-contract system in the British coal industry. In L. S. Pressnell, ed., *Studies in the Industrial Revolution*. London: Athone Press.

Teitelbaum, Michael S. 1984. *The British Fertility Decline: Demographic Transition in the Crucible of the Industrial Revolution*. Princeton: Princeton University Press.

Teitelbaum, Michael S., and Jay M. Winter. 1985. *The Fear of Population Decline*. New York: Academic Press.

Tenfelde, Klaus. 1981. *Sozialgeschichte der Bergarbeiterschaft an der Ruhr im 19 Jahrhundert*. Bonn: Verlag Neue Gesellschaft.

Terrier, Didier, and Philippe Toutain. 1979. Pression démographique et marché due travail à Comines au xviiie siècle. *Revue du Nord*, 61, 19–26.

Terrisse, Michel. 1974. Méthode de recherches démographiques en milieu urbain ancien (xviie–xviiie). In *Annales de démographie historique*. Paris and The Hague: Mouton.

Tesniere, L. 1928. Statistique des langues de L'Europe. In A. Meillet, ed., *Les Langues dans l'Europe Nouvelle*. Paris: Payot.

Thane, Patricia. 1982. *The Foundations of the Welfare State*. London: Longman.

Tholfsen, Trygve R. 1977. *Working-Class Radicalism in Mid-Victorian England*. New York: Columbia University Press.

Thomas, Keith. 1971. *Religion and the Decline of Magic*. New York: Scribners.

Thompson, Paul. 1967. *Socialists, Liberals and Labour: The Struggle for London, 1885–1914*. London: Routledge.

Thompson, Warren S. 1929. Population. *American Journal of Sociology*, 34, 959–75.

Tilly, Charles. 1973. Population and pedagogy in France. *History of Education Quarterly*, 13, 113–27.

—. 1975. Reflections on the history of European state-making. In Charles Tilly, ed., *The Formation of National States in Western Europe*. Princeton: Princeton University Press.

—. 1978a. The historical study of vital processes. In Charles Tilly, ed. *Historical Studies of Changing Fertility*. Princeton: Princeton University Press.

—. 1978b. Migration in modern European history. In William McNeill and Ruth Adams, eds., *Human Migration: Patterns and Policies*. Bloomington: Indiana University Press.

—. 1978c. Questions and conclusions. In Charles Tilly, ed., *Historical Studies of Changing Fertility*. Princeton: Princeton University Press.

—. 1981. *As Sociology Meets History*. New York: Academic Press.

—. 1984. Demographic origins of the European proletariat. In David Levine, ed., *Proletarianization and Family History*. Orlando Fla.: Academic Press.

Tilly, Louise. 1985. Coping with company paternalism: family strategies of coal miners in nineteenth-century france. *Theory and Society*, 14, 403–17.

—. 1992. *Politics and Class in Milan, 1880–1901*. New York: Oxford University Press.

Tilly, Louise, and Joan Scott. 1978. *Women, Work and Family*. New York: Holt, Rinehart & Winston.

Tilly, Louise; Joan Scott; and Miriam Cohen. 1976. Nineteenth century European fertility patterns and women's work. *Journal of Interdisciplinary History*, 6, 447–76.

Titmuss, Richard, M. 1950. *Problems of Social Policy*. London: His Majesty's Stationery Office.

Tocqueville, Alexis de. 1983 [1835]. Memoir on pauperism. *Public Interest*, 70, 102–20.

Todd, Emmanuel. 1975. Mobilité géographique et cycle de vie en Artois et en Toscane au XVIIIᵉ siècle. *Annales: Economies, Sociétés, Civilisations*, 30, 726–44.

—. 1985. *The Explanation of Ideology: Family Structure and Social Systems*. London: Basil Blackwell.

Tolnay, Stewart E.; Stephen N. Graham; and Avery M. Guest. 1982. Own-child estimates of U. S. white fertility, 1886–1899. *Historical Methods*, 15, 127–38.

Tomas, François. 1963. Quelques traits de l'histoire agraire de la plaine du Forez. *Revue Géographique de Lyon*, 38, 131–61.

Toulemon, André. 1945. Note. *Revue de l'Alliance Nationale contre la Dépopulation*, 369, 2.

Trainor, Richard. 1982. Peers on an industrial frontier: the earls of Dartmouth and of Dudley in the Black Country, c. 1810 to 1914. In David Cannadine, ed., *Patricians, Power and Politics in Nineteenth-Century Towns*. Leicester: Leicester University Press.

Treffers, P. E. 1967. Abortion in Amsterdam. *Population Studies*, 20, 295–309.

Trudgill, Peter. 1983. *Sociolinguistics: An Introduction to Language and Society*. Harmondsworth: Penguin.

Tucker, M. J. 1974. The child as beginning and end: fifteenth and sixteenth century English childhood. In Lloyd de Mause, ed., *The History of Childhood*. New York: Psychohistory Press.

Tufte, Virginia, and Barbara Myerhoff. 1979. Introduction. In Tufte and Myerhoff, eds. *Changing Images of the Family*. New Haven: Yale.

Ungari, Paolo. 1970. *Il diritto di famiglia in Italia*. Bologna: Il Mulino.

United Nations. 1953. Department of Economic and Social Affairs. *The Determinants and Consequences of Population Trends*. New York: United Nations.

—. 1973. *The Determinants and Consequences of Population Trends: New Summary of Findings on Interaction of Demographic, Economic and Social Factors*. New York: United Nations.

Urlanis, Boris. 1971. *Wars and Population*. Moscow: Century Publishing House.

van de Walle, Etienne. 1974. *The Female Population of France in the Nineteenth Century*. Princeton: Princeton University Press.

—. 1980. Motivations and technology in the decline of French fertility. In Robert Wheaton and Tamara Hareven, eds., *Family and Sexuality in French History*. Philadelphia: University of Pennsylvania Press.

—. 1986. La Fécondité française au XIXe siècle. *Communications*, 44, 35–45.

van Gennep, Arnold. 1960. *The Rites of Passage*. Chicago: University of Chicago Press.

Veblen, Thorstein. 1967 [1899]. *Theory of the Leisure Class*. New York: Viking.

Verdery, Katherine. 1976. Ethnicity and local systems: the religious organization of wellness. In C. A. Smith, ed., *Regional Analysis*, vol. 2. New York: Academic Press.

Vries, Jan de. 1984. *European Urbanization, 1500–1800*. Cambridge: Harvard University Press.

Walsh, J. H. 1857. *A Manual of Domestic Economy Suited to Families Spending from £100 to £1000 a Year*. London: Routledge.

Wareing, John. 1975. Migration to London and transatlantic emigration of indentured servants, 1683–1775. *Journal of Historical Geography*, 7, 356–78.

Warner, Marina. 1985. *Monuments and Maidens: The Allegory of the Female Form*. London: Picador.

Watkins, Susan Cotts. 1980. Variation and persistence in nuptiality: age-patterns of marriage in Europe, 1870–1960. Ph.D. diss., Princeton University.

—. 1981. Regional patterns of nuptiality in Europe. *Population Studies*, 35, 199–215.

—. 1986. Conclusions. In Ansley J. Coale and Susan Cotts Watkins, eds., *The Decline of Fertility in Europe*. Princeton: Princeton University Press.

—. 1990. From local communities to national communities. *Population and Development Review*, 16, no. 2, 241–72.

—. 1991. *From Provinces into Nations: The Demographic Integration of Western Europe, 1870–1960*. Princeton: Princeton University Press.

Watterson, P. A. 1986. The role of the environment in the decline of infant mortality: an analysis of the 1911 census of England and Wales. Journal of Biosocial Science, 18, 457–70.

—. 1988. Infant mortality by father's occupation from the 1911 census of England and Wales. *Demography*, 25, 289–306.

Wautier, Diane. 1981. L'Image de la femme dans les caricatures des grands quotidiens janvier 1914–juin 1919. M. A. thesis, University of Paris I.

Webb, Sidney. 1907. *The Decline of the Birth-Rate, Fabian Tract No. 131*. London: The Fabian Society.

Weber, Adna. 1967. *The Growth of Cities in the Nineteenth Century*. 1899. Ithaca. Cornell University Press.

Weber, Eugen. 1976. Peasants into Frenchmen: The Modernization of Rural France, 1870–1914. Stanford: Stanford University Press.

Weber-Kellermann, Ingeborg. 1974. *Die deutsche Familie*. Frankfurt am Main: Suhrkamp.

Wehler, Hans-Ulrich. 1969. *Bismarck und der Imperialismus*. Cologne and Berlin: Kiepenheuer und Witsch.

Weinberg, Ian. 1976. The problem of convergence of industrial societies: a critical look at the state of a theory. In Cyril E. Black, ed., *Comparative Modernization*. New York: Free Press.

Weir, David Rangeler. 1982. Fertility transition in rural France, 1740–1829. Ph.D. diss., Stanford University.

Weiss, John. 1983. Origins of the French welfare state: poor relief in the Third Republic, 1871–1914. *French Historical Studies*, 13, 47–78.

White, Paul E. 1989. Migration in later nineteenth- and twentieth-century France: the social and economic Context. In Paul E. White and Philip Ogden, eds., *Migrants in Modern France: Population Mobility in the Later Nineteenth and Twentieth Centuries*. London: Unwin Hyman.

Wickham, James. 1983. Working-class movement and working-class life: Frankfurt-am-Main during the Weimar Republic. *Social History*, 8, 313–43.

Williamson, Jeffrey G. 1965. Regional inequality and the process of national development: a description of the patterns. *Economic Development and Cultural Change*, 12, 3–84.

Wilson, Adrian. 1985. Participant or patient? Seventeenth century childbirth from the mother's point of view. In Roy Porter, ed., *Patients and Practitioners: Lay Perception of Medicine in Pre-Industrial Societies*. Cambridge: Cambridge University Press.

Wilson, Chris. 1986. The proximate determinants of marital fertility in England, 1600–1799. In Lloyd Bonfield, Richard Smith, and Keith Wrightson, eds., *The World We Have Gained*. New York: Basil Blackwell.

Winter, Jay M. 1985. *The Great War and the British People*. London: Macmillan.

—. 1986. Demographic consequences of the Second World War. In H. Smith, ed., *War and Social Change*. Manchester: Manchester University Press.

—. 1988. Some paradoxes of the Great War. In Richard Wall and Jay M. Winter, eds., *The Upheaval of War, Family, Work, and Welfare in Europe 1914–1918*. Cambridge: Cambridge University Press.

—. 1989. Socialist and social democratic approaches to population questions in Europe. In Michael S. Teitelbaum and Jay M. Winter, eds., *Population and Resources in Western Intellectual Traditions*. New York: Cambridge University Press.

Wohl, Anthony S. 1983. *Endangered Lives: Public Health in Victorian Britain*. London: J. M. Dent & Sons.

Woods, Robert. 1985. The fertility transition in nineteenth-century England and Wales: a social class model? *Tijdschrift voor Economische en Sociale Geografie*, 76, 180–91.

—. 1987. Approaches to the fertility transition in Victorian England. *Population Studies*, 41, 283–311.

Woods, Robert, and P. R. A. Hinde. 1985. Nuptiality and age at marriage in nineteenth-century England. *Journal of Family History*, 10, 119–44.

Woods, Robert, and C. W. Smith. 1983. The decline of marital fertility in the late nineteenth century: the case of England and Wales. *Population Studies*, 37, 207–25.

Woodside, Moya. 1963. Attitude of women abortionists. *Howard Journal*, 11, 93–112.

Woycke, James. 1984. The diffusion of birth control in Germany, 1871–1933. Ph.D. diss., University of Toronto.

——. 1988. *Birth Control in Germany, 1871–1933*. London. Routledge.

Wray, Joe D. 1978. Maternal nutrition, breast-feeding and infant survival. In W. Henry Mosley, ed., *Nutrition and Human Reproduction*. New York: Plenum Press.

Wrigley, E. Anthony. 1965. The fall in marital fertility in nineteenth century France. *Historical Social Research*, 34, 4–21.

——. 1967. A simple model of London's importance in changing English society and economy, 1650–1750. *Past and Present*, 37, 44–70.

——. 1969. *Population and History*. London: Jonathan Cape; New York: McGraw-Hill.

——. 1983. The growth of population in eighteenth-century England: a conundrum resolved. *Past and Present*, 98, 121–50.

——. 1985. The fall of marital fertility in nineteenth century France: exemplar or exeption? *European Journal of Population*, 1, 31–60, 141–77.

Wrigley, E. Anthony, and Roger Schofield. 1981. *The Population History of England, 1541–1871: A Reconstruction*. Cambridge: Cambridge University Press.

Wylie, Laurence. 1964. *Village in the Vaucluse: An Account of Life in a French Village*. New York: Harper & Row.

——. 1966. *Chanzeaux: A Village in Anjou*. Cambridge: Harvard University Press.

Young, Michael, and Peter Wilmott. 1957. *Family and Kinship in East London*. London: Routledge & Kegan Paul.

Zanuso, Lorenza. 1983. La segregazione occupazionale: I dati di lungo periodo (1901–1971). In Giuseppe Barile, ed., *Lavoro femminile, sviluppo technologico e segregazione occupazionale*. Milan: Franco Angeli.

Zariski, Raphael. 1972. *Italy: The Politics of Uneven Development*. Hinsdale, Ill. Dryden Press.

Zelizer, Viviana A. 1985. *Pricing the Priceless Child*. New York: Basic Books.

Zeller, Olivier. 1983. *Les Recensements lyonnais de 1597 et 1636: Démographie historique et géographie sociale*. Lyon: Presses universitaires de Lyon.

Index